Emerging Concepts in MR Angiography

Guest Editors

WILLIAM J. WEADOCK, MD

THOMAS L. CHENEVERT, PhD

MAGNETIC RESONANCE IMAGING CLINICS OF NORTH AMERICA

www.mri.theclinics.com

February 2009 • Volume 17 • Number 1

SAUNDERS an imprint of ELSEVIER, Inc.

W.B. SAUNDERS COMPANY
A Division of Elsevier Inc.

1600 John F. Kennedy Boulevard • Suite 1800 • Philadelphia, Pennsylvania 19103-2899

http://www.theclinics.com

MRI CLINICS OF NORTH AMERICA Volume 17, Number 1
February 2009 ISSN 1064-9689, ISBN 13: 978-1-4377-0497-6, ISBN 10: 1-4377-0497-2

Editor: Barton Dudlick
Developmental Editor: Theresa Collier

Magnetic Resonance Imaging Clinics of North America (ISSN 1064-9689) is published quarterly by Elsevier Inc., 360 Park Avenue South, New York, NY 10010-1710. Months of issue are February, May, August, and November. Business and Editorial Offices: 1600 John F. Kennedy Blvd., Suite 1800, Philadelphia, PA 19103-2899. Customer Service Office: 11830 Westline Industrial Drive, St. Louis, MO 63146. Periodicals postage paid at New York, NY and additional mailing offices. Subscription prices are $276.00 per year (domestic individuals), $414.00 per year (domestic institutions), $134.00 per year (domestic students/residents), $308.00 per year (Canadian individuals), $520.00 per year (Canadian institutions), $400.00 per year (international individuals), $520.00 per year (international institutions), and $194.00 per year (international and Canadian students/residents). International air speed delivery is included in all *Clinics* subscription prices. All prices are subject to change without notice. **POSTMASTER:** Send address changes to *Magnetic Resonance Imaging Clinics*, 11830 Westline Industrial Drive, St. Louis, MO 63146. Customer Service (orders, claims, online, change of address): Elsevier Periodicals Customer Service, 11830 Westline Industrial Drive, St. Louis, MO 63146. Tel: 1-800-654-2452 (U.S. and Canada). Fax: 314-523-5170. E-mail: journalscustomerservice-usa@elsevier.com (for print support); journalsonlinesupport-usa@elsevier.com (for online support).

Reprints. For copies of 100 or more of articles in this publication, please contact the Commercial Reprints Department, Elsevier Inc., 360 Park Avenue South, New York, NY 10010-1710. Tel.: 212-633-3812; Fax: 212-462-1935; E-mail: reprints@elsevier.com.

Magnetic Resonance Imaging Clinics of North America is covered in the *RSNA Index of Imaging Literature, MEDLINE/PubMed (Index Medicus),* and *EMBASE/Excerpta Medica.*

Printed and bound by CPI Group (UK) Ltd, Croydon, CR0 4YY

Transferred to Digital Print 2011

Contributors

GUEST EDITORS

WILLIAM J. WEADOCK, MD
Associate Professor of Radiology, Department of Radiology, University of Michigan Health System, Ann Arbor, Michigan

THOMAS L. CHENEVERT, PhD
Professor of Radiology, Department of Radiology, University of Michigan Health System, Ann Arbor, Michigan

AUTHORS

SAMUEL R.S. BARNES, MS
Research Assistant, Department of Radiology, Loma Linda University Medical Center, Loma Linda, California

MAURICIO CASTILLO, MD
Professor and Chief of Neuroradiology, Department of Radiology, University of North Carolina School of Medicine, Chapel Hill, North Carolina

THOMAS L. CHENEVERT, PhD
Professor of Radiology, Department of Radiology, University of Michigan Health System, Ann Arbor, Michigan

TAYLOR CHUNG, MD
Associate Director, Department of Diagnostic Imaging, Children's Hospital and Research Center Oakland, Oakland, California

NANCY DUDEK, BS
Department of Radiology, University of Michigan Health System, Ann Arbor, Michigan

CHRISTOPHER J. FRANÇOIS, MD
Assistant Professor, Department of Radiology, University of Wisconsin, Madison, Wisconsin

DHEERAJ GANDHI, MD
Department of Radiology, University of Michigan Health System, Ann Arbor, Michigan; Johns Hopkins Hospital, Baltimore, Maryland

LIESBETH GEERTS, PhD
Philips Healthcare, MR Clinical Science, Best, The Netherlands

MICHAEL GRIFFIN, PhD
Department of Radiology, University of Wisconsin, Madison, Wisconsin

THOMAS M. GRIST, MD
Professor and Chair, Department of Radiology, University of Wisconsin, Madison, Wisconsin

E. MARK HAACKE, PhD
Professor, Department of Radiology, Wayne State University; and Professor, Department of Biomedical Engineering, Wayne State University, MRI Institute for Biomedical Engineering, Detroit, Michigan

ELIZABETH M. HECHT, MD
Assistant Professor, Department of Radiology, New York University School of Medicine, New York, New York

KARIN A. HERRMANN, MD
Institute for Clinical Radiology, University Hospital Munich, Munich, Germany

R. HOOGEVEEN, PhD
Philips Healthcare, MR Clinical Science, Best, The Netherlands

BENJAMIN Y. HUANG, MD, MPH
Assistant Professor, Department of Radiology, University of North Carolina School of Medicine, Chapel Hill, North Carolina

MARKO K. IVANCEVIC, PhD
MR Clinical Scientist, Philips Healthcare, MR Clinical Science, Cleveland, Ohio; Department of Radiology, University of Michigan Health System, Ann Arbor, Michigan

SEBASTIAN KELLE, MD
Division of Cardiology, Department of Medicine, German Heart Institute, Berlin, Germany; Division of Magnetic Resonance Research, Department of Radiology, Johns Hopkins University School of Medicine, Baltimore, Maryland

HARALD KRAMER, MD
Institute for Clinical Radiology, University Hospital Munich, Munich, Germany

RAJESH KRISHNAMURTHY, MD
Clinical Assistant Professor of Radiology and Pediatrics (Cardiology), Baylor College of Medicine; Associate Radiologist, Edward B. Singleton Department of Diagnostic Imaging, Texas Children's Hospital, Houston, Texas

PHILLIP H. KUO, MD, PhD
Associate Professor, Department of Medicine, Section of Hematology/Oncology, University of Arizona; Staff Radiologist, Department of Radiology, Southern Arizona Veterans Administration Hospital, Tucson, Arizona

JEFFREY H. MAKI, MD, PhD
Associate Professor, Department of Radiology, University of Washington; Department of Radiology, Puget Sound Veterans Affairs Health Care System, Seattle, Washington

S.K. MUKHERJI, MD
Department of Radiology, University of Michigan Health System, Ann Arbor, Michigan

RAJA MUTHUPILLAI, PhD
MR Imaging Physicist/Scientist, Department of Diagnostic Radiology, St. Luke's Episcopal Hospital, Houston, Texas

KONSTANTIN NIKOLAOU, MD
Institute for Clinical Radiology, University Hospital Munich, Munich, Germany

HEMANT PARMAR, MD
Department of Radiology, University of Michigan Health System, Ann Arbor, Michigan

MAXIMILIAN F. REISER, MD
Institute for Clinical Radiology, University Hospital Munich, Munich, Germany

ANDREW ROSENKRANTZ, MD
Body/Cardiovascular MRI Fellow, Department of Radiology, New York University School of Medicine, New York, New York

WIELAND SOMMER, MD
Institute for Clinical Radiology, University Hospital Munich, Munich, Germany

MATTHIAS STUBER, PhD
Division of Magnetic Resonance Research, Department of Radiology, Johns Hopkins University School of Medicine; Division of Cardiology, Department of Medicine; Department of Electrical and Computer Engineering, Johns Hopkins University, Baltimore, Maryland

WILLIAM J. WEADOCK, MD
Associate Professor of Radiology, Department of Radiology, University of Michigan Health System, Ann Arbor, Michigan

JEFFREY C. WEINREB, MD
Professor of Radiology, Department of Diagnostic Radiology, Yale University School of Medicine; Director of Imaging Services, and Chief of Body Imaging and MRI, Yale-New Haven Hospital, New Haven, Connecticut

ROBERT G. WEISS, MD
Division of Magnetic Resonance Research, Department of Radiology, Johns Hopkins University School of Medicine; Division of Cardiology, Department of Medicine, Johns Hopkins University, Baltimore, Maryland

GREGORY J. WILSON, PhD
Affiliate Assistant Professor, Department of Radiology, University of Washington, Seattle, Washington; Philips Healthcare, Cleveland, Ohio

Contents

> Magnetic resonance provides a wide variety of possibilities for arterial and venous blood vessel imaging in all vascular territories. This article provides a brief review of the technical principles of MR angiography. The first section is dedicated to non–contrast-enhanced angiography techniques and includes several distinct approaches: time-of-flight, phase contrast, triggered angiography non–contrast-enhanced, and balanced steady-state free precession. The second section relates to the contrast-enhanced and time-resolved contrast-enhanced MR angiography methods. The latest technical developments in MR imaging hardware, sequences and software, coil technology, and reconstruction capability allow dynamic MR angiography performance similar to CT angiography, without risks of iodine contrast agent and ionizing radiation exposure.

> Balanced steady-state free precession (Bal-SSFP) techniques produce excellent anatomic images of renal arteries without the use of contrast agents and are relatively flow-insensitive. Electrocardiography (ECG)-triggered and non–ECG-triggered sequences have been shown to be quite sensitive for detection of regional arterial stenosis (RAS), and the already high specificity is likely to increase with further refinement of the techniques. Bal-SSFP sequences can be used as a screening tool or as an alternative to contrast-enhanced (CE) magnetic resonance angiography (MRA) when contrast agents are contraindicated. In addition to morphologic imaging of RAS, non-CE techniques can be used in functional assessment of hemodynamic significance. The complimentary tools can be used alone or in combination with CE-MRA for MR imaging of renal vascular hypertension.

> The primary advantage of high field strength MR imaging over imaging on modern 1.5 Tesla (T) systems is increased signal-to-noise ratio, which can be used to improve image quality or shorten scan acquisition time. In the years since 3.0T scanners were first approved for clinical use, one of the areas which has benefited greatly from its introduction is neurovascular MR angiography (MRA). Early experience has shown significant improvements in resolution and image quality. Whether high field strength MRA is robust or accurate enough to replace digital subtraction angiography in the foreseeable future remains to be seen. This article discusses the current state of neurovascular MRA at 3.0T, basic physical differences between MR imaging at 1.5T and 3.0T, and their effects on MRA sequences. The literature regarding the efficacy of 3.0T MRA techniques for diagnosing specific neurovascular pathologies and carotid steno occlusive disease is reviewed.

artery occlusive disease has changed substantially in the last few years. Recent technical developments such as the introduction of new image reconstruction algorithms and dedicated contrast agents have pushed the limits of MR angiography toward higher spatial resolution and image quality and have enabled time-resolved imaging. This article discusses various techniques of peripheral MR angiography, including step-by-step, hybrid, continuous table movement, and non–contrast-enhanced MR angiography.

This article discusses the role of magnetic resonance angiography (MRA) in evaluating the pulmonary arterial system. For depiction of pulmonary arterial anatomy and morphology, MRA techniques are compared with CT angiography and digital subtraction x-ray angiography. Perfusion, flow, and function are emphasized, as the integrated MR examination offers a comprehensive assessment of vascular morphology and function. Advances in MR technology that improve spatial and temporal resolution and compensate for potential artifacts are reviewed as they pertain to pulmonary MRA. Current and emerging gadolinium contrast-enhanced and non–contrast-enhanced MRA techniques are discussed. The role of pulmonary MRA, clinical protocols, imaging findings, and interpretation pitfalls are reviewed for clinical indications.

Vascular pathology in children is commonplace and involves every organ system; however, the powerful, noninvasive, and rapid three-dimensional imaging capability offered by MR angiography is underutilized in children. The success of pediatric MR angiography depends on modifying the MR angiography on the basis of patient size, hemodynamic status, and clinical indications in children, and requires an adequate understanding of pediatric-specific hardware, software, and equipment requirements. This article provides an overview of general pediatric MR angiography techniques, common indications for body MR angiography in children, and the complementary role of MR angiography to other vascular imaging modalities in children, including CT angiography, Doppler ultrasound, and catheter angiography.

Coronary MR imaging is a promising noninvasive technique for the combined assessment of coronary artery anatomy and function. Anomalous coronary arteries and aneurysms can reliably be assessed in clinical practice using coronary MR imaging and the presence of significant left main or proximal multivessel coronary artery disease detected. Technical challenges that need to be addressed are further improvements in motion suppression and abbreviated scanning times aimed at improving spatial resolution and patient comfort. The development of new and specific contrast agents, high-field MR imaging with improved spatial resolution, and continued progress in MR imaging methods development will undoubtedly lead to further progress toward the noninvasive and comprehensive assessment of coronary atherosclerotic disease.

Jeffrey C. Weinreb and Phillip H. Kuo

There seems to be an association between exposure to intravenous gadolinium-based contrast agents (GBCAs) and nephrogenic systemic fibrosis (NSF), a debilitating and sometimes fatal disease. This article addresses the relationship between GBCAs and NSF and answers some common questions. The policy deployed at Yale-New Haven Hospital for prevention of NSF and screening for patients at risk is delineated and discussed along with recommendations by the Food and Drug Administration.

Magnetic Resonance Imaging Clinics of North America

RELATED INTEREST

Radiologic Clinics of North America January 2009 (Vol. 47, No. 1)
Advances in MDCT
Dushyant Sahani, MD and Vahid Yaghami, MD, *Guest Editors*

THE CLINICS ARE NOW AVAILABLE ONLINE!

Access your subscription at:
www.theclinics.com

GOAL STATEMENT

The goal of *Magnetic Resonance Imaging Clinics of North America* is to keep practicing physicians up to date with current clinical practice by providing timely articles reviewing the state of the art in patient care.

ACCREDITATION

The *Magnetic Resonance Imaging Clinics of North America* is planned and implemented in accordance with the Essential Areas and Policies of the Accreditation Council for Continuing Medical Education (ACCME) through the joint sponsorship of the University of Virginia School of Medicine and Elsevier. The University of Virginia School of Medicine is accredited by the ACCME to provide continuing medical education for physicians.

The University of Virginia School of Medicine designates this educational activity for a maximum of 15 *AMA PRA Category 1 Credits*™. Physicians should only claim credit commensurate with the extent of their participation in the activity.

The American Medical Association has determined that physicians not licensed in the US who participate in this CME activity are eligible for 15 *AMA PRA Category 1 Credits*™.

Credit can be earned by reading the text material, taking the CME examination online at: http://www.theclinics.com/home/cme, and completing the evaluation. After taking the test, you will be required to review any and all incorrect answers. Following completion of the test and evaluation, your credit will be awarded and you may print your certificate.

FACULTY DISCLOSURE/CONFLICT OF INTEREST

The University of Virginia School of Medicine, as an ACCME accredited provider, endorses and strives to comply with the Accreditation Council for Continuing Medical Education (ACCME) Standards of Commercial Support, Commonwealth of Virginia statutes, University of Virginia policies and procedures, and associated federal and private regulations and guidelines on the need for disclosure and monitoring of proprietary and financial interests that may affect the scientific integrity and balance of content delivered in continuing medical education activities under our auspices.

The University of Virginia School of Medicine requires that all CME activities accredited through this institution be developed independently and be scientifically rigorous, balanced and objective in the presentation/discussion of its content, theories and practices.

All authors/editors participating in an accredited CME activity are expected to disclose to the readers relevant financial relationships with commercial entities occurring within the past 12 months (such as grants or research support, employee, consultant, stock holder, member of speakers bureau, etc.). The University of Virginia School of Medicine will employ appropriate mechanisms to resolve potential conflicts of interest to maintain the standards of fair and balanced education to the reader. Questions about specific strategies can be directed to the Office of Continuing Medical Education, University of Virginia School of Medicine, Charlottesville, Virginia.

The faculty and staff of the University of Virginia Office of Continuing Medical Education have no financial affiliations to disclose.

The authors/editors listed below have identified no professional or financial affiliations for themselves or their spouse/ partner:
Samuel R.S. Barnes, MS; Mauricio Castillo, MD, FACR; Thomas L. Chenevert, PhD (Guest Editor); Taylor Chung, MD; Eduard de Lange, MD (Test Author); Nancy Dudek, BS; Dheeraj Ghandi, MD; Michael Griffin, PhD; Elizabeth M. Hecht, MD; Karin A. Herrmann, MD; Benjamin Y. Huang, MD, MPH; Sebastian Kelle, MD; Harald Kramer, MD; Rajesh Krishnamurthy, MD; Konstantin Nikolaou, MD; Maximiliam F. Reiser, MD; Barton Dudlick (Acquisitions Editor); Andrew Rosenkrantz, MD; Wieland H. Sommer, MD; William J. Weadock, MD (Guest Editor); and Robert G. Weiss, MD.

The authors/editors listed below identified the following professional or financial affiliations for themselves or their spouse/partner:
Christopher J. François, MD is a consultant for GE.
Liesbeth Geerts, PhD is employed by and owns stock in Philips Healthcare.
Thomas M. Grist, MD is an industry funded research/investigator for, owns a patent with, and serves on the Speakers Bureau for GE Healthcare, owns stock in Cellector, and is a consultant for Bayer.
E. Mark Haacke, PhD is an industry funded research/investigator for Siemens Medical Solutions.
Romhild M. Hoogeveen, PhD is employed by Philips Healthcare.
Marko K. Ivancevic, PhD is employed by Philips Healthcare.
Phillip H. Kuo, MD, PhD received a one-time honorarium from Bracco in June 2008.
Jeffrey H. Maki, MD, PhD serves on the Speakers Bureau for Bracco Diagnostics.
Suresh K. Mukherji, MD is a consultant for Bracco, Bayer, Philips, and Xoran Technologies.
Raja Muthupillai, PhD is an industry funded research/investigator for and owns stock in Philips Medical Systems.
Hemant Parmar, MD is an industry funded research/investigator for Bayer Healthcare.
Matthias Stuber, PhD is the founder of Diagnosoft, Inc., and was a consultant with Philips Medical Systems until 2007.
Jeffrey C. Weinreb, MD, FACR is an industry funded research/investigator and consultant for GE Healthcare and Bayer Pharmaceuticals and serves on the Speakers Bureau for GE Healthcare.
Gregory J. Wilson, PhD is employed by Philips Healthcare.

Disclosure of Discussion of non-FDA approved uses for pharmaceutical products and/or medical devices:
The University of Virginia School of Medicine, as an ACCME provider, requires that all faculty presenters identify and disclose any "off label" uses for pharmaceutical and medical device products. The University of Virginia School of Medicine recommends that each physician fully review all the available data on new products or procedures prior to instituting them with patients.

TO ENROLL

To enroll in the Magnetic Resonance Imaging Clinics of North America Continuing Medical Education program, call customer service at 1-800-654-2452 or visit us online at: www.theclinics.com/home/cme. The CME program is available to subscribers for an additional fee of $99.95.

Preface

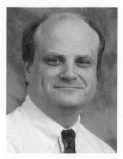 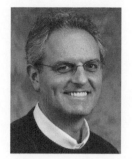

William J. Weadock, MD   Thomas L. Chenevert, PhD

Guest Editors

Over the past 15 years, there have been numerous significant advances in magnetic resonance angiography (MRA). Developments in software and hardware have created the ability to image in near real time and at high resolution. Theoretic improvement in signal to noise of 3T systems is being realized in imaging of small vessels in the head, neck, and abdomen. Combined with parallel imaging and multichannel coils, four dimensional imaging is not only possible, but also is becoming common practice for many clinical applications.

This issue is a combination of clinical MRA examples and fundamental physics concepts that form the basis of MRA methods. Most of the techniques are Introduced in the first article and are reinforced throughout the issue to give the reader an appreciation of how they work.

Contrast-enhanced MRA suffered a setback with the recognition of intravenous gadolinium administration's association with nephrogenic systemic fibrosis (NSF). Closer analysis seems to indicate that not all gadolinium contrast agents convey the same risk of developing NSF. Patients who have an estimated glomerular filtration rate of less than 30 mL/min/1.73 m^2 may be affected with NSF, which has no known treatment or cure.

Renewed interest in non–contrast-enhanced techniques has also increased as a result of NSF. Techniques used for cine cardiac imaging can also be applied to other parts of the body with success. While there have been improvements in time of flight and phase contrast imaging, newer techniques, such as steady state free precession, have made non–contrast MRA a valuable tool in the MRA armamentarium.

Authors of the articles in this issue are recognized leaders in the advancement of MRA throughout the body. We thank them for their insight into this exciting field. This issue is a snapshot in time of MRA applications, and we hope the reader gains an appreciation of current state of the art and future technological trends.

William J. Weadock, MD

Thomas L. Chenevert, PhD
Department of Radiology
University of Michigan Health System
1500 East Medical Center Drive
Ann Arbor, MI 48109-5030, USA

E-mail addresses:
weadock@umich.edu (W.J. Weadock)
tlchenev@umich.edu (T.L. Chenevert)

doi:10.1016/j.mric.2009.02.005
1064-9689/09/$

mri.theclinics.com

Technical Principles of MR Angiography Methods

Marko K. Ivancevic, PhD[a,b],*, Liesbeth Geerts, PhD[c],
William J. Weadock, MD[b], Thomas L. Chenevert, PhD[b]

KEYWORDS

- MR angiography • Contrast-enhanced
- Time-resolved • 4D-TRAK

In the last 20 years, MR imaging has been increasingly used to image vascular lumens in a large variety of anatomies: intracranial, carotids, head and neck, spine, chest, renal arteries, peripheral arteries. MR angiography is gaining ground as a safer and noninvasive alternative to X-ray digital subtracted angiography with inherent risks of ionizing radiation, catheterization, and iodine contrast media.

Because of high sensitivity of MR imaging to motion, flow-sensitive, noncontrast methods were the basis for original MR angiography methods. These approaches remain in use today; however, these early techniques suffer from a number of flow-related artifacts and other limitations. Consequently, original noncontrast MR angiography methods have been augmented by three-dimensional contrast-enhanced (CE) techniques. Since the association of intravenous gadolinium administration and nephrogenic systemic sclerosis, however, new and improved noncontrast techniques have stimulated renewed interest.

This article provides a brief review of the technical principles of MR angiography. The first section is dedicated to non-CE angiography techniques and includes several distinct approaches: time-of-flight (TOF), phase contrast, triggered angiography non-CE, and balanced steady-state free precession. The second section relates to the use of intravenous gadolinium-based contrast material for CE and time-resolved CE MR angiography methods.

NONCONTRAST METHODS
Time-of-Flight MR Angiography

TOF angiography was introduced in the late 1980s[1,2] and continues to undergo significant refinement even today. It was initially based on the spin-echo sequence.[1] In the spin-echo TOF sequence, selective 90- and 180-degree radiofrequency pulses are used at different slice locations. In static tissue no echo is generated. For blood flowing at just the right velocity, however, the blood protons experience both 90- and 180-degree pulses and generate an echo. This spin-echo approach was prone to error, and the gradient echo TOF was introduced later and has become the common element in modern TOF-based MR angiography. The basic concept with the gradient echo method is that static tissue experiencing a rapid series of slice-selective radiofrequency pulses at a TR shorter than tissue T1 loses most of its signal because of T1 saturation (**Fig. 1**). Flowing blood that has not experienced these radiofrequency pulses, however, enters the slice fully magnetized and has exceptionally strong signal relative to saturated background tissue. The standard two-dimensional TOF technique is based on relatively thin two-dimensional slice-selective

a Philips Healthcare, MR Clinical Science, 595 Miner Road, Cleveland, OH 44143, USA
b Department of Radiology, University of Michigan Health System, 1500 East Medical Center Drive, Ann Arbor, MI 48109-5030, USA
c Philips Healthcare, MR Clinical Science, 5680 DA, Veenpluis 4–6, Best, The Netherlands
* Corresponding author. Philips Healthcare, MR Clinical Science, 595 Miner Road, Cleveland, OH 44143.
E-mail address: markoi@med.umich.edu (M.K. Ivancevic).

Magn Reson Imaging Clin N Am 17 (2009) 1–11
doi:10.1016/j.mric.2009.01.012

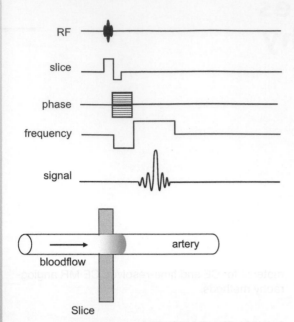

Fig. 1. Time-of-flight sequence diagram with schematic slice saturation and fresh blood inflow.

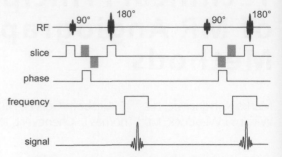

Fig. 2. Phase-contrast sequence diagram with velocity-encoding gradients in the slice direction.

gradient echo sequence with additional spatial saturation of flow from undesired directions. Three-dimensional TOF methods provide greater spatial resolution at the expense of partial saturation of flow remaining in the thick three-dimensional volume for many radiofrequency pulses. This effect is mitigated by the "multiple overlapping thin slab acquisition" technique where thin three-dimensional volumes are acquired and overlapped to achieve the inflow benefit of two-dimensional TOF along with the resolution and signal-to-noise ratio (SNR) gain of three-dimensional TOF. This method is often used for intracranial vasculature imaging.[3,4]

Phase-Contrast Angiography

Phase-contrast angiography (PCA)[5] applies additional gradient pulses to induce a phase shift that is directly proportional to flow velocity along the gradient direction. This bipolar gradient is turned on in one direction for a given time, then an opposite gradient is applied for the same amount of time (Fig. 2). The first gradient dephased spins, and the second one rephases the spins as long as they are not moving. That is, stationery spins have a zero phase shift. In reality, a reference image is acquired in addition to the velocity-encoded scan and is subtracted from the flow-sensitive images to remove phase errors unrelated to flow. The end result is to have flowing spins accumulate phase proportional to the velocity of flow:

$$\phi = \gamma G v \tau^2 \qquad \text{(Eq 1)}$$

where γ is the gyromagnetic ratio, G the gradient amplitude, τ the gradient duration, and v the flow velocity component parallel to the applied gradient direction. Flow encoding can be applied in one, two, or three perpendicular directions with scan duration proportional to the number of selected flow directions. In addition, several image types can be generated to display flow velocity, speed, or various composites to yield a PCA (Fig. 3).

Because phase is proportional to flow velocity, an image can be generated where pixel intensity directly relates to flow velocity; this is the "phase" image. The accepted convention for phase images is to display flow in the same direction as the biplolar gradient as positive values (ie, bright pixels) and flow in the opposite direction as negative (ie, dark pixels) relative to static tissue having zero phase (ie, gray pixels). Often, one desires an image of flow speed without concern of flow direction. To generate this, the "absolute value" of phase images for three orthogonal flow-encoding directions are combined; this is a "speed" image (Fig. 4). Ideally, speed images display flow regardless of direction as bright pixels in high contrast to dark static tissues. To accurately map pixel values to a desired range of flow speed, the maximum flow speed is entered into the PCA scan parameters and is referred to as the "velocity encoding" value or phase sensitivity value. A velocity encoding well above the true maximum flow speed has reduced sensitivity to slow flow near the edge of vessel lumen. Conversely, a velocity encoding too low for the given flow speeds may "alias" high flow and map to low pixel values or other artifacts may occur.

A composite PCA is used for vascular morphology visualization, and a reference gradient echo image magnitude image for soft tissue detail. With the image contrast being sensitive to flow velocity, an adequate velocity encoding should be selected depending on the flow velocity of the vessel of interest. It is important for the velocity encoding to be reasonably matched to the true maximum flow velocity, to avoid phase aliasing

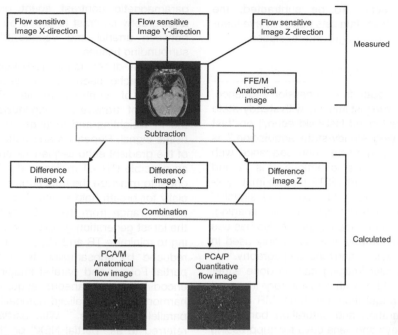

Fig. 3. Image combination used to generate anatomic flow phase-contrast angiography (PCA) image (magnitude) and the quantitative flow PCA image (phase).

artifacts resulting in reversing flow and decreased signal intensity while maintaining good sensitivity to the desired flow speed. PCA acquisition can be synchronized to the heart cycle by cardiac gating, and performed as a cine-PCA providing images at different times of the cardiac cycle.

Triggered Three-Dimensional Turbo Spin-Echo Non–Contrast-Enhanced Angiography

Blood acceleration during the high-flow systolic part of the cardiac cycle leads to a flow void caused by spin dephasing.[6] In venous flow with less acceleration, spin dephasing is less prominent, and veins retain most of their signal. This property can be used for vessel imaging with

a turbo spin-echo sequence, and typically is used in the peripheral vasculature.[7–9] When acquired in systole, at peak of blood flow, arteries appear dark and veins bright. In diastole, however, with constant flow and no acceleration, signal in the vessel remains high (Fig. 5). By subtracting data sets acquired in diastole and systole, the static tissue and venous blood are suppressed, and only the arterial signal difference stays apparent (Fig. 6).

Cardiac triggering is required to align the acquisition with systole and diastole. To determine the times of systolic peak and diastolic plateau for proper trigger delays in the subsequent three-dimensional turbo spin-echo MR angiography scan, it is recommended to acquire a cine

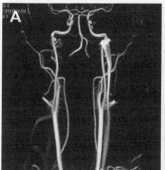
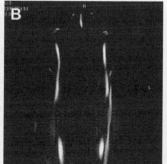
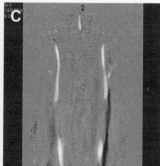

Fig. 4. Set of neck PCA images. (A) PCA maximum intensity projection. (B) Magnitude PCA speed image. (C) Phase PCA velocity image.

phase-contrast scan. To be subtracted, the systolic and diastolic data sets need to have identical field of view, coverage, and resolution.

Balanced Steady State Free Precession

Balanced steady-state free precession sequence, also known as "true fast imaging with steady-state precession," "balanced fast-field echo," or "fast imaging employing steady-state acquisition," is a free precession gradient echo sequence with balanced gradients in all directions. It is T2 and T1 weighted; uses short TR/TE (approximately 2-3/1–1.5 milliseconds); yields high fluid signal;[10] and has been used extensively in cardiac imaging. By virtue of its bright blood signal, it also has use for non-CE angiography. It is commonly used in coronary,[11] thoracic,[12] and renal angiography.[13,14] Abdominal vascular imaging can be done either during breath hold or with a respiratory-triggered free-breathing acquisition. For renal MR angiography, fat saturation and saturation bands are used over kidneys and vena cava for suppressing high signal. In addition, a slice-selective inversion pulse can be used to suppress background signal, whereas noninverted inflowing blood yields high signal. Moreover, it has been reported that the increased sensitivity to oxygenation at 3 T allows higher contrast between arteries and veins.[15] Balanced steady-state free precession applications are discussed elsewhere in this issue.

CONTRAST-ENHANCED MR ANGIOGRAPHY
T1-Weighted Three-Dimensional Gradient Echo MR Angiography

CE MR angiography is based on the concept of blood T1 shortening after the injection of the

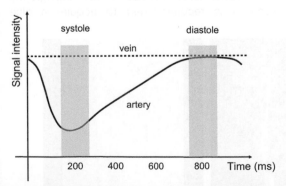

Fig. 5. Arterial and venous signal intensities throughout the cardiac cycle. Maximum signal difference occurs in systole and minimum difference in diastole.

paramagnetic contrast agent gadolinium. MR angiography contrast is based on T1 differences between arterial and venous blood, and the surrounding tissues.

A three-dimensional radiofrequency-spoiled gradient echo sequence is used following the injection of contrast media. Radiofrequency spoiling of transverse magnetization increases the T1 weighting and reduces some background tissue signal. Repetition and echo times (TR, TE) of the gradient echo sequences are kept as short as possible (TR <4 milliseconds, TE <3 milliseconds) to minimize the total acquisition time, especially for breath hold scans. The total scan times usually range from 10 to 30 seconds. Besides the latest generation gradient performance allowing to minimize TR and TE, scan times are further reduced by subsampling techniques, such as partial Fourier and parallel imaging:[16] sensitivity encoding,[17] simultaneous acquisition of spatial harmonics,[18] generalized autocalibration partially parallel acquisitions.[19] With partial Fourier, also referred to as "partial NEX" or "halfscan," over half of k-space is acquired (typically 60%), and the remaining part synthesized by complex conjugation. With the current development of multiple channels radiofrequency coils, overall parallel acceleration of six times or higher can be achieved without substantial loss of image quality. Typical volumes of chest MR angiography can be acquired in breath hold times below 20 seconds.

Unlike CT, MR imaging acquires a full three-dimensional volume before Fourier transform reconstruction. A three-dimensional magnetic resonance acquisition does not suffer slice misregistration in case of slight patient motion, but the artifact is spread out through the entire k-space, and the resulting artifact is not too severe in case of minor motion. In the case of severe motion, all images in the three-dimensional volume may be compromised. The SNR of a three-dimensional acquisition is higher compared with two-dimensional because signal from each voxel is sampled throughout the entire scan. Interpolation is often used in the reconstruction to enhance vessel appearance, but it does not improve true resolution. With the latest acceleration techniques (reviewed later), the performance of three-dimensional MR angiography is approaching that of multislice CT in terms of resolution and speed.

K-space sampling
MR signal is collected as spatial frequencies, known as "k-space," and images are reconstructed by Fourier transform. The central part of k-space, containing low spatial frequencies,

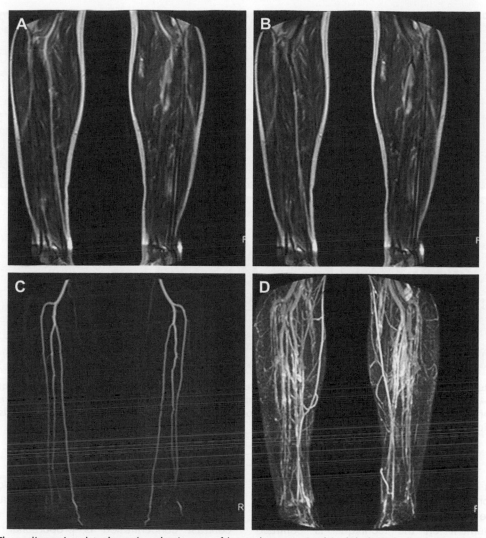

Fig. 6. Three-dimensional turbo spin-echo image of lower legs acquired in (*A*) diastole (high signal artery and veins) and (*B*) systole (low signal arteries, high signal veins). (*C*) Subtracted image disastole-systole with high arterial signal. (*D*) Maximum intensity projection of the systolic phase showing a venogram.

constitutes the dominant determinant of image contrast, whereas the higher frequencies at the periphery of k-space provide the high-resolution detail (**Fig. 7**). The k-space temporal sampling of the three-dimensional acquisition can be sequential (or linear), starting from one edge of k-space, progressing through the center, then to the other edge. In centric temporal sampling, the acquisition starts in the center of k-space and then alternatively fills in toward the periphery. For three-dimensional imaging, there are two phase encoding directions and a single frequency direction. The same concepts of centric ordering can be applied to three-dimensional imaging in either phase encoding direction or both directions for elliptic-centric ordering. Centric or elliptic-centric

sampling order is most commonly used for MR angiography.[20] Following gadolinium administration, the timing of the arrival of the contrast bolus is aligned with the peak of a centric acquisition. The peak of contrast enhancement is captured early, and edge-enhancement artifacts are avoided.[21] To capture the arterial phase, low k-space frequencies have to be acquired precisely at the peak of arterial enhancement, well before the contrast arrives in the veins. Interestingly, the contrast may arrive in the veins toward the end of the acquisition without severe consequence of venous contamination. The presence of gadolinium in a structure during acquisition of the center of k-space is the key determinant of the final image contrast.

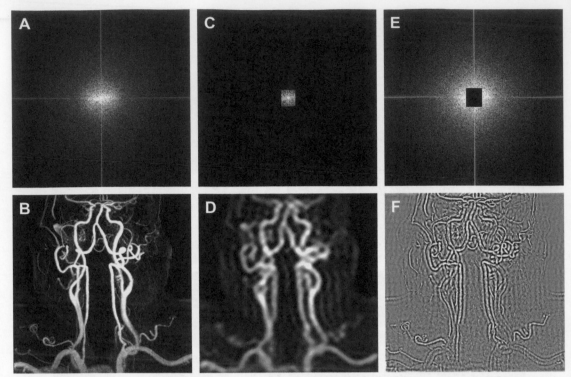

Fig. 7. Representation of low and high spatial k-space frequencies, and their effect on the image. Fully acquired k-space (*A*) and the Fourier reconstructed image (*B*). Fourier transforming only the center of k-space (*C*) results in high-contrast features and low-resolution image (*D*). Fourier transforming of k-space periphery (*E*) results in fine resolution detail (*F*).

With centric encoding, the precise timing from injection to scan delay is extremely important to capture the peak contrast enhancement. An improvement on the technique is contrast-enhanced timing-robust angiography.[22] With contrast-enhanced timing-robust angiography, the first few seconds of the central elliptic k-space zone are sampled randomly to create a larger time window of the arterial phase. This decreases the sensitivity of the center of k-space acquisition to the contrast enhancement peak.

Timing, contrast dose, injection rate
The T1 is related to the gadolinium contrast concentration through the following relation:

$$1/T1 = 1/T1_0 + r1 \times [Gd] \qquad (Eq\ 2)$$

where $T1_0$ is the T1 before contrast arrival, r1 the agent relaxivity expressed in $mM^{-1}s^{-1}$, and [Gd] the gadolinium concentration expressed in millimolars.

It is essential to inject a sufficient dose of contrast agent to shorten the T1 of blood well below surrounding tissues, thereby increasing the SNR in the vessels. In abdominal MR angiography it is desired to have the blood T1 to be less than the T1 of fat, which has a native T1 of 270 milliseconds at 1.5 T. The arterial contrast concentration is proportional to the ratio of injection rate (milliliter per second) and inversely proportional to the cardiac output (milliliter):

$$Arterial\ [Gd]\ Concentration \propto$$
$$injection\ rate/cardiac\ output \qquad (Eq\ 3)$$

Combining equations (2) and (3) gives the following relationship between the blood T1, cardiac output, and the injection rate:

$$T1 \propto (cardiac\ output)/(injection\ rate \times r1) \qquad (Eq\ 4)$$

The relationship between the blood T1 and injection rate in **Fig. 8** has been established by Maki and colleagues.[23]

With the gadolinium relaxivity of 4.5 mmol/L-1s-1 it is estimated that the gadolinium arterial blood concentration should be at least 1 mmol/L. Usual doses for conventional agents (0.5 M) and injection rates of contrast are

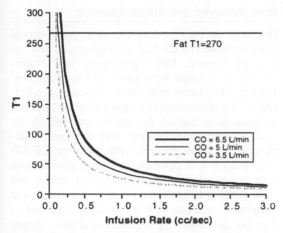

Fig. 8. Blood T1 versus infusion rate relation for different cardiac outputs. (*From* Maki JH, Prince MR, Chenevert TC. Optimizing three-dimensional gadolinium-enhanced magnetic resonance angiography. Invest Radiol 1998;33:528–37; with permission.)

0.2 mmol per kg of body weight at 2 to 3 mL/s, or 20 to 30 mL regardless of body weight. With the possible risk of nephrogenic systemic sclerosis associated with gadolinium, the tendency is to reduce contrast dose, especially if scanning is performed at 3 T. Contrast agent can be injected by hand, but is mostly done by power injector that delivers a precise, reproducible dose and injection rate, and is followed by a saline flush to clear the injection line and to avoid bolus dispersion.

Timing of injection and acquisition is critical to capture the contrast enhancement in the vascular territory optimally. The center of k-space should ideally be acquired when the contrast arrives into the vessel of interest. The time of contrast arrival can be determined by test bolus, automatic triggering on contrast agent arrival, or "fluoroscopic" real-time monitoring (**Fig. 9**). Test bolus is a low volume injected before the MR angiography sequence. A signal versus time curve is plotted for an area of interest, and the time to bolus peak (TTP) is determined. The scan delay for the

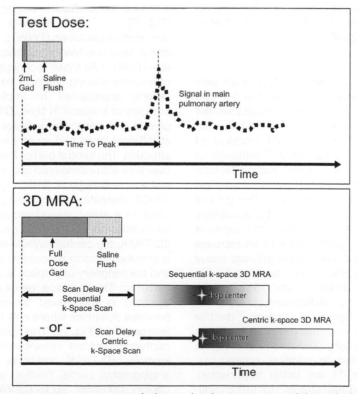

Fig. 9. Time-to-peak measurement on a test bolus and subsequent scan delay calculation for the three-dimensional MR angiography contrast agent injection.

subsequent MR angiography scan can be calculated as follows:

$$scan\ delay = TTP + \frac{injection\ duration}{2} - \frac{scan\ duration}{2}$$

for sequential k-space ordered scan. Alternatively, for centric ordered acquisition,

$$scan\ delay = TTP + \frac{injection\ duration}{2}$$

Often an additional few seconds to account for bolus rise time are added to the scan delay to avoid "ringing artifact" if the scan starts too early relative to agent arrival (ie, it is better to be a little late than a little early).[21] With contrast-enhanced timing-robust angiography, the additional rise-time delay is not necessary, because a central ellipse of k-space is randomly sampled during rise time.

Inadequate timing of center of k-space acquisition can result in suboptimal arterial-venous contrast.[24,25] Another method is the fluoroscopic-like real-time imaging of a thick slab, usually in the coronal and sagittal plane at a rate of two scans per second. The full contrast dose is injected during that scan. As the contrast arrives in the area of interest, the subsequent MR angiography scan is started either by user interaction or by an automated algorithm.

Field strength

To date, most MR angiography has been performed on 1.5-T magnets. The advent of 3-T field strength into clinical practice has brought several advantages to both noncontrast and CE MR angiography. First, a theoretical SNR increase of approximately 90% is expected,[26] although in practice not fully used because of multiple factors, such as flip angle reduction for specific absorption rate limitation and T1 prolongation. The gain of signal can be used to increase spatial resolution, or acquisition speed, or to reduce the contrast dose. The T1 prolongation refers to an increase in T1 of tissue at 3 T, decreasing intrinsic tissue T1 contrast. Lu and colleagues[27] reported a 15% to 30% increase of tissue T1 and 10% to 20% decrease in T2*, but the relative contrast enhancement by gadolinium injection is stronger,[28] despite a reduction of 4% to 7% in relaxivity at 3 T.[29] Three Tesla MR angiography benefits from higher contrast-to-noise ratio. In addition, nonvascular tissues with longer T1 are better suppressed. The advantage of 3-T field strength for MR angiography was reported in multiple studies.[30–34]

Time-Resolved MR Angiography

The scan duration of fully sampled conventional three-dimensional CE MR angiography is still too long for dynamic MR angiography, and is performed as a single time point MR angiography. The lack of dynamic information, however, is a limitation. The application of k-space sharing between multiple time frames (ie, dynamics) allows for kinetic CE MR angiography, and provides hemodynamic flow information. With dynamic CE MR angiography it is possible to depict phenomena with short arterial-to-venous transit times and distinguish arterial from venous structures and determine direction of flow. Dynamic information can be assessed by visual inspection, simple subtraction of time frames, creation of contrast arrival time maps,[35] or more advanced postprocessing methods.[36] By acquiring a precontrast mask for subtraction from the dynamic series, all the surrounding nonvascular tissue is removed and the vasculature is better visualized. The requirements of time-resolved MR angiography are high spatial and temporal resolution, accurate sampling of contrast transit curves, and acceptable reconstruction and reformatting times.

Time-resolved CE MR angiography techniques are mostly known by acronyms: time-resolved imaging of contrast kinetics (TRICKS),[37] time-resolved echo-shared angiographic technique (TREAT),[19,38] time-resolved imaging with stochastic trajectories (TWIST),[39] and four-dimensional time-resolved angiography using keyhole (4D-TRAK).[40] All these techniques use some form of k-space sharing, such as keyhole.[41] There are several approaches to implementing sharing portions of k-space in time. Different sections of central and peripheral k-space can be acquired at different times and recombined for final reconstruction. The central part of k-space is resampled over time with interleaved updates of more peripheral k-space regions (TRICKS) or lines (TREAT). TWIST alternates central and peripheral k-space parts in a spiral, pseudostochastic way, based on radial distance from the center of k-space. In 4D-TRAK, the central keyhole ellipsoid of k-space is acquired at each successive dynamic time point and the periphery of k-space is acquired at the last dynamic. The k-space periphery from the last dynamic is then used to reconstruct all the previous dynamics where only the central keyhole was acquired (**Fig. 10**). This optimizes the speed of capturing contrast enhancement. In addition to keyhole, 4D-TRAK combines CE timing-robust angiography, partial Fourier, and sensitivity encoding. Currently, up to 63-fold acceleration (6x keyhole, 8x sensitivity encoding, and 1.33x partial

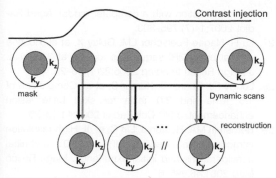

Fig. 10. Schematic representation of partial dynamic k-space keyhole acquisition, full mask and reference acquisition, and reconstruction dynamics from k-space periphery from the reference at the end of dynamic series.

Fourier) is possible with 4D-TRAK. This results in a subsecond temporal resolution and a reconstructed spatial resolution of 1.15 × 1.15 × 1.5 mm^3. In the beginning of the dynamic scan, a precontrast fully sampled mask can be acquired, which may be subtracted from subsequent dynamics to help remove residual background tissue signal. Adding view-sharing to keyhole can in addition double the temporal resolution to the order of 500 milliseconds per dynamic with the same spatial resolution. In view sharing portions of two successive keyholes are combined together to create an intermediate time point. Each of the previously mentioned approaches makes a trade-off between spatial and temporal resolution, and the temporal resolution could be limited for some anatomies and injection rates.[42] Additionally, each image contains information acquired before or after the nominal time point.

The main difference between the TRICKS, TREAT, TWIST, and 4D-TRAK is in the size of the central k-space portion, and the way it is combined with k-space periphery. With TRICKS the k-space is subdivided into fixed portions, and a part of peripheral k-space is updated for every keyhole dynamic. TRICKS and TREAT use rectangular keyhole acquiring full length of k-space lines. In 4D-TRAK and TWIST the keyhole portion of k-space is elliptic and the keyhole size is adjustable. TWIST partially updates the k-space periphery, whereas with 4D-TRAK the k-space periphery is acquired at the end of the scan.

SUMMARY

Magnetic resonance provides a wide variety of possibilities for arterial and venous blood vessel imaging in all vascular territories, from two-dimensional or three-dimensional nonexogenous contrast techniques to three-dimensional CE time-resolved MR angiography. This article reviews the basic technical concepts of TOF, PCA, triggered three-dimensional turbo spin-echo, balanced steady-state free precession, and three-dimensional CE and time-resolved three-dimensional CE MR angiography. The latest technical developments in MR imaging hardware, sequences and software, coil technology, and reconstruction capability allow dynamic MR angiography performance similar to CT angiography, without risks of iodine contrast agent and ionizing radiation exposure.

REFERENCES

1. Nishimura DG. Time-of-flight MR angiography. Magn Reson Med 1990;14:194–201.
2. Laub GA, Kaiser WA. MR angiography with gradient motion refocusing. J Comput Assist Tomogr 1988; 12(3):377–82.
3. Miyazaki M, Lee VS. Nonenhanced MR angiography. Radiology 2008;248(1):20–43, Review.
4. Eissa AM, Wilman AH. Effects of RF inhomogeneity at 3.0T on ramped RF excitation: application to 3D time-of-flight MR angiography of the intracranial arteries. J Magn Reson Imaging 2007;25(3).466–72.
5. Dumoulin CL, Souza SP, Walker MF, et al. Three-dimensional phase contrast angiography. Magn Reson Med 1989;9:139–49.
6. Wehrli FW, Shaw D, Kneeland JB. Biomedical magnetic resonance imaging: principles, methodology, and applications. New York: VCH Publishers; 1988.
7. Wedeen VJ, Meuli RA, Edelman RR, et al. Projective imaging of pulsatile flow with magnetic resonance. Science 1985;230:946–8.
8. Meuli RA, Wedeen VJ, Geller SC, et al. MR gated subtraction angiography: evaluation of lower extremities. Radiology 1986;159:411–8.
9. Miyazaki M, Sugiura S, Tateishi F, et al. Non-contrast-enhanced MR angiography using 3D ECG-synchronized half-Fourier fast spin echo. J Magn Reson Imaging 2000;12:776–83.
10. Scheffler K, Lehnhardt S. Principles and applications of balanced SSFP techniques. Eur Radiol 2003;13(11):2409–18, Epub 2003 Aug 20, Review.
11. Deshpande VS, Shea SM, Laub G, et al. 3D magnetization-prepared true-FISP: a new technique for imaging coronary arteries. Magn Reson Med 2001; 46:494–502.
12. Krishnam MS, Tomasian A, Deshpande V, et al. Non-contrast 3D steady-state free-precession magnetic resonance angiography of the whole chest using nonselective radiofrequency excitation over a large field of view: comparison with single-phase 3D

contrast-enhanced magnetic resonance angiography. Invest Radiol 2008;43(6):411–20.

13. Wyttenbach R, Braghetti A, Wyss M, et al. Renal artery assessment with nonenhanced steady-state free precession versus contrast-enhanced MR angiography. Radiology 2007;245(1):186–95.

14. Potthast S, Maki JH. Non-contrast-enhanced MR imaging of the renal arteries. Magn Reson Imaging Clin N Am 2008;16(4):573–84, vii, Review.

15. Brittain JH, Shimakawa A, Johnson JW, et al. SSFP Non-contrast-enhanced MR angiography at 3.0T: improved arterial-venous contrast with increased TR [abstract]. Proceedings of the Thirteenth Meeting of the International Society for Magnetic Resonance in Medicine, Miami, FL, May 7–13, 2005.

16. Wilson GJ, Hoogeveen RM, Willinek WA, et al. Parallel imaging in MR angiography. Top Magn Reson Imaging 2004;15(3):169–85, Review.

17. Pruessmann KP, Weiger M, Scheidegger MB, et al. SENSE: sensitivity encoding for fast MRI. Magn Reson Med 1999;42(5):952–62.

18. Sodickson DK, Manning WJ. Simultaneous acquisition of spatial harmonics (SMASH): fast imaging with radiofrequency coil arrays. Magn Reson Med 1997;38(4):591–603.

19. Griswold MA, Jakob PM, Heidemann RM, et al. Generalized autocalibrating partially parallel acquisitions (GRAPPA). Magn Reson Med 2002;47(6):1202–10.

20. Huston J, Fain SB, Wald JT, et al. Carotid artery: elliptic centric contrast-enhanced MR angiography compared with conventional angiography. Radiology 2001;218:138–43.

21. Maki JH, Prince MR, Londy FJ, et al. The effects of time varying intravascular signal intensity and k-space acquisition order on three-dimensional MR angiography image quality. J Magn Reson Imaging 1996;6(4):642–51.

22. Willinek WA, Gieseke J, Conrad R, et al. Randomly segmented central k-space ordering in high-spatial-resolution contrast-enhanced MR angiography of the supraaortic arteries: initial experience. Radiology 2002;225:583–8.

23. Maki JH, Prince MR, Chenevert TC. Optimizing three-dimensional gadolinium-enhanced magnetic resonance angiography. Invest Radiol 1998;33(9):528–37.

24. Zhang H, Maki JH, Prince MR. 3D contrast-enhanced MR angiography. J Magn Reson Imaging 2007;25(1):13–25, Review.

25. Prince MR, Chenevert TL, Foo TK, et al. Contrast-enhanced abdominal MR angiography: optimization of imaging delay time by automating the detection of contrast material arrival in the aorta. Radiology 1997;203(1):109–14.

26. Merkle EM, Dale BM, Barboriak DP. Gain in signal-to-noise for first-pass contrast-enhanced abdominal MR angiography at 3 Tesla over standard 1.5 Tesla: prediction with a computer model. Acad Radiol 2007;14(7):795–803.

27. Lu H, Nagae-Poetscher LM, Golay X, et al. Routine clinical brain MRI sequences for use at 3.0 Tesla. J Magn Reson Imaging 2005;22(1):13–22.

28. Londy FJ, Rohrer S, Kumar S, et al. Comparison of 1.5 Tesla and 3.0 Tesla for skull base lesion enhancement. J HK Coll Radiol 2008;11:19–23.

29. Bernstein MA, Huston J, Lin C, et al. High-resolution intracranial and cervical MRA at 3.0T: technical considerations and initial experience. Magn Reson Med 2001;46:995–6.

30. Allkemper T, Heindel W, Koojman H, et al. Effect of field strengths on magnetic resonance angiography: comparison of an ultrasmall superparamagnetic iron oxide blood-pool contrast agent and gadobenate dimeglumine in rabbits at 1.5 and 3.0 Tesla. Invest Radiol 2006;41:97–104.

31. Leiner T, de Vries M, Hoogeveen R, et al. Contrast-enhanced peripheral MR angiography at 3.0 Tesla: initial experience with a whole-body scanner in healthy volunteers. J Magn Reson Imaging 2003;17(5):609–14.

32. Willinek WA, Bayer T, Gieseke J, et al. High spatial resolution contrast-enhanced MR angiography of the supraaortic arteries using the quadrature body coil at 3.0T: a feasibility study. Eur Radiol 2007;17(3):618–25.

33. Willinek WA, Schild HH. Clinical advantages of 3.0 T MRI over 1.5 T. Eur J Radiol 2008;65(1):2–14, Review.

34. Kuhl CK, Träber F, Gieseke J, et al. Whole-body high-field-strength (3.0-T) MR imaging in clinical practice. Part II. Technical considerations and clinical applications. Radiology 2008;247(1):16–35.

35. Du J, Thornton FJ, Mistretta CA, et al. Dynamic MR venography: an intrinsic benefit of time-resolved MR angiography. J Magn Reson Imaging 2006;24(4):922–7.

36. Bock M, Schoenberg SO, Floemer F, et al. Separation of arteries and veins in 3D MR angiography using correlation analysis. Magn Reson Med 2000;43(3):481–7.

37. Korosec FR, Frayne R, Grist TM, et al. Time-resolved contrast-enhanced 3D MR angiography. Magn Reson Med 1996;36(3):345–51.

38. Pinto C, Hickey R, Carroll TJ, et al. Time-resolved MR angiography with generalized autocalibrating partially parallel acquisition and time-resolved echosharing angiographic technique for hemodialysis arteriovenous fistulas and grafts. J Vasc Interv Radiol 2006;17:1003–9.

39. Lim RP, Shapiro M, Wang EY. 3D time-resolved MR angiography (MRA) of the carotid arteries with time-resolved imaging with stochastic trajectories: comparison with 3D contrast-enhanced bolus-chase MRA and 3D time-of-flight MRA. AJNR Am J Neuroradiol 2008;29(10):1847–54.

40. Willinek WA, Hadizadeh DR, von Falkenhausen M, et al. 4D time-resolved MR angiography with keyhole (4D-TRAK): more than 60 times accelerated MRA using a combination of CENTRA, keyhole, and SENSE at 3.0T. J Magn Reson Imaging 2008;27(6): 1455–60.

41. van Vaals JJ, Brummer ME, Dixon WT, et al. Keyhole method for accelerating imaging of contrast agent uptake. J Magn Reson Imaging 1993;3:671–5.

42. Carroll TJ, Korosec FR, Swan JS, et al. The effect of injection rate on time-resolved contrast-enhanced peripheral MRA. J Magn Reson Imaging 2001;14(4):401–10.

Non–Contrast-Enhanced MR Imaging of Renal Artery Stenosis at 1.5 Tesla

Gregory J. Wilson, PhD[a,b],*, Jeffrey H. Maki, MD, PhD[a,c]

KEYWORDS

- Non–contrast-enhanced MR imaging
- Magnetic resonance angiography
- Renal artery stenosis
- Renal vascular hypertension
- Steady state free precession

Renal artery stenosis (RAS) is the number one cause of secondary hypertension, with a prevalence of 3% to 5% in hypertensive patients.[1–3] Seventy percent to 90% of significant RAS is caused by atherosclerosis and typically occurs near the renal ostium in the proximal renal artery (RA). Ten percent to 30% is attributable to fibromuscular dysplasia (FMD) often affecting distal RAs, presenting with a "bead-like" appearance on angiography.[4–6] Accurate diagnosis of renal vascular hypertension (RVH) relies on the ability to characterize the hemodynamic significance of stenoses. Historically, this diagnosis is based on measurement of percent stenosis by angiography. Effective treatment of RVH includes medical therapy, revascularization with percutaneous transluminal renal angioplasty with or without stent placement, or a combination of medical therapy and revascularization. Timely detection and treatment of significant RAS can cure or improve hypertension and preserve renal function.

Current diagnostic tests for grading RAS include diagnostic intra-arterial digital subtraction angiography (IA-DSA), color Doppler ultrasound (US), CT angiography (CTA), and magnetic resonance angiography (MRA).[7,8] IA-DSA is considered the "gold standard" imaging technique for detecting RAS, providing high spatial resolution lumenograms with the added benefit of directly measuring the pressure gradient across stenosis to characterize the degree of disease further. In addition, IA-DSA can be converted to a revascularization procedure during the same treatment session. With IA-DSA, a luminal diameter reduction of more than 50% to 70% (typically measured with two-dimensional [2D] projections) is the standard diagnostic criterion for hemodynamically significant RAS. If measured, a transstenotic pressure differential of 10 mm Hg (mean) or 20 mm Hg (peak) can be used to define hemodynamic significance further.[9] Color Doppler US is often used to characterize stenoses because it is readily available and low cost; however, it has a high rate of technical failure and interobserver variability and has been shown to be less accurate than CTA and contrast-enhanced (CE) MRA.[8] Despite using ionizing radiation to produce images of similar diagnostic efficacy to CE-MRA, CTA is gaining in popularity. CTA also uses injection of iodinated contrast, which is often a problem in patients with coexistent renal insufficiency. The present state-of-the-art MRA technique is gadolinium (Gd)-chelate

[a] Department of Radiology (AA010-J), University of Washington, 1959 NE Pacific Street, Seattle, WA 98195, USA

[b] Philips Healthcare, Cleveland, OH, USA

[c] Department of Radiology (S113), Puget Sound Veterans Affairs Health Care System, 1660 South Columbian Way, Seattle, WA 98108, USA

* Corresponding author. Department of Radiology (AA010-J), University of Washington, 1959 NE Pacific Street, Seattle, WA 98195.

E-mail address: gregory.wilson@philips.com (G.J. Wilson).

Magn Reson Imaging Clin N Am 17 (2009) 13–27

doi:10.1016/j.mric.2009.01.002

CE-MRA, which can be combined with additional MR imaging techniques to provide complimentary functional information (further described elsewhere in this article).

IA-DSA is infrequently used for the primary diagnosis of RAS. This invasive procedure requires arterial puncture, ionizing radiation, and nephrotoxic and potentially allergenic contrast material, often mandating a costly hospital stay. In addition, IA-DSA is constrained to 2D projections that limit the ability to characterize eccentric atherosclerotic stenoses and has been shown to have high inter-reader variability for diagnosis of RAS.[10–12] Thus, despite its gold standard status, IA-DSA is an invasive and imperfect reference standard and is considered a poor choice for first-line diagnosis of RAS.

Because of its noninvasive nature, excellent soft tissue contrast, and diversity of useful contrast mechanisms, a comprehensive MR imaging evaluation of RAS is not limited to anatomic CE-MRA lumenography alone. MR imaging evaluation of RAS typically includes volume measurements of the kidneys, usually performed with T_1-weighted scans, and additional functional information provided by correlation with poststenotic dephasing in phase-contrast angiography (PCA), quantitative flow measurements, and quantitative or qualitative Gd perfusion imaging.[13–15] Combinations of these techniques contribute to determining the "hemodynamic significance" of RAS.

This unique combined anatomic and functional capability of MR imaging brings into focus one ultimate goal in the diagnostic workup of hemodynamically significant RAS, namely, predicting the response to revascularization.[7,16] CE-MRA alone has been shown to be a costly and relatively ineffective diagnostic procedure in a poorly screened referral population.[17] The effectiveness of a comprehensive MR imaging evaluation of RAS is improved by combining stenosis measurements with functional information and further screening patients continuing to CE-MRA, however. If a comprehensive MR imaging examination combining prescreening, morphology, and functional assessment is used, a more cost-effective and better predictor of therapy response may be realized.

As mentioned previously, prescreening the referred patient population is critical for cost-effective use of MR imaging for diagnosis of RVH. Two studies[18,19] showed an approximately 20% prevalence of angiographically proved RAS when appropriate prescreening is performed using standard clinically accepted clues (eg, bruit; other vascular occlusive disease; malignant, accelerating, or sudden worsening of hypertension; unilateral small kidney; hypertension with unexplained impairment of renal function; hypertension in a child or young adult or refractory to a three-drug regimen; impairment of renal function in response to an angiotensin-converting enzyme inhibitor) for the presence of RAS.[5] Further screening with non–CE-MRA could increase the prevalence of RAS in patients moving on to CE-MRA and further improve the cost-effectiveness of MR imaging examinations. In addition, prescreening with non–CE-MRA can facilitate prescription of subsequent CE-MRA, resulting in more effective CE-MRA examinations. For example, by providing a high-quality scout view of the RAs using non–CE-MRA, the CE-MRA volume can be reduced, resulting in higher resolution or shorter breath-hold durations. Thus, non–CE-MRA has a potential role as a screening tool before CE-MRA.

CONTRAST-ENHANCED RENAL MAGNETIC RESONANCE ANGIOGRAPHY

CE-MRA of RAs is acquired with a radiofrequency spoiled gradient echo acquisition synchronized to the passage of a contrast agent bolus.[20] Sequence timing can be determined with a test bolus, automatic detection of the bolus,[21] or "fluoroscopic" triggering using real-time monitoring.[22] State-of-the-art acquisitions typically use elliptic centric ordering[23] to capture peak arterial signal, eliminate overlapping venous signal, and minimize effects of motion. Respiratory motion is reduced by breath-hold acquisition; however, this limits scan duration, and thus acquired resolution.

As reported in a 2001 meta-analysis of diagnostic tests for RAS,[8] several researchers have evaluated CE-MRA for characterization of RAS using DSA as the standard of reference.[24–29] Reported sensitivities and specificities for the individual studies range from 88% to 100% and from 75% to 100%, respectively. A recent large multicenter study by Vasbinder and colleagues[18] evaluated 356 patients and reported much lower sensitivity and specificity (62% and 84%, respectively) when compared with IA-DSA, however. Limitations of the study include the use of IA-DSA as the standard of reference, an unusually high prevalence of FMD (38% of stenoses), and dependence on CE-MRA stenosis measurements alone rather than on a more comprehensive MR imaging examination. Moreover, CE-MRA techniques have improved during and subsequent to the study.

Nevertheless, as made clear by Vasbinder and colleagues,[8] CE-MRA does have limitations. Most notably, resolution of CE-MRA in RAs is limited by bolus profile and motion. The RAs are subject to respiratory- and cardiac-related motion. Respiratory motion primarily affects more distal branches of the RAs and is not entirely eliminated by breath-holding.[30] Cardiac-related motion is most pronounced in the proximal RA, the site of most atherosclerotic RAS.[31] Respiratory motion limits the nominal acquired resolution by limiting scan time to a breath-hold, and, more importantly, bolus profile and uncompensated motion limit the realized image resolution by blurring vessel edges.[30,32] In addition, CE-MRA image quality can be degraded by poststenotic intravoxel dephasing, leading to poststenotic luminal signal voids,[33] and depiction of distal RAs may be obscured by parenchymal enhancement.

Notable improvements to CE-MRA image quality are provided by reduced field of view (FOV) imaging[34] and use of parallel imaging techniques.[35–38] Both techniques allow more rapid image acquisition, leading to higher nominal resolution and reduction of motion and bolus artifacts. The highest potential for improvement may be the combination of luminal imaging (eg, CE-MRA or non–CE-MRA) with functional MR imaging scans to provide a comprehensive evaluation of the hemodynamic significance of RAS, however.[15]

CONTRAST-ENHANCED PERFUSION OF KIDNEYS

Several researchers have reported efforts to measure kidney perfusion using Gd-enhanced MR imaging.[39–45] This effort is warranted, because accurate measurement of kidney perfusion could provide a direct measure of the hemodynamic significance of RAS. Quantitative and reproducible measurement of kidney perfusion is complicated by several technical issues, however, including motion of the kidneys, accurate determination of arterial input function (including inflow effects),[46] and T_1 and T_2^* dependence on contrast agent concentration. Moreover, extracellular Gd-chelate contrast agents are cleared by glomerular filtration (most 100%) and do not remain in the blood pool, further complicating analysis of Gd perfusion measurements.

Developments in this area are ongoing. For example, a recent study of 56 patients who had renovascular disease used a low-dose (Gd-chelate, 2 mL) protocol to semiquantitatively evaluate renal perfusion.[43] After bolus injection, a three-dimensional (3D) volume covering the kidneys was acquired at multiple time points with a minimal temporal resolution of 7 seconds. This small-bolus technique can be immediately followed by CE-MRA without compromising image quality; however, the small bolus failed in several patients (9 of 56) when no enhancement was seen in the cortex. The perfusion technique showed a significantly reduced cortical-aortic

peak enhancement ratio and time delay in severely stenosed RAs. Furthermore, model-based methods can be used to give additional quantitative perfusion measures. Gd-perfusion measurements are a potentially valuable but contrast-based method to provide functional information in a comprehensive evaluation of RAS. Non-CE methods for assessment of kidney function are described next.

NON–CONTRAST-ENHANCED TECHNIQUES FOR EVALUATION OF RENAL ARTERY STENOSIS

Non–CE-MRA techniques have been around for many years but are re-emerging as potential compliments, prescreening tools, or replacements for CE-MRA. Using non–CE-MRA as a screening step before CE-MRA potentially increases the cost-effectiveness of CE-MRA as a diagnostic test by increasing the prevalence of RAS in patients who proceed to CE-MRA, decreasing the number of patients requiring contrast agent administration, and improving the volume-planning efficiency of any subsequent CE-MRA. As mentioned previously, non–CE-MRA may also provide benefit in combination with measures of kidney function, such as low-dose Gd-based kidney perfusion or other non-CE measurements of function (described elsewhere in this article). Moreover, the recent discovery of a link between specific Gd-chelate contrast agents and nephrogenic systemic fibrosis and nephrogenic fibrosing dermopathy mandates judicious use of contrast agents.[47] Although the incidence of this complication is rare, the likelihood increases in patients with compromised renal function. Updated US Food and Drug Administration (FDA) guidelines for the use of Gd-chelate contrast agents are available on the Web[48] and also in an article elsewhere in this issue.

Non-CE MR imaging techniques for the evaluation of RAS include measures of morphology and function. Time of flight (TOF), phase contrast angiography (PCA), arterial spin labeling (ASL), and balanced steady-state free precession (Bal-SSFP) angiography have been used for morphologic characterization of RAS. Dephasing in PCA, quantitative flow (QFlow), and ASL perfusion have been investigated for assessment of renal function. An overview of each technique is provided in this article, with a thorough review of the recent Bal-SSFP techniques for characterizing RA morphology.

TIME OF FLIGHT

TOF angiography relies on the saturation of background signal in the imaging slab while inflowing fresh blood appears bright when entering the imaging volume.[49] The technique is often limited by saturation of in-plane flowing blood. This saturation is particularly problematic for imaging the RAs because they lie nearly orthogonal to the aorta. Several developments have improved TOF image quality, including decreasing the 3D imaging slab thickness by using multiple overlapping thin-slab acquisitions[50] and use of variable excitation angles (tilt-optimized non-saturated excitation)[51] to reduce saturation of inflowing blood. These techniques are particularly successful for evaluation of the intracranial vasculature.

In the hands of expert users, 3D TOF techniques have been shown to be fairly accurate for grading RAS. A recent (2001) meta-analysis of diagnostic tests for RAS[8] included six publications reporting 3D TOF comparison to IA-DSA for evaluation of RAS. In these studies, sensitivity ranged from 54% to 100% and specificity ranged from 73% to 96%. Limitations of TOF in the RAs include long scan times, saturation of in-plane flow, poststenotic signal voids, and respiratory motion artifacts. Although TOF is used effectively in other anatomies, such as carotid, intracranial, and peripheral (calf) arteries, it is not routinely used for evaluation of RAS.

PHASE CONTRAST ANGIOGRAPHY

PCA uses flow-encoding gradients to create a phase difference between flowing blood and stationary tissue.[52] A map of the phase difference can be displayed as an angiogram, because only flowing blood accumulates the phase variation. For primary morphologic evaluation, this technique is limited by signal voids created by poststenotic turbulent flow causing intravoxel phase dispersion. The previously mentioned 2001 meta-analysis[8] included three publications of PCA comparisons to IA-DSA. In these three studies, sensitivities ranged from 90% to 100% and specificities ranged from 65% to 99%. As a consequence of poststenotic signal voids, RAS tends to be overcalled on PCA; therefore, PCA is infrequently used for primary morphologic assessment of RAS.

Phase contrast techniques, however, are an effective adjunct to CE-MRA to help grade the hemodynamic significance, with PCA and QFlow techniques used in this regard. Hemodynamic significance of RAS can be defined as a transstenotic pressure drop of functional significance. Poststenotic signal voids in PCA correlate with pressure gradients, and therefore can be used to predict hemodynamic significance.[53] In 1997,

Prince and colleagues[13] published an outcome study correlating poststenotic dephasing in PCA with patient response to therapy. These researchers' recommendation was to perform CE-MRA and PCA for evaluation of RAS. A severe stenosis appeared occluded on PCA and occluded or stenotic on CE-MRA, whereas a moderate stenosis appeared stenotic on both sequences (ie, incomplete flow void with PCA). This stenosis grading, combined with measures of renal length, parenchymal thickness, loss of corticomedullary differentiation, asymmetry of enhancement, and poststenotic dilatation, is used to predict the hemodynamic significance of the stenosis. In this way, signal dephasing in PCA provides an additional qualitative measure of the hemodynamic significance of RAS.

QUANTITATIVE FLOW

QFlow imaging uses the same principle of phase contrast flow encoding to create quantitative maps of blood flow velocity in a single slice (2D) orthogonal to a vessel. Typically, the acquisition is triggered by electrocardiography (ECG) and acquired in multiple heart phases (cine QFlow) displaying hemodynamic flow patterns throughout the cardiac cycle. For evaluation of RAS, the imaging plane is prescribed just distal to the stenosis and orthogonal to the RA. This noncontrast MR imaging technique has potential for quantitative evaluation of blood flow across a stenosis; however, application in the RA has been limited by achievable spatial resolution and respiratory motion.[54,55]

Respiratory-compensated techniques do not produce adequate temporal resolution for analysis of hemodynamic flow patterns but have been shown to produce accurate measures of mean flow.[56] Alternatively, nonrespiratory compensated techniques can have higher temporal resolution but have respiratory motion-related blurring.[57] These higher temporal resolution techniques can be used to differentiate flow patterns throughout the cardiac cycle (eg, early systolic peak, midsystolic maximum flow), however. Recently, investigations by Schoenberg and colleagues[15] have shown high correlation with IA-DSA when CE-MRA is combined with high temporal resolution (25–32 milliseconds) cine QFlow for grading RAS. Severe stenosis was marked by a featureless flow pattern, in contrast to a normal RA flow pattern, which displays an early systolic peak and a midsystolic maximum. In combination with CE-MRA, this comprehensive diagnostic approach achieved greater agreement with

IA-DSA than CE-MRA alone (33 of 34 patients versus 28 of 34 patients, using a binomial classification of significance) and significantly higher interobserver agreement (median κ = 0.75) than CE-MRA (median κ = 0.7) or IA-DSA alone (median κ = 0.67).

Recent developments in MR imaging, such as parallel imaging, radial imaging, and undersampling in the spatial and temporal domains, have been applied to phase contrast and QFlow measurements, potentially increasing their effectiveness in characterizing RAS. In 2005, Baltes and colleagues[58] applied k-t broad-use linear acquisition speed-up technique to QFlow measurements in the aorta, providing a fivefold acceleration with no significant difference in flow measurements. The 2D sequence acquired 1.3 mm in-plane resolution with 30 to 32 cardiac phases. In 2007, Lum and colleagues[59] applied phase contrast vastly undersampled isotropic projection reconstruction[60] in a swine model for evaluation of arterial stenoses in the carotid arteries, iliac arteries, and RAs, including QFlow and pressure gradient measurements. The transstenotic pressure gradients correlated well (r = 0.952, P<.001) with endovascular pressure-sensing guide wires in the carotid and iliac arteries; however, imaging of the RAs was problematic because of respiratory motion in this animal model. Despite the current respiratory motion complication for imaging RAs, the continued acceleration of QFlow imaging holds promise for MR imaging measurement of transstenotic pressure gradients that may soon become applicable to comprehensive MR imaging evaluation of RAS.

ARTERIAL SPIN-LABELING PERFUSION

In ASL, inflowing blood is "labeled" by spin inversion upstream from the imaging volume. After a "labeling delay," the volume of interest is imaged using a fast readout (eg, Bal-SSFP, echo-planar imaging). By subtracting "labeled" acquisitions from "nonlabeled" acquisitions, maps of blood flow are created. Many variations of this technique have been investigated for brain perfusion, and a few have been reported for evaluation of kidney perfusion.[61,62] In 2006, Fenchel and colleagues[63] reported strong correlation (r = 0.83) between an ASL technique and scintigraphic perfusion for evaluation of renal perfusion in 18 patients. This initial study used flow-sensitive alternating inversion recovery ASL labeling with Bal-SSFP readout. Although larger studies are needed to evaluate the efficacy of such techniques, ASL perfusion holds promise as a tool in evaluating RVH without the need for contrast agents.

ARTERIAL SPIN-LABELING MAGNETIC RESONANCE ANGIOGRAPHY

In a similar way, ASL can be used to create bright-blood images of arterial anatomy. In ASL perfusion, the labeling delay is adjusted to allow labeled blood to perfuse the tissue of interest. Alternatively, to create morphologic maps of arteries, the labeling delay is decreased so that the labeled blood is still in the arteries during signal acquisition. Two techniques have been described in the literature for ASL MRA in RAs. The first uses signal targeting with alternating radiofrequency.[64] This technique has been demonstrated in human RAs[65] and in an animal model combined with ASL perfusion.[62]

The second ASL angiography technique applied to the RAs uses a "pencil-beam" 2D excitation pulse to label aortic blood selectively. This technique can be respiratory navigator-gated to eliminate respiratory motion artifacts and ECG-triggered to reduce cardiac motion and artifacts from pulsatile flow. The technique was evaluated in human subjects (8 controls and 7 patients)[66] and in an animal model.[67] Both ASL techniques report promising initial results with good depiction of RAs. Further evaluation is needed to evaluate efficacy in patients, particularly because these techniques are relatively flow-dependent.

BALANCED STEADY-STATE FREE PRECESSION MAGNETIC RESONANCE ANGIOGRAPHY

Several investigators have reported encouraging results using Bal-SSFP sequences for MRA of RAs.[68–74] Bal-SSFP is fast, is weighted by T_2/T_1 ratio, provides bright blood signal, and is relatively flow-insensitive.[75,76] Bal-SSFP is a gradient echo sequence with short repetition time (TR) and echo time (TE) (TE = $\frac{1}{2}$ TR) and complete gradient refocusing to provide high signal-to-noise images. Bal-SSFP has been applied extensively in cardiac imaging, including evaluation of cardiac function using bright-blood cine imaging and bright-blood coronary imaging. Non-CE coronary imaging sequences typically use ECG triggering, prospective respiratory navigator-gating, and magnetization preparation (eg, T_2 preparation).[77] Bal-SSFP can be combined with a variety of fat suppression and other magnetization preparation techniques.

The prospective respiratory navigator employed in several of the RA studies uses a 2D pencil-beam excitation to track the position of the diaphragm during respiration.[78–81] The navigator position is specified during sequence planning by the operator and is typically placed near the dome of the liver. The sequence periodically (eg, each heart beat) determines the position of the lung-dia-phragm interface and accepts only data acquired during end expiration. End-expiratory position is determined automatically by the scanner during sequence preparation. Data acquired at other points during the respiratory cycle are rejected, resulting in reduced scan efficiency (typically around 50%). Thus, respiratory motion compensation is achieved during the free-breathing scan.

In the eight published studies of RA imaging with Bal-SSFP, several combinations of ECG triggering, respiratory navigator-gating, breath-holding, and fat saturation have been investigated. These studies are described next.

ELECTROCARDIOGRAPHY-TRIGGERED BALANCED STEADY-STATE FREE PROCESSION

In 2004, Katoh and colleagues[68] reported Bal-SSFP for RA MRA using ECG triggering, respiratory navigator-gating, and slab-selective inversion for background signal suppression. After the inversion, a user-defined delay (inversion time [TI]) allows flow of fresh blood into the imaging slab. The trigger delay (Td) is adjusted so that inversion occurs just before systolic flow and acquisition occurs during diastolic flow in the RAs to allow maximum inflow of the noninverted blood. As in coronary imaging, this timing also reduces the effect of cardiac-related motion during the acquisition, because diastole is typically the period of most quiescent motion. The reported study compared sequences with slab-selective inversion, nonselective inversion, and no inversion and found that the slab-selective inversion provided the desired bright-blood signal with good background suppression.

Sequence parameters are summarized in **Table 1** (Katoh, 2004) for the slab-selective technique. The sequence acquired a 3D volume of a 320-mm FOV with 40-mm cranial-caudal coverage. The slab is oriented near transverse, with double obliquity to cover the desired RA anatomy efficiently. Resolution of 1.25 mm × 1.25 mm × 4.0 mm was acquired with reconstruction to 0.6 mm × 0.6 mm × 2.0 mm. The sequence used three regional saturation pulses: one inferior to suppress signal from the inferior vena cava (IVC) and two anterior for suppression of abdominal wall. Scan time was 3 minutes, with approximately 50% navigator efficiency.

Results are summarized in **Table 2** (Katoh, 2004). Eight patients were evaluated, with 15 main RAs, 3 high-grade stenoses, and 3 low-grade stenoses. All stenoses were correctly identified by the Bal-SSFP technique.

Table 1
Electrocardiography-triggered navigator-gated steady-state free precession: sequence parameters

	Katoh, 2004 (Slab-Selective IR)	Katoh, 2005 (Cartesian)	Wyttenbach
Technique	3D IR Bal-TFE	3D IR Bal-TFE	3D IR Bal-TFE
FOV (mm³) (RL × AP × FH)	320 × 320 × 40	390 × 390 × 32	360 × 360 × 40
Acquired resolution (mm) (RL × AP × FH)	1.25 × 1.25 × 4.0	1.0 × 1.0 × 3.6	0.9 × 1.2 × 2.0
Scan time (min:sec)	3:00 (with 50% navigator-gated eff.)	2:05	4:00 (with 50% navigator-gated eff.)
TR (ms)	4.4	5.2	5.4
TE (ms)	2.2	2.6	2.7
Excitation angle	85	85	85
Turbo factor	—	—	—
Averages	—	—	2
Fat suppression	None	None	SPIR
Cardiac triggering	ECG-triggered	ECG-triggered	ECG-triggered
Respiratory gating	Navigator-gated (5 mm)	Navigator-gated (5 mm)	Navigator-gated (5 mm)
Additional prepulse	Slab-selective IR	Slab-selective IR	Slab-selective IR (TI = 325 milliseconds)
REST slabs	2 anterior, 1 inferior	2 anterior, 1 inferior	1 inferior

Abbreviations: AP, anterior-posterior; eff, efficiency; FH, foot-head; IR, inversion recovery; REST, regional saturation pulse; RL, right-left; TFE, turbo field echo.

Table 2
Electrocardiography-triggered navigator-gated steady-state free precession: results

	Katoh, 2004	Katoh, 2005	Wyttenbach
Patients, years (average age)	8 (53)	10 (42.9)	57 (58)
No. main RAs in patient study	15	23 (main + accessories)	108
No. accessory RAs	—	—	26
No. stenoses	3 high-grade, 3 low-grade	2 high-grade, 2 low/moderate-grade, 5 FMD	20 high-grade, 22 low-grade
Sensitivity	100%	100%	95%/100%[a]
Specificity	100%	100%	93%/95%[a]
NPV	100%	100%	99%/100%[a]
	—	—	—

[a] Reader 1/reader 2. Patient-by-patient statistics: sensitivity, 100%/100%; specificity, 92%/95%; NPV, 100%/100%.

In 2005, Katoh and colleagues[69] reported further modification and evaluation of the technique. This study compared three variations of the technique, including a modification of the previous Cartesian acquisition, implementation of a Cartesian acquisition with water-selective excitation, and a radial acquisition with water-selective excitation. Each acquisition used ECG triggering, respiratory navigator-gating, and slab-selective inversion as in the previous study. Of the three sequences evaluated, the Cartesian acquisition was preferred for overall image quality and reduction of artifacts.

The preferred sequence acquired has a 390-mm FOV with 32-mm cranial-caudal coverage. The acquired resolution was 1.0 mm × 1.0 mm × 3.6 mm (reconstructed to 0.76 mm × 0.76 mm × 1.8 mm), which was slightly greater than the previous study. Scan time was just longer than 2 minutes. Sequence parameters are summarized in **Table 1** (Katoh, 2005). This study evaluated 10 patients with 23 total (main + accessory) RAs. Two high-grade stenoses, 2 low-grade stenoses, and 5 cases of FMD were correctly characterized. Results are summarized in **Table 2** (Katoh, 2005).

A larger patient study using a similar ECG-triggered Bal-SSFP sequence was reported by Wyttenbach and colleagues[70] in 2007. This study evaluated 57 patients with a blind comparison to CE-MRA. Sequence parameters are shown in **Table 1** (Wyttenbach). The sequence used ECG triggering with similar definition of TI and Td, respiratory navigator-gating, and slab-selective inversion. The investigators used a 2D cine QFlow prescan to measure the blood flow in the aorta at the level of the RAs and determine the patient-dependent trigger delay used in the MRA acquisition. A spectral presaturation with inversion recovery (SPIR) was added to the sequence for fat suppression, and only one saturation band

was used (inferiorly). A 360-mm FOV was acquired with 40-mm cranial-caudal coverage. Acquired resolution was 0.9 mm × 1.2 mm × 2.0 mm (reconstructed to 0.7 mm × 0.7 mm × 1.0 mm). The free-breathing scan required 4 minutes with 50% navigator efficiency. A diagram of sequence timing is shown in **Fig. 1**.

The patient study evaluated 108 main RAs and 26 accessories. Results are summarized in **Table 2** (Wyttenbach). The reference standard CE-MRA found 20 high-grade and 22 low-grade stenoses. Two blinded readers evaluated the ECG-triggered Bal-SSFP and CE-MRA scans. The sensitivity, specificity, and negative predictive value (NPV) for detection of high-grade stenoses for reader 1 and reader 2 were 95%, 93%, and 99% and 100%, 95%, and 100%, respectively, on a per-RA basis. On a per-patient basis, the values were 100%, 92%, and 100% and 100%, 95%, and 100%, respectively. Example images from a patient with normal RAs are presented in **Fig. 2**, and example images from a patient who had high-grade stenosis are presented in **Fig. 3**.

The high sensitivity, specificity, and NPV reported in this study of 57 patients (19% prevalence of high-grade stenosis per RA) are encouraging for use of the technique as a screening tool and suggest high diagnostic value for primary evaluation of RAS. The CE-MRA used for comparison is of high quality; however, as the authors acknowledge, CE-MRA alone is an imperfect reference standard for grading RAS. Further study is warranted, perhaps with combined CE-MRA and functional MR imaging as a reference standard.

ECG-triggered Bal-SSFP techniques provide a means to suppress cardiac and respiratory motion during a free-breathing scan. ECG triggering does require some additional time for planning (2D QFlow) and patient preparation in terms

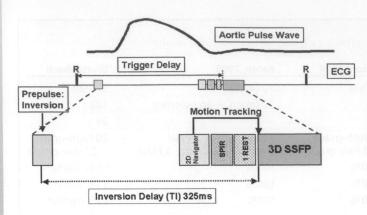

Fig. 1. Schematic illustration of elements for cardiac-triggered navigator-gated SSFP renal MRA sequence combined with a slab-selective inversion prepulse. The slab-selective inversion prepulse was applied before the data acquisition and after the aortic pulse wave by adjusting the trigger delay individually after 2D phase contrast flow measurement in the abdominal aorta. The inversion delay of 325 milliseconds allowed suppression of the renal parenchyma and renal vein signals. Spectral fat saturation (SPIR) was applied, and use of an inferior regional saturation pulse (REST) slab suppressed the signal from the IVC. Prospective real-time navigator technology was used to suppress respiratory motion. (*From* Wyttenbach R, Braghetti A, Wyss M, et al. Renal artery assessment with nonenhanced steady-state free precession versus contrast-enhanced MR angiography. Radiology 2007;245:188; with permission.)

of ECG lead placement. If ultimately used in place of CE-MRA, however, patient preparation time may perhaps be on par, because the need for intravenous access is obviated. As seen in **Fig. 3**, there is some sensitivity to flow, particularly in poststenotic RAs. The appearance of this effect is different than that of the poststenotic intravoxel dephasing seen in some CE-MRA and PCA scans. As evidenced by the clinical study, the flow dependence does not seem to have a negative impact on diagnostic value.

NON–ELECTROCARDIOGRAPHY-TRIGGERED BALANCED STEADY-STATE FREE PRECESSION

A series of additional publications reports the use of Bal-SSFP without the use of ECG triggering and without an inversion prepulse. These techniques have used breath-holding or navigator-gating for respiratory motion compensation. Various methods of fat suppression have been reported.

Coenegrachts and colleagues[71] (2004) used a multiple breath-hold Bal-SSFP sequence to acquire multiple overlapping 3D slabs covering the superior mesenteric artery to the aortic bifurcation, with a single slab centered over the main RAs. Sequence parameters are summarized in **Table 3** (Coenegrachts). The sequence required 21 seconds per breath-hold and was repeated as required to obtain the desired cranial-caudal coverage. The FOV was 300 mm × 105 mm, and the acquired resolution was 1.25 mm × 1.25 mm × 3.0 mm (reconstructed to 0.59 mm × 0.59 mm × 1.5 mm). Water-only binomial excitation was used to suppress fat, and three saturation bands were used to suppress unwanted inflowing signal from the renal veins and IVC.

Twenty-five patients were evaluated with DSA comparison. Results are summarized in **Table 4**

(Coenegrachts). Fifty main RAs, 11 accessories, and 11 high-grade stenoses (22% prevalence per RA) were identified. Three experienced vascular radiologists independently read each study twice (2-week delay between readings), with randomized patient ordering. The sensitivity, specificity, and NPV were 100%, 98%, and 100%, respectively.

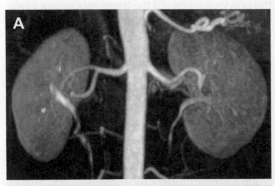
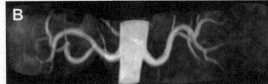

Fig. 2. Coronal CE-MRA (3.8/1.3, 35° flip angle) (*A*) and nonenhanced SSFP MRA (5.4/2.7, 85° flip angle) (*B*) Maximum-intensity projections (MIPs) in a 54-year-old patient with hypertension and normal RAs. Note the sharp delineation of the main and peripheral RAs in *B* because of suppression of cardiac and respiratory motion by means of cardiac triggering and navigator-gating. (*From* Wyttenbach R, Braghetti A, Wyss M, et al. Renal artery assessment with nonenhanced steady-state free precession versus contrast-enhanced MR angiography. Radiology 2007;245:189; with permission.)

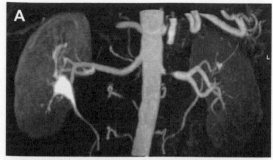

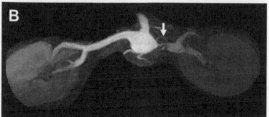

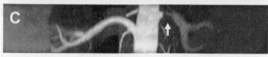

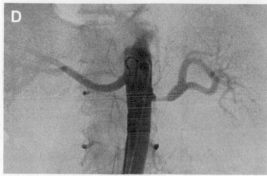

Fig. 3. (A) Coronal CE-MRA maximum-intensity projection (MIP) (3.8/1.3, 35° flip angle) in 56-year-old patient who had 80% stenosis of proximal left RA. Transverse (B) and coronal (C) nonenhanced SSFP MIPs (5.4/2.7, 85° flip angle) in the same patient show correct grading of the RAS (*arrow*), which was confirmed on the DSA image (D). In B and C, note the substantially decreased signal intensity distal to the RAS, which still enables visualization of the distal left RA. (*From* Wyttenbach R, Braghetti A, Wyss M, et al. Renal artery assessment with nonenhanced steady-state free precession versus contrast-enhanced MR angiography. Radiology 2007;245:190; with permission.)

In 2006, Herborn and colleagues[72] reported their experience with fat-saturated, breath-hold, 3D Bal-SSFP for grading RAS. The right-left FOV was 380 mm with multiple 3D slab acquisition (23-second breath-hold per 3D slab). A spectral fat saturation pulse (SPIR) was used, and the reported voxel size was 1.2 mm × 1.4 mm × 1.6

mm. Sequence parameters are summarized in **Table 3** (Herborn).

In 21 patients, 3D Bal-SSFP was compared with CE-MRA as the reference standard. Thirty-nine of 41 RAs were detected by Bal-SSFP. The study subjects included only 2 patients who had high-grade stenosis (prevalence of 5% per RA). Both (2 of 2) high-grade stenoses were correctly characterized. Two other low-grade stenoses (2 of 2) were overcalled as high-grade stenoses, and a single case of FMD was called high-grade stenosis. The investigators report a sensitivity of 92% (95% confidence interval [CI]: 0.6, 0.98) and a specificity of 81% (95% CI: 0.4, 0.95). Results are summarized in **Table 4** (Herborn).

In 2007, Maki and colleagues[73] reported comparison of three Bal-SSFP techniques for characterization of RAs. Twenty patients were imaged with (1) single breath-hold, single 3D slab; (2) three breath-hold, three 3D slab; and (3) respiratory navigator-gated, two 3D slab acquisitions. All sequences used the three-saturation band technique of Coenegrachts and colleagues[71] for suppression of inflowing venous signal. Sequence parameters for the three sequences can be found in the original reference. The parameters in **Table 3** from the subsequent clinical study[74] are similar to those used in this comparison.

In this substudy, the three Bal-SSFP sequences were compared in 20 subjects from the 40-patient clinical evaluation described elsewhere in the article.[74] Two readers graded image quality, sharpness of the RA, and reader certainty. The navigator-gated sequence was deemed superior to the two breath-hold sequences in each category. Complete clinical results are summarized elsewhere in this article. Of note for this comparison study, the single breath-hold Bal-SSFP scan missed one additional accessory artery because of reduced cranial-caudal coverage (36 mm). The three breath-hold (50 mm) and navigator-gated (48 mm) sequences covered a larger volume and detected this accessory artery.

Subsequently, Maki and colleagues[74] reported a clinical comparison of single breath-hold Bal-SSFP and navigator-gated Bal-SSFP versus CE-MRA in 40 patients with suspicion of RAS. Sequence parameters are presented in **Table 3** (Maki: BH and Nav). Each patient was scanned with single breath-hold Bal-SSFP, navigator-gated Bal-SSFP, and CE-MRA. Breath-hold Bal-SSFP covered 300 mm × 105 mm × 36 mm with 1.3 mm × 1.3 mm × 3.0 mm acquired resolution (reconstructed to 0.6 mm × 0.6 mm × 1.5 mm) in 18 seconds. Navigator-gated Bal-SSFP covered

Table 3
Non–electrocardiography-triggered steady-state free precession: sequence parameters

	Coenegrachts	Herborn	Maki (BH)	Maki (Nav)
Technique	3D Bal-TFE	3D SSFP	3D Bal-TFE	3D Bal-TFE
FOV (mm³) (RL × AP × FH)	300 × 105 × (variable)	380 (LR) × 48 (FH)	300 × 105 × 36	300 × 105 × 48
Acquired resolution (mm) (RL × AP × FH)	1.25 × 1.25 × 3.0	1.4 × 1.2 × 1.6	1.3 × 1.3 × 3.0	1.3 × 1.3 × 2.0
Scan time (min:sec)	0:21 per slab	0:23	0:18	3:24 (with 50% navigator-gated efficiency)
TR (ms)	6.9	3.8	6.4	6.4
TE (ms)	3.45	1.55	3.2	3.2
Excitation angle	80	65	80	80
Turbo factor	—	—	64	64
Averages	2 (foldover suppression)	—	4	4
Fat suppression	Water-only excitation	Fat saturated	Water-only excitation	Water-only excitation
Cardiac triggering	None	None	None	None
Respiratory gating	Exhalation BH per 3D slab	BH per 3D slab	Exhalation BH	Navigator-gated (5 mm)
Additional prepulse	None	None	None	None
REST slabs	Bilateral sagittal over kidney, and inferior	—	Bilateral sagittal over kidney, and inferior	Bilateral sagittal over kidney, and inferior

Abbreviations: AP, anterior-posterior; BH, breath-hold; FH, foot-head; RL, right-left.

300 mm × 105 mm × 48 mm with 1.3 mm × 1.3 mm × 2.0 mm acquired resolution (reconstructed to 0.6 mm × 0.6 mm × 1.0 mm) in 3 minutes 24 seconds with approximately 50% navigator efficiency. Both Bal-SSFP techniques used a water-only binomial excitation pulse and the three-saturation band technique[71] to suppress inflowing venous signal.

Both Bal-SSFP sequences were successfully performed in 38 of the 40 patients. In two cases,

Table 4
Non–electrocardiography-triggered steady-state free precession: results

	Coenegrachts	Herborn	Maki
Patients, years (average age)	25 (72)	19 (60.1)	40 (median = 67)
No. main renal arteries in patient study	50	41 (main + accessories)	83
No. accessory RAs	11		20
No. stenoses	11	2 high-grade, 2 low-grade, 1 FMD	20
Sensitivity	100%	92%	100%[a]
Specificity	98%	81%	82%[a]
NPV	100%	—	100%[a]

[a] Patient-by-patient statistics: sensitivity, 100%; specificity, 84%; NPV, 100%.

the navigator-gated sequence was not performed, once because of patient anxiety and once because of respiratory drift. When performed successfully, navigator-gated Bal-SSFP was used for Bal-SSFP read. Otherwise (in the two cases described previously), breath-hold Bal-SSFP was performed successfully and used for Bal-SSFP read. In total, 83 of 83 main RAs and 19 of 20 accessory RAs were identified by Bal-SSFP. The missed accessory RA contained moderate stenosis, and was thus more difficult to detect by Bal-SSFP. CE-MRA detected significant stenosis (>50%) in 20 of 83 main RAs (24% prevalence per RA) and in 15 of 40 patients (38% prevalence per patient). When a 45% stenosis threshold was used for Bal-SSFP, the sensitivity, specificity, and NPV were 100%, 82%, and 100%, respectively, per RA (100%, 84%, and 100%, respectively, per patient). Results are summarized in **Table 4** (Maki). Image examples are shown in **Figs. 4** and **5**.

Preliminary experience in imaging RAs with Bal-SSFP and Dixon subtraction for fat suppression was reported by Stafford and colleagues[82] in 2008. The technique was investigated at 3 T and acquired in in-phase and opposed-phase images in separate breath-holds. Implementation of an elliptic centric view order allowed relatively long acquisition times per breath-hold and high spatial resolution (mean = 2.83 mm^3). Image quality was evaluated in five normal volunteers, and results suggest good visualization of proximal RAs. This technique represents an interesting alternative to fat suppression in non–CE-MRA of RAs. Further study is required to evaluate the clinical utility of this technique.

Non–ECG-triggered Bal-SSFP techniques have been compared with reference standard DSA and CE-MRA in 84 patients with extremely high sensitivity (92%–100%) and good specificity (81%–98%).[71–74] These techniques offer simplified and shorter examination times than the ECG-triggered options. A direct comparison between ECG-triggered and non–ECG-triggered techniques for image quality (eg, sharpness) and diagnostic value has not been reported, however. The high diagnostic value of non–ECG-triggered scans likely indicates insignificance or effective averaging of cardiac-related motion for these techniques.

Both breath-hold and free-breathing non–ECG-triggered techniques produce images with high diagnostic value. In the only direct comparison of breath-hold and navigator-gating,[73] the navigator-gated sequence produced better image quality. Of potential concern is misregistration of breath-hold acquisitions in the multiple–breath-

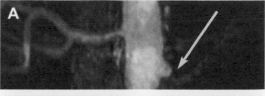
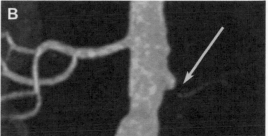
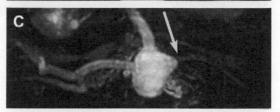
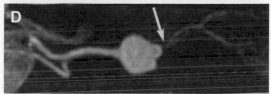

Fig. 4. A 68-year-old man with suspected RVH. Coronal and axial subvolume maximum intensity projections (MIPs) from navigator-gated (Nav) SSFP MRA (A, C) and CE-MRA (B, D) show concordance for normal right RA (0% on CE-MRA, 11% on Nav SSFP MRA) and high-grade left RAS (arrows) of 95% on CE-MRA and 82% on Nav SSFP. (A) Note that there seems to be more than 11% stenosis on Nav SSFP in the right RA secondary to MIP artifact from overlapping signal in the IVC. Stenosis measurements were obtained from thin-slice reformatted images rather than from MIPs. (From Maki JH, Wilson GJ, Eubank WB, et al. Navigator-gated MR angiography of the renal arteries: a potential screening tool for renal artery stenosis. AJR Am J Roentgenol 2007;188:W542; with permission.)

hold techniques. Furthermore, Maki and colleagues[74] reported decreased signal intensity distal to some stenoses, apparently attributable to the partial inflow dependence of Bal-SSFP. Non–ECG-triggered techniques have been successfully implemented with three different fat suppression techniques: water-only binomial excitation, spectrally selective fat saturation prepulse, and Dixon subtraction. Although each technique

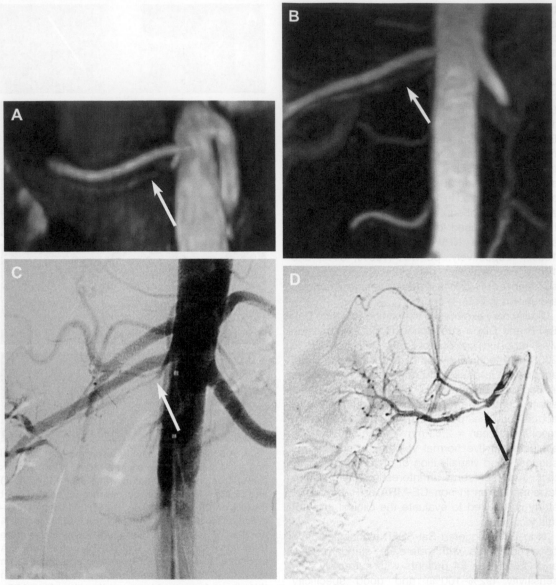

Fig. 5. A 33-year-old man with suspected RVH. Coronal subvolume maximum intensity projections from navigator-gated (Nav) SSFP MRA (*A*) and CE-MRA (*B*) with DSA correlation show injection of the aorta (*C*) and accessory RAs (*D*). Nav SSFP and CE-MRA agreed that both main arteries were nondiseased. Arrows represent the accessory artery, which was seen and thought to be diseased on Nav SSFP MRA and CE-MRA. The accessory artery was believed to represent intimal fibroplasia (an atypical form of FMD) and to be responsible for the patient's hypertension. (*From* Maki JH, Wilson GJ, Eubank WB, et al. Navigator-gated MR angiography of the renal arteries: a potential screening tool for renal artery stenosis. AJR Am J Roentgenol 2007;188:W544; with permission.)

offers potential advantages, no direct comparison of fat suppression techniques has been reported.

SUMMARY

Bal-SSFP techniques produce excellent anatomic images of RAs without the use of contrast agents and are relatively flow-insensitive. ECG-triggered

and non–ECG-triggered sequences have been shown to be quite sensitive (range: 92%–100%) for detection of RAS, and the already high specificity (range: 81%–100%) is likely to increase with further refinement of the techniques. Further study is warranted to compare techniques and increase specificity through technical improvements. ECG-triggered sequences, although more difficult to perform and inherently more flow-sensitive, have excellent background suppression and may ultimately provide sharper images. Bal-SSFP sequences can be used as a screening tool or as an alternative to CE-MRA when contrast agents are contraindicated.

In addition to morphologic imaging of RAS, non-CE techniques can be used in functional assessment of hemodynamic significance. In particular, the phase contrast techniques PCA and QFlow add valuable functional characterization of stenoses without the use of contrast agents. Future refinement and evaluation of these techniques may lead to further incorporation in MR imaging evaluation of hemodynamically significant RAS. Non-CE techniques provide valuable tools for morphologic and functional assessment of RAS. The complimentary tools can be used alone or in combination with CE-MRA in a comprehensive MR imaging evaluation of RVH.

ACKNOWLEDGMENTS

The authors thank Dr. Rolf Wyttenbach for providing figures for the ECG-triggered Bal-SSFP technique and Dr. Silke Potthast for helpful discussion.

REFERENCES

1. Hillman BJ. Imaging advances in the diagnosis of renovascular hypertension. AJR Am J Roentgenol 1989;153:5–14.
2. Derkx FH, Schalekamp MA. Renal artery stenosis and hypertension. Lancet 1994;344:237–9.
3. Eardley KS, Lipkin GW. Atherosclerotic renal artery stenosis: is it worth diagnosing? J Hum Hypertens 1999;13:217–20.
4. Safian R, Textor S. Renal-artery stenosis. N Engl J Med 2001;344:431–2.
5. Detection, evaluation, and treatment of renovascular hypertension. Working Group on Renovascular Hypertension. Arch Intern Med 1987;147:820–9.
6. Slovut DP, Olin JW. Fibromuscular dysplasia. N Engl J Med 2004;350:1862–71.
7. Leiner T, de Haan MW, Nelemans PJ, et al. Contemporary imaging techniques for the diagnosis of renal artery stenosis. Eur Radiol 2005;15:2219–29.
8. Vasbinder G, Nelemans P, Kessels A, et al. Diagnostic tests for renal artery stenosis in patients suspected of having renovascular hypertension: a meta-analysis. Ann Intern Med 2001;135:401–11.
9. Yim PJ, Cebral JR, Weaver A, et al. Estimation of the differential pressure at renal artery stenoses. Magn Reson Med 2004;51:969–77.
10. Schreij G, de Haan MW, Oei TK, et al. Interpretation of renal angiography by radiologists. J Hypertens 1999;17:1737–41.
11. van Jaarsveld BC, Pieterman H, van Dijk LC, et al. Interobserver variability in the angiographic assessment of renal artery stenosis. J Hypertens 1999;17:1731–6.
12. Paul JF, Cherrak I, Jaulent MC, et al. Interobserver variability in the interpretation of renal digital subtraction angiography. Am J Roentgenol 1999;173:1285–8.
13. Prince M, Schoenberg S, Ward J, et al. Hemodynamically significant atherosclerotic renal artery stenosis: MR angiographic features. Radiology 1997;205:128–36.
14. Michaely HJ, Schoenberg SO, Rieger JR, et al. MR angiography in patients with renal disease. Magn Reson Imaging Clin N Am 2005;13:131–51.
15. Schoenberg S, Knopp M, Londy F, et al. Morphologic and functional magnetic resonance imaging of renal artery stenosis: a multireader tricenter study. J Am Soc Nephrol 2002;13:158–69.
16. Binkert CA, Debatin JF, Schneider E, et al. Can MR measurement of renal artery flow and renal volume predict the outcome of percutaneous transluminal renal angioplasty? Cardiovasc Intervent Radiol 2001;24:233–9.
17. van Helvoort-Postulart D, Dirksen CD, Nelemans PJ, et al. Renal artery stenosis: cost-effectiveness of diagnosis and treatment. Radiology 2007;244:505–13.
18. Vasbinder G, Nelemans P, Kessels A, et al. Accuracy of computed tomographic angiography and magnetic resonance angiography for diagnosing renal-artery stenosis. Ann Intern Med 2004;141:674–82.
19. Krijnen P, van Jaarsveld B, Steyerberg E, et al. A clinical prediction rule for renal artery stenosis. Ann Intern Med 1998;129:705–11.
20. Prince M, Yucel E, Kaufman J, et al. Dynamic gadolinium-enhanced three-dimensional abdominal MR arteriography. J Magn Reson Imaging 1993;3:877–81.
21. Foo T, Saranathan M, Prince M, et al. Automated detection of bolus arrival and initiation of data acquisition in fast, three-dimensional, gadolinium-enhanced MR angiography. Radiology 1997;203(1):275–80.
22. Riederer S, Fain S, Kruger D, et al. 3D contrast-enhanced MR angiography using fluoroscopic triggering and an elliptical centric view order. Int J Cardiovasc Imaging 1999;15:117–29.
23. Wilman A, Riederer S. Performance of an elliptical centric view order for signal enhancement and motion artifact suppression in breath-hold three-dimensional gradient echo imaging. Magn Reson Med 1997;38:793–802.
24. Reiumont M, Kaufman J, Geller S, et al. Evaluation of renal artery stenosis with dynamic gadolinium-enhanced MR angiography. Am J Roentgenol 1997;169:39–44.
25. Leung DA, Pelkonen P, Hany TF, et al. Value of image subtraction in 3D gadolinium-enhanced MR

angiography of the renal arteries. J Magn Reson Imaging 1998;8:598–602.

26. Thornton J, O'Callaghan J, Walshe J, et al. Comparison of digital subtraction angiography with gadolinium-enhanced magnetic resonance angiography in the diagnosis of renal artery stenosis. Eur Radiol 1999;9:930–4.

27. Bongers V, Bakker J, Beutler JJ, et al. Assessment of renal artery stenosis: comparison of captopril renography and gadolinium-enhanced breath-hold MR angiography. Clin Radiol 2000;55:346–53.

28. de Cobelli F, Venturini M, Vanzulli A, et al. Renal arterial stenosis: prospective comparison of color Doppler US and breath-hold, three-dimensional, dynamic, gadolinium-enhanced MR angiography. Radiology 2000;214:373–80.

29. Korst M, Joosten F, Postma C, et al. Accuracy of normal-dose contrast-enhanced MR angiography in assessing renal artery stenosis and accessory renal arteries. Am J Roentgenol 2000;174: 629–34.

30. Vasbinder G, Maki J, Nijenhuis R, et al. Motion of the distal renal artery during 3D contrast-enhanced breath-hold MRA. J Magn Reson Imaging 2002;16: 685–96.

31. Kaandorp D, Vasbinder G, de Haan M, et al. Motion of the proximal renal artery during the cardiac cycle. J Magn Reson Imaging 2000;12:924–8.

32. Fain S, Riederer S, Bernstein M, et al. Theoretical limits of spatial resolution in elliptical-centric contrast-enhanced 3D-MRA. Magn Reson Med 1999;42:1106–16.

33. Evans AJ, Richardson DB, Tien R, et al. Poststenotic signal loss in MR angiography: effects of echo time, flow compensation, and fractional echo. AJNR Am J Neuroradiol 1993;14:721–9.

34. Fain S, King B, Breen J, et al. High-spatial-resolution contrast-enhanced MR angiography of the renal arteries: a prospective comparison with digital subtraction angiography. Radiology 2001;218: 481–90.

35. Weiger M, Pruessmann K, Kassner A, et al. Contrast-enhanced 3D MRA using SENSE. J Magn Reson Imaging 2000;12:671–7.

36. Chen Q, Quijano CV, Mai VM, et al. On improving temporal and spatial resolution of 3D contrast-enhanced body MR angiography with parallel imaging. Radiology 2004;231:893–9.

37. Schoenberg S, Rieger J, Weber C, et al. High-spatial-resolution MR angiography of renal arteries with integrated parallel acquisitions: comparison with digital subtraction angiography and US. Radiology 2005;235:687–98.

38. Wilson GJ, Eubank WB, Vasbinder GBC, et al. Utilizing SENSE to reduce scan duration in high-resolution contrast-enhanced renal MR angiography. J Magn Reson Imaging 2006;24:873–9.

39. Ros P, Gauger J, Stoupis C, et al. Diagnosis of renal artery stenosis: feasibility of combining MR angiography, MR renography, and gadopentetate-based measurements of glomerular filtration rate. Am J Roentgenol 1995;165:1447–51.

40. Miller S, Schick F, Duda SH, et al. Gd-enhanced 3D phase-contrast MR angiography and dynamic perfusion imaging in the diagnosis of renal artery stenosis. Magn Reson Imaging 1998;16: 1005–112.

41. Prasad PV, Goldfarb J, Sundaram C, et al. Captopril MR renography in a swine model: toward a comprehensive evaluation of renal arterial stenosis. Radiology 2000;217:813–8.

42. Lee VS, Rusinek H, Johnson G, et al. MR renography with low-dose gadopentetate dimeglumine: feasibility. Radiology 2001;221:371–9.

43. Gandy SJ, Sudarshan TAP, Sheppard DG, et al. Dynamic MRI contrast enhancement of renal cortex: a functional assessment of renovascular disease in patients with renal artery stenosis. J Magn Reson Imaging 2003;18:461–6.

44. Hacklander T, Mertens H, Stattaus J, et al. Evaluation of renovascular hypertension. J Comput Assist Tomogr 2004;28:823–31.

45. Michoux N, Montet X, Pechere A, et al. Parametric and quantitative analysis of MR renographic curves for assessing the functional behaviour of the kidney. Eur J Radiol 2005;54:124–35.

46. Ivancevic MK, Zimine I, Montet X, et al. Inflow effect correction in fast gradient-echo perfusion imaging. Magn Reson Med 2003;50:885–91.

47. Grobner T. 2006 gadolinium—a specific trigger for the development of nephrogenic fibrosing dermopathy and nephrogenic systemic fibrosis? Nephrol Dial Transplant 2006;21:1104–8.

48. Available at: http://www.fda.gov/cder/drug/infopage/gcca/default.htm. Accessed February 15, 2009.

49. Dumoulin C, Cline H, Souza S, et al. Three-dimensional time-of-flight magnetic resonance angiography using spin saturation. Magn Reson Imaging 1989;11:35–46.

50. Parker D, Yuan C, Blatter D. MR angiography by multiple thin slab 3D acquisition. Magn Reson Med 1991;17:434–51.

51. Laub G, Purdy D. Variable tip-angle slab selection for improved three-dimensional acquisition: preliminary clinical experience in 80 patients. New York (NY): Proceedings of the SMRI; 1992. p. 25.

52. Dumoulin C, Souza S, Walker M, et al. Three-dimensional phase contrast angiography. Magn Reson Med 1989;9:139–49.

53. Mustert BR, Williams DM, Prince MR. In vitro model of arterial stenosis: correlation of MR signal dephasing and trans-stenotic pressure gradients. Magn Reson Imaging 1998;16:301–10.

54. Thomsen C, Cortsen M, Sondergaard L, et al. A segmented k-space velocity mapping protocol for

quantification of renal artery blood flow during breath-holding. J Magn Reson Imaging 1995;5:393–401.

55. Maier SE, Scheidegger MB, Liu K, et al. Renal artery velocity mapping with MR imaging. J Magn Reson Imaging 1995;5:669–76.

56. de Haan MW, Kouwenhoven M, Kessels AGH, et al. Renal artery blood flow: quantification with breath-hold or respiratory triggered phase-contrast MR imaging. Eur Radiol 2000;10:1133–7.

57. Schoenberg SO, Knopp MV, Bock M, et al. Renal artery stenosis: grading of hemodynamic changes with cine phase-contrast MR blood flow measurements. Radiology 1997;203:45–53.

58. Baltes C, Kozerke S, Hansen MS, et al. Accelerating cine phase-contrast flow measurements using k-t BLAST and k-t SENSE. Magn Reson Med 2005;54:1430–8.

59. Lum DP, Johnson KM, Paul RK, et al. Transstenotic pressure gradients: measurement in swine—retrospectively ECG-gated 3D phase-contrast MR angiography versus endovascular pressure-sensing guidewires. Radiology 2007;245:751–60.

60. Gu T, Korosec FR, Block WF, et al. PC VIPR: a high-speed 3D phase-contrast method for flow quantification and high-resolution angiography. AJNR Am J Neuroradiol 2005;26:743–9.

61. Roberts DA, Detre JA, Bolinger L, et al. Renal perfusion in humans: MR imaging with spin tagging of arterial water. Radiology 1995;196:281–6.

62. Prasad PV, Kim D, Kaiser AM, et al. Noninvasive comprehensive characterization of renal artery stenosis by combination of STAR angiography and EPISTAR perfusion imaging. Magn Reson Med 1997;38:776–87.

63. Fenchel M, Martirosian P, Langanke J, et al. Perfusion MR imaging with FAIR true FISP spin labeling in patients with and without renal artery stenosis: initial experience. Radiology 2006;238:1013–21.

64. Edelman RR, Siewert B, Adamis M, et al. Signal targeting with alternating radiofrequency (STAR) sequences: application to MR angiography. Magn Reson Med 1994;31:233–8.

65. Wielopolski PA, Adamis M, Prasad P, et al. Breath-hold 3D STAR MR angiography of the renal arteries using segmented echo planar imaging. Magn Reson Med 1995;33:432–8.

66. Spuentrup E, Manning WJ, Bornert P, et al. Renal arteries: navigator-gated balanced fast field-echo projection MR angiography with aortic spin labeling: initial experience. Radiology 2002;225:589–96.

67. Spuentrup E, Buecker A, Meyer J, et al. Navigator-gated free-breathing 3D balanced FFE projection renal MRA: comparison with contrast-enhanced breath-hold 3D MRA in a swine model. Magn Reson Med 2002;48:739–43.

68. Katoh M, Buecker A, Stuber M, et al. Free-breathing renal MR angiography with steady-state free-precession (SSFP) and slab-selective spin inversion: initial results. Kidney Int 2004;66:1272–8.

69. Katoh M, Spuentrup E, Stuber M, et al. Free-breathing renal magnetic resonance angiography with steady-state free-precession and slab-selective spin inversion combined with radial k-space sampling and water-selective excitation. Magn Reson Med 2005;53:1228–33.

70. Wyttenbach R, Braghetti A, Wyss M, et al. Renal artery assessment with nonenhanced steady-state free precession versus contrast-enhanced MR angiography. Radiology 2007;245:186–95.

71. Coenegrachts K, Hoogeveen R, Vaninbroukx J, et al. High-spatial-resolution 3D balanced turbo field-echo technique for MR angiography of the renal arteries: initial experience. Radiology 2004;231:237–42.

72. Herborn C, Watkins D, Runge V, et al. Renal arteries: comparison of steady-state free precession MR angiography and contrast-enhanced MR angiography. Radiology 2006;239:263–8.

73. Maki JH, Wilson GJ, Eubank WB, et al. Steady-state free precession MRA of the renal arteries: breath-hold and navigator-gated techniques vs. CE-MRA. J Magn Reson Imaging 2007;26:966–73.

74. Maki JH, Wilson GJ, Eubank WB, et al. Navigator-gated MR angiography of the renal arteries: a potential screening tool for renal artery stenosis. AJR Am J Roentgenol 2007;188:W540–6.

75. Duerk J, Lewin J, Wendt M, et al. Remember true FISP? A high SNR, near 1-second imaging method for T2-like contrast in interventional MRI at 2 T. J Magn Reson Imaging 1998;8:203–8.

76. Foo T, Ho V, Marcos H, et al. MR angiography using steady-state free precession. Magn Reson Med 2002;48:699–706.

77. Stuber M, Weiss RG. Coronary magnetic resonance angiography. J Magn Reson Imaging 2007;26:219–34.

78. Nehrke K, Bornert P, Groen J, et al. On the performance and accuracy of 2D navigator pulses. Magn Reson Imaging 1999;17:1173–81.

79. Stuber M, Botnar R, Danias P, et al. Submillimeter three-dimensional coronary MR angiography with real-time navigator correction: comparison of navigator locations. Radiology 1999;212:579–87.

80. Spuentrup E, Manning WJ, Botnar RM, et al. Impact of navigator timing on free-breathing submillimeter 3D coronary magnetic resonance angiography. Magn Reson Med 2002;47:196–201.

81. Spuentrup E, Bornert P, Botnar R, et al. Navigator-gated free-breathing three-dimensional balanced fast field echo (TrueFISP) coronary magnetic resonance angiography. Invest Radiol 2002;37:637–42.

82. Stafford RB, Sabati M, Haakstad MJ, et al. Unenhanced MR angiography of the renal arteries with balanced steady-state free precession Dixon method. AJR Am J Roentgenol 2008;191:243–6.

Neurovascular Imaging at 1.5 Tesla Versus 3.0 Tesla

Benjamin Y. Huang, MD, MPH*, Mauricio Castillo, MD

KEYWORDS

- 3.0 Tesla • Head and neck MRA • Carotid MR angiography
- Time-of-flight MR angiography
- Contrast-enhanced MR angiography

When 3.0 Tesla (T) MR imaging systems were first approved for clinical use in the United States, they were received with much excitement and fanfare, and they brought the promise of higher quality images and considerably shorter acquisition times compared with 1.5T systems. Nearly a decade later, there have been significant gains in some areas as a result of 3.0T imaging (eg, functional brain imaging); while in other applications, improvements have been less noticeable. One area that has seen a dramatic improvement because of 3.0T MR imaging systems is MR angiography (MRA).

Because all MRA techniques are inherently reliant on high signal-to-noise ratio (SNR) to provide sufficient vascular contrast and resolution for depiction of pathology, these techniques are expected to benefit substantially from the higher signal available at 3.0T, and current experience seems to confirm this. On the other hand, application of existing MRA techniques to 3.0T systems has been hindered to some degree by competing properties of high field strength systems, such as higher radiofrequency (RF) energy deposition. Pulse sequences which may have been optimized for 1.5T MR imaging units, through years of research and clinical application, may not translate seamlessly, if at all, into use at 3.0T.

In this article, the authors discuss the current state of MRA techniques at 3.0T. Basic physical differences between MR imaging at 1.5T and at 3.0T, and their effects, both positive and negative, on MRA sequences. At the conclusion of the article, existing literature on the efficacy of 3.0T MRA techniques for diagnosing specific neurovascular pathologies, including aneurysms, arteriovenous malformations, and carotid steno-occlusive disease, is reviewed.

MR IMAGING AT 3.0 TESLA VERSUS 1.5 TESLA

The principle advantage of 3.0T imaging is improved intrinsic signal compared with 1.5T. Magnetization increases with the square of the field strength, while noise increases only linearly. Therefore, SNR should double as field strength is increased from 1.5T to 3.0T.[1] This theoretical twofold increase in SNR has been confirmed in phantom models and in some tissues such as cerebrospinal fluid.[2] In other tissues, including white matter and gray matter, SNR gains at 3.0T have proven to be more modest (only 30% to 60%). This observation is likely because of a combination of decreased signal from changes in relaxation rates and increased susceptibility-induced signal loss caused by iron contained within these tissues.[1] Nevertheless, the increase in tissue SNR at 3.0T remains substantial and can be used to improve spatial resolution, shorten scan time, or some combination of both.

Increased SNR has also proven beneficial in the application of parallel imaging techniques. Parallel imaging takes advantage of the spatial-encoding properties of high SNR multichannel phased-array coils to decrease the number of phase-encoding steps (ie, lines of k-space) required to complete

Department of Radiology, University of North Carolina School of Medicine, CB#7510, 101 Manning Drive, Chapel Hill, NC 27599, USA
* Corresponding author.
E-mail address: bhuang@med.unc.edu (B.Y. Huang).

Magn Reson Imaging Clin N Am 17 (2009) 29–46
doi:10.1016/j.mric.2008.12.005
1064-9689/08/$ – see front matter © 2009 Elsevier Inc. All rights reserved.

mri.theclinics.com

an image. As a result, scan times are significantly reduced without a loss of resolution; alternatively, resolution and coverage can be improved without increasing scan time. Data lost due to k-space undersampling from parallel imaging is made up for by using reconstruction algorithms which use the additional information provided by the sensitivity patterns of the specific phased-array coil.[3] These reconstruction techniques fall into two main categories: (1) those applied in the frequency domain, such as SMASH (simultaneous acquisition of spatial harmonics)[4] and GRAPPA (generalized auto-calibrating partially parallel acquisition);[5] and (2) those applied in the image domain, such as SENSE (sensitivity encoding).[6] Regardless of the specific type of reconstruction used, all parallel imaging techniques suffer from a progressive loss of SNR as acceleration factors increase, owing to the corresponding decrease in the number of k-space lines being acquired. At 1.5T, signal loss scales with the square root of the parallel imaging factor.[3] Thus, a parallel imaging acceleration factor of four would result in a 50% reduction in SNR. This SNR penalty can be an important obstacle to applying parallel imaging to MR studies requiring high spatial resolution, such as MRA. In general, the use of these techniques is limited to a maximum acceleration factor of approximately two for most applications at 1.5T.[7] What makes parallel imaging particularly well suited to 3.0T imaging is that SNR gains at higher field strengths offset signal loss due to k-space undersampling,[1,3] which means that higher acceleration factors can be used at 3.0T than at 1.5T. As a result, additional improvements in spatial resolution, scan coverage, and scan time can be achieved at 3.0T through parallel imaging.

An additional phenomenon observed with increasing field strengths which impacts MRA is a corresponding increase in the longitudinal relaxation times (T1) of tissues. The T1 of water in brain parenchyma increases by roughly 25% to 40% from 1.5T to 3.0T (more so in gray matter than white matter). Furthermore, the relative differences in T1 between gray and white matter are decreased at the higher field strength.[1,2,8–10] In conventional spin-echo T1 weighted imaging, this phenomenon has the undesired effect of reducing contrast between gray and white matter at 3.0T,[11,12] but for certain MRA applications, this prolongation of T1 times is advantageous, as discussed below.

Imaging at higher field strengths is not without its drawbacks, chief among which is significantly increased RF energy deposition. With all else equal, specific absorption rate (SAR) increases with the square of the RF transmission frequency which is, in turn, directly proportional to magnetic field strength.[2,13] Therefore, a twofold increase in field strength from 1.5T to 3.0T leads to a fourfold increase in SAR. This effect becomes problematic for pulse sequences which are very RF intensive. A few simple strategies for lowering SAR at 3.0T include use of gradient recalled echo (GRE) sequences, increasing repetition time (TR), and reducing flip angle (FA).[14]

Additional drawbacks of imaging at 3.0T are more exaggerated magnetic susceptibility and chemical shift artifacts compared with 1.5T.[1,14] Chemical shift is proportional to magnetic field strength; therefore the difference in frequencies of fat and water increases from 220 Hz at 1.5T to 440 Hz at 3.0T. As chemical shift is inversely related to bandwidth, one can counter the effects of greater chemical shift at 3.0T by doubling the receiver bandwidth. Unfortunately, increasing the bandwidth on a scan carries with it the undesirable effect of reducing signal.[14] By doubling bandwidth, one reduces the potential SNR improvement at 3.0T from a twofold gain to only a 40% increase.[2,14] Fortunately, chemical shift effects in neuroimaging tend to be less dramatic than they are in other parts of the body (eg, abdominal imaging); therefore, some choose not to adjust bandwidth to preserve SNR.

The above differences between 1.5T and 3.0T MR imaging will affect MRA to a greater or lesser degree depending on the specific technique being used. That said, one should keep in mind that the main factor affecting all MRA techniques at 3.0T is higher SNR.

MR ANGIOGRAPHY TECHNIQUES AT 1.5 TESLA AND 3.0 TESLA

The chief prerequisites for any MRA study are high spatial resolution, high vessel-to-background contrast, sufficient anatomic coverage, and reasonably short scan time. Existing techniques each have their relative advantages and disadvantages when it comes to addressing these demands. The three main MRA techniques currently used for neurovascular imaging are time-of-flight (TOF) MRA, contrast-enhanced (CE) MRA, and phase-contrast (PC) MRA. Of these, TOF MRA and CE MRA are the most widely used, so the authors will primarily focus on these two techniques. As was alluded to in the introduction, potential improvements in resolution and scan time are signal limited for all MRA techniques. That is, for a given amount of signal, there is only a finite amount by which one can improve resolution or reduce scan time before image quality is degraded by signal loss. It is, therefore, not surprising that MRA techniques benefit significantly from the higher signal available with an increase in magnetic field strength.

Time-of-Flight MR Angiography

TOF techniques derive contrast from flow-related enhancement, which occurs when unsaturated or fully magnetized blood enters an imaging volume in which the magnetization of stationary tissue has been presaturated. TOF MRA pulse sequences typically consist of GRE which can be acquired using a two-dimensional (2D) technique (obtained as a stack of contiguous or slightly overlapped 2D sections) or a three-dimensional (3D) technique (in which one or more overlapping 3D volumes are acquired). For intracranial arterial imaging, 3D TOF MRA is perhaps the most widely accepted technique, whereas 2D TOF techniques are primarily used for evaluation of the cervical carotids and for intracranial MR venography (MRV). The primary advantages of 3D TOF MRA are its excellent spatial resolution and its use of the intrinsic contrast from flowing blood which obviates the need for injected contrast agents. 3D TOF MRA is not as well-suited to cervical imaging because of long acquisition times (usually several minutes), which makes the technique more susceptible to degradation because of motion from swallowing and breathing.

At 3.0T, TOF techniques benefit from the two field strength dependent phenomena which were described earlier: (1) higher SNR and (2) increased tissue T1 relaxation times.[2,9,10,15] Although the actual improvement in SNR at 3.0T is variable depending on the properties of the tissues being imaged, in vivo experiments comparing intracranial 3D TOF MRA at 1.5T and 3.0T have demonstrated that SNR measured in arteries actually improves twofold at 3.0T.[9,16] Because imaging matrix size is limited by SNR, increased matrix sizes can be used at 3.0T with the end results being higher spatial resolution and reduced partial volume artifact within voxels due to smaller voxel size.[2] Acquired voxel sizes as small as 0.07 mm^3 have been described for 3D TOF MRA at 3.0T.[15]

The second phenomenon which makes 3D TOF MRA at 3.0T attractive is the increase in longitudinal relaxation times seen at high field strengths. As discussed above, the T1 of brain parenchyma is roughly 25% to 40% longer at 3.0T than it is at 1.5T, while the T1 of blood increases by a much smaller amount (less than 10%) from 1.5T to 3.0T.[1,2,9,10] The differences in T1 between blood and background brain parenchyma are, therefore, larger at 3.0T than they are at 1.5T, which translates into improved blood-to-background contrast (better background suppression) at the higher field strength.[1] Not surprisingly, side-by-side comparisons of 3D TOF MRA at 1.5T and 3.0T have consistently shown a significant improvement in subjective image quality and distal vessel depiction at 3.0T due to the combination of higher SNR and better background suppression (Fig. 1).[9,10,16–18] In addition, the higher SNR available at 3.0T allows use of higher parallel imaging factors which translates into further improvements in spatial resolution and imaging time (Table 1).[1]

Improved background suppression on TOF MRA can also be achieved through use of magnetization transfer contrast (MTC). In MTC, an off-resonance RF pulse is applied to suppress the signal from brain parenchyma through the transfer of magnetization from selectively saturated

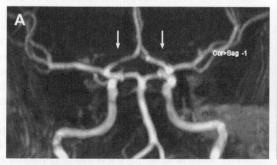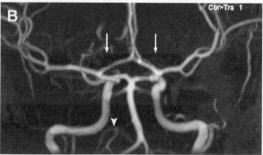

Fig. 1. Intracranial 3D TOF multiple overlapping thin slab acquisition MRA of the circle of Willis at 1.5T and 3.0T. (A) 1.5T and (B) 3.0T frontal maximum intensity projection from the same patient. Image parameters for the 1.5T MRA are: TR 37 milliseconds, echo time (TE) 7.15 milliseconds, FA 25°, field of view (FOV) 200 × 200 mm^2, matrix 512 × 256, and acquisition time 7:12. Parameters for the 3.0T MRA are: TR 32 milliseconds, TE 3.69 milliseconds, FA 25°, FOV 200 × 175 mm^2, matrix 512 × 224, and acquisition time 6:23. Notice the improvement in vessel sharpness and background suppression on the 3.0T image. Small vessels such as the M3 branches of the middle cerebral arteries, the superior cerebellar arteries, and the posterior inferior cerebellar arteries (arrowhead) are also better depicted on the 3.0T image. Notice the more pronounced "venetian blind" artifact (arrows) at 3.0T.

Table 1
Literature reporting use of intracranial three dimensional time-of-flight MR angiograph at 3.0 Tesla

Study (Year)	TE/TR (ms)	Parallel Imaging Factor	Voxel Volume (mm³)[a]	Acquisition Time (min:sec)
Bernstein et al. (2001)[9]	3.4/38	N/A	0.70	8:04
Al-Kwifi et al. (2002)[10]	6.9/36	N/A	0.31	9:48
Willinek et al. (2003)[16]	3.4/26	N/A	0.13	7:57
Gaa et al. (2004)[18]	3.8/24	2	0.08	7:35
Gibbs et al. (2004)[17]	3.4/38	N/A	0.53	8:04
Majoie et al. (2005)[66]	4/21	1.5	0.24	7:14
Villablanca et al. (2006)[35]	3.2/20	2	0.27	5:40
Heidenreich et al. (2007)[79]	4.4/30	N/A	0.31	11:30
Anzalone et al. (2008)[38]	3.5/23	2.5	1.0	5:40
Urbach et al. (2008)[68]	3.5/25	2	0.28	6:52

Abbreviation: N/A, not applicable.
[a] Before reconstruction.

macromolecule bound protons to free water protons within tissue.[19] Addition of MTC to TOF MRA has been shown to substantially improve small vessel conspicuity at 1.5T, as blood is less affected by MTC pulses than brain tissue,[20] and many centers routinely use MTC for MRA at 1.5T. Application of MTC to clinical 3.0T MRA has been hindered by concerns over exceeding SAR limits—as MTC is a RF-intensive technique—necessitating that MTC pulses be modified for 3.0T imaging. Thomas and colleagues[13] have successfully applied MTC to 3D TOF MRA at 3.0T without exceeding SAR guidelines by using a modulated MTC scheme which selectively uses the full MTC pulse over the 30% of acquisition corresponding to the central portion of k-space. Applying this technique, they found that contrast and distal artery visualization was consistently better on 3.0T TOF MRA with MTC compared with MRA performed at 3.0T without MTC and MRA performed at 1.5T with or without MTC.

Among the disadvantages of TOF MRA, perhaps most important is the effect of in-plane blood saturation. As blood travels through an imaging slab, it progressively loses magnetization, resulting in variations in blood-to-background contrast within the slab. This phenomenon is particularly problematic when thick slabs are used in 3D TOF MRA, as the amount of time it takes blood to traverse a slab increases with slab thickness. If a slab is too thick, then blood at the exiting edge of the slab may become saturated. In addition, flow saturation can hinder visualization of long in-plane vessel segments and giant aneurysms (due to slow turbulent flow within the aneurysm sacs) (**Fig. 2**). Strategies employed to reduce

the effects of in-plane blood saturation include reducing slab thickness, prolonging TR, or decreasing FA.[2,15,21] None of these solutions is perfect, as the trade-off for using thinner slabs is decreased coverage, and increasing TR and raising the FA both have the undesirable effect of reducing background suppression. Therefore, optimization of these parameters requires a compromise between coverage, blood saturation, and background suppression. For 3D TOF imaging, the TR generally ranges from 20 to 50 milliseconds, and FAs typically range from 15° to 35°.[2] Because of inherent improvements in background suppression provided by increased tissue T1 at higher field strengths, longer TRs and smaller FAs can be used at 3.0T to reduce in-plane saturation effects while maintaining a similar degree of background suppression compared with scans acquired at 1.5T. In addition, because of the increased signal available with higher field strengths, blood can be pulsed more often at 3.0T before becoming fully saturated.[2] Al-Kwifi and colleagues[10] found that at 3.0T, for a TR of 36 ms, a FA of 22o provided the best compromise between visualization of smaller intracranial vessels and proximal vessel SNR.

One common strategy to overcome in-plane saturation effects while maintaining coverage in 3D TOF MRA is to acquire the imaging volume as multiple 3D slabs (instead of as a single large slab) using a technique referred to as multiple overlapping thin slab acquisition (MOTSA).[22,23] Because MOTSA reconstructs the MRA image from multiple slabs, it decreases sensitivity to the effects of blood saturation, similar to a 2D TOF technique, while preserving the improved

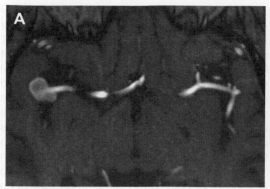
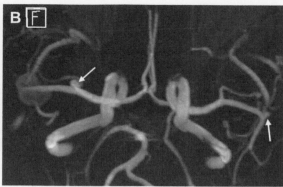

Fig. 2. Flow saturation effect on 3D TOF MRA. (*A*) Axial source image and (*B*) maximum intensity projection (MIP) from a 3D TOF MRA performed at 3.0T (TR 32 milliseconds, TE 3.69 milliseconds, FA 25°, field of view 200 × 175 mm², matrix 576 × 256, acquisition time 6:23) demonstrate reduced flow-related enhancement within a large right middle cerebral artery bifurcation aneurysm. Notice the difference in signal within that aneurysm compared with the two smaller aneurysms seen on the MIP image (*arrows*).

resolution of a 3D technique. One of the drawbacks to using MOTSA for 3D TOF MRA is the so-called "venetian blind artifact," which is seen when images are viewed as maximum intensity projection (MIP) reconstructions. This artifact is caused primarily by nonuniform distribution of FA across a slice as well as by the nonuniform signal intensity of blood across a slab owing to spin saturation.[24] Because of the differences in background tissue T1, venetian blind artifacts tend to be more conspicuous at 3.0T than at 1.5T (**Fig. 1**).[2]

Another artifact noted to be more pronounced at 3.0T is pulsatile flow artifact, which is due to flow-induced phase shifts[2,9,15] It has been speculated that these flow artifacts are worse at 3.0T because of greater artifact-to-noise ratio which occurs as an unwanted byproduct of higher SNR.[2,9] This artifact can be partially offset through the use of a technique known as flow compensation (also referred to as gradient moment rephasing),[2] but to implement this technique, higher echo times (TE) are needed to ensure sufficient time to apply the necessary flow compensation gradients between the excitation and readout pulses. Because 3D TOF MRA is best performed with water and fat out of phase (to reduce signal from fat), and chemical shift differs at 1.5T and 3.0T, the TE typically used for 3D TOF MRA at 3.0T (roughly 3.4 milliseconds) is approximately half of what is generally used at 1.5T (6.9 milliseconds). Therefore, at 3.0T, choosing to use an out-of-phase TE means that less time is available to apply flow compensation gradients.[2] Furthermore, the effects of increasing TE to allow application of flow compensation can be counterproductive as increasing TE can result in decreased SNR, increased susceptibility artifacts,

and increased sensitivity to complex flow-related signal loss.[15]

Contrast-Enhanced MR Angiography

CE MRA relies on the lumen-filling characteristics of intravenously injected contrast to create intravascular enhancement, making this technique analogous to conventional catheter-based angiography and computed tomography angiography.[25] CE MRA has a number advantages over TOF MRA and PC MRA. The principal ones are shorter acquisition times (typically under a minute and often within a single breath-hold), significantly improved coverage (from aortic arch to the top of the head), and significantly decreased susceptibility to artifacts caused by pulsatility and flow. These advantages make CE MRA particularly well suited to evaluation of the cervical arteries, and many institutions now use CE MRA as the first-line imaging tool for extracranial neurovascular imaging.

The primary shortcomings of conventional CE MRA techniques are limited spatial resolution compared with TOF MRA and the potential for significant venous contamination owing to the transient arterial phase. Early attempts at CE MRA used imaging times and contrast infusions which lasted several minutes and, as a result, suffered from significant venous contamination and motion artifacts.[26] Rapid time resolved first-pass imaging techniques were subsequently developed to overcome these problems. In turn, they brought shortcomings of their own, including persistent limitations in spatial resolution and problems related to matching the timing of acquisition with the contrast bolus. A number of techniques have been proposed to optimize visualization of arterial structures while limiting venous contamination. One strategy involves performing temporally resolved CE MRA, in which multiple short (5–10 seconds) 3D acquisitions are acquired after the initiation of the contrast bolus.[27,28] With temporally resolved CE MRA, it is not necessary to accurately time the contrast bolus with the image acquisition, however the short acquisition time for each set of images comes at the cost of limited spatial resolution.[29,30]

An alternative to temporally resolved CE MRA is to use a bolus timing technique. These techniques include the use of test boluses to estimate arrival time or the use of real-time triggering methods (line scan method or 2D fluoroscopic monitoring) to initiate the 3D scan.[31,32] Real-time triggered techniques use an elliptic centric view order, in which the central portions of k-space are acquired at the peak of arterial contrast enhancement, effectively suppressing out venous signal, even with acquisition times exceeding 40 seconds.[30,33] In addition, the longer imaging times used with bolus timing techniques allow improved resolution compared with time-resolved techniques,[33] with voxel volumes on the order of 1 mm^3 or less at 1.5T.[2,26,29,34]

The introduction of 3.0T systems has significantly improved the performance of CE MRA,

with respect to spatial resolution, speed of acquisition, and coverage,[35] again as a result of higher SNR. Experiments comparing CE MRA at 1.5T and 3.0T have shown a significant improvement in overall image quality and depiction of distal vessel segments (**Fig. 3**).[36] In general, large field of view (FOV) CE-MRA protocols at 3.0T produce voxels which are 25% to 40% smaller than those used at 1.5T, with typical acquired voxel volumes at 3.0T being roughly on the order of 0.3 to 0.7 mm^3 (**Table 2**).[7,9,15,35–38] Furthermore, as with TOF MRA, the ability to use higher parallel imaging factors at 3.0T results in additional improvements in resolution and scan time. Nael and colleagues[7] compared parallel imaging factors of 2 (iPAT-2) and 4 (iPAT-4) for a breath-hold, high-resolution CE MRA of the carotids and found that spatial resolution at iPAT-4 was 1.7 higher than that at iPAT-2. Actual voxel volume at iPAT-4 was 0.50 mm^3 compared with a voxel volume of 0.87 mm^3 at iPAT-2, and the investigators noted no detrimental effect on image interpretation caused by the SNR loss at the higher acceleration factor.

Time-resolved CE MRA techniques have also benefited from higher SNR at 3.0T. Temporal resolutions as low as 2.9 seconds have been described for neurovascular imaging at 1.5T,[39,40] but this has come at the cost of dramatically reduced spatial resolution and anatomic coverage. At 3.0T, higher

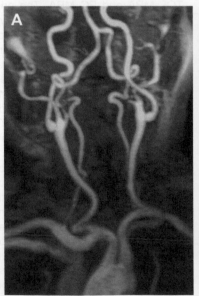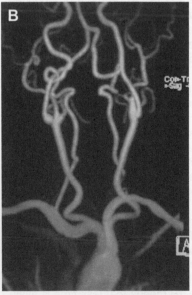

Fig. 3. Standard CE cervical MRA at 1.5T (A) and 3.0T (B) using elliptic centric phase ordering. MIP images demonstrate better image quality and resolution at 3.0T (B). Notice improved depiction of the right vertebral artery and external carotid artery branches on the 3.0T study. For the 1.5T study, the imaging parameters were: TR 3.06 milliseconds, TE 1.17 milliseconds, FA 25°, FOV 280 × 210 mm^2, matrix 256 × 154, acquisition time 7.45 seconds. For the 3.0T study, the imaging parameters were: TR 2.43 milliseconds, TE 1.12 milliseconds, FA 17°, FOV 280 × 184 mm^2, matrix 320 × 105, acquisition time 7 seconds.

Table 2
Literature reporting use of high-resolution craniocervical contrast-enhanced MR angiograph at 3.0Tesla

Study (Year)	TE/TR (ms)	Parallel Imaging Factor	Voxel Volume (mm³)ᵃ	Acquisition Time (Sec)
Bernstein et al. (2001)[9]	1.5/6.7	N/A	0.62–0.72	51
Gibbs et al. (2005)[17]	1.5/6.7	N/A	0.62	51
Markl et al. (2006)[37]	1.11/3.15	3	0.65	21
Nael et al. (2006)[7]	1.2/3.0	4	0.37	20
Nael et al. (2006)[56]	1.2/3.0	4	0.34	20
Villablanca et al. (2006)[35]	1.2/3.0	4	0.39	20
Anzalone et al. (2008)[38]	1.8/5.9	3	0.41	24
Saleh et al. (2008)[85]	1.1/3.1	4	0.45	22

Abbreviation: N/A, not applicable.
ᵃ Before reconstruction.

signal can be used not only for improving spatial resolution, but alternatively for shortening scan times. As a result, more dynamic MRA frames can be acquired over a given period of time at 3.0T while preserving both coverage and spatial resolution. In addition, use of parallel imaging techniques, partial Fourier imaging, and recently developed view-sharing techniques such as keyhole,[41] TRICKS (time-resolved imaging of contrast kinetics)[27] and TREAT (time-resolved echo-shared angiography technique),[42] have further improved the temporal resolution of CE MRA at 3.0T—which is now on the order of 1 to 2 seconds for cerebrovascular imaging encompassing the supra-aortic vessels and circle of Willis—with only minor losses in spatial resolution due to the faster frame rates (**Table 3**).[36,43–45] As hardware and software applications tailored to 3.0T systems become increasingly available, further improvements in temporal and spatial resolution will be achieved with CE MRA at 3.0T. In the last year Willinek and colleagues[46] described a protocol using a combination of centric phase order, keyhole imaging, and SENSE to acquire time resolved MRAs with a temporal resolution of 608 milliseconds and a spatial resolution of 1.1 × 1.4 × 1.1 mm³.

Phase-Contrast MR Angiography

For the sake of completeness, the authors briefly mention PC MRA, although it is the least widely used of existing MRA techniques. PC MRA generates image contrast through the application of bipolar velocity-encoding gradients of a predetermined value (known as VENC). For each RF excitation, these gradients are applied twice, with opposing polarity, so that stationary tissues do not acquire any phase. The result is a phase shift

arising only in moving spins that is dependent on the direction and velocity of flow. Because signal in PC MRA is proportional to the velocity of flowing blood, hemodynamic information can also be obtained from these sequences. In addition, PC imaging provides better background suppression than TOF MRA techniques. The factors preventing conventional PC MRA from being widely used in neurovascular imaging are lower resolution, much longer acquisition times, and more degradation by pulsatile flow compared with TOF and CE MRA.[15]

Two-dimensional PC techniques are used primarily in the assessment of the venous system as an adjunct to TOF MRV.[2] Three-dimensional PC techniques are primarily of use in the setting of intracranial hemorrhage and following prior administration of gadolinium. In these cases, T1 shortening from hematoma or gadolinium results in poorer background suppression on TOF sequences; in addition, intravenous gadolinium can cause venous contamination on TOF MRA.[2,15]

New techniques which overcome the present limitations of PC MRA are currently under investigation. Gu and colleagues[47] recently described a 3D PC MRA technique at 1.5T which uses a k-space sampling algorithm known as "vastly undersampled isotropic projection reconstruction" (VIPR).[48] The VIPR technique can be used to reduce scan time significantly without compromising coverage or resolution. Compared to conventional 3D PC MRA, PC-VIPR provides improved coverage, better spatial resolution, and shorter imaging times, while demonstrating less ghosting artifact due to pulsatile flow. In addition, flow velocities can be calculated in any vessel in the image volume without additional imaging. PC-VIPR has also been shown in animal models to be potential useful in assessing hemodynamic effects of carotid stenoses[49] and determining

Table 3
Literature reporting use of time-resolved craniocervical contrast-enhanced MR angiograph at 3.0Tesla

Study (Year)	TE/TR (ms)	Parallel Imaging Factor	Voxel Volume (mm³)[a]	Temporal Resolution (sec)
Ziyeh et al. (2005)[45]	1.62/4.31	2	3.84	1.5
Nael et al. (2006)[44]	1/2.16	3	5.59	1.8
Cashen et al. (2006)[36]	1.3/3.2	2	3.03	2.5
Frydrychowicz et al. (2006)[43]	0.87–1.02/2.1–2.39	4	2.71–3.03	2.9
Saleh et al. (2008)[85]	1.1/2.6	3	4.80	1.5
Willinek et al. (2008)[46]	0.9/2.2	8	2.16	0.61

Abbreviation: N/A, not applicable.
[a] Before reconstruction.

pressure gradients within cerebral aneurysms,[50] neither of which are possible with TOF or CE-MRA techniques.

To date, there is a scarcity of published work on the PC MRA at 3.0T. PC techniques, like TOF and CE MRA, do appear to benefit from signal gains at 3.0T. PC MRA performed on 1.5T and 3.0T systems are equally accurate with respect to flow measurements, and in vitro studies have demonstrated that noise measured as a percentage of VENC is substantially lower at 3.0T.[51] This means that there is greater built-in tolerance for the choice of the VENC at 3.0T than at 1.5T. As a result, one can select a higher VENC at 3.0T to reduce aliasing artifacts in regions of high flow, while maintaining the ability to detect vessels with relatively slow flow.[2,51]

MR ANGIOGRAPHY OF SPECIFIC PATHOLOGIES AT 3.0 TESLA VERSUS 1.5 TESLA

As promising as high field strength MR imaging may seem in theory, the ultimate determinant of its usefulness remains whether its theoretical advantages translate into significant improvements in clinical diagnostic accuracy. For most neurovascular pathologies, including intracranial aneurysms, arteriovenous malformations (AVMs), arteriovenous fistulas (AVFs), and carotid atherosclerotic disease, the gold standard for diagnosis and characterization arguably continues to be digital subtraction angiography (DSA). Numerous studies have evaluated noninvasive imaging techniques, such as MRA, CT angiography, and ultrasound, as potential replacements for DSA, but none of these noninvasive techniques can match DSA in terms of its spatial and temporal resolution. Nonetheless, most institutions now use noninvasive techniques as first-line studies for the detection of the most neurovascular disorders. In this section, the authors discuss the state of MRA

imaging at 1.5T for evaluating each of the above-listed neurovascular pathologies and review the literature on imaging of these entities at 3.0T.

Aneurysms

At 1.5T, MRA techniques have been shown to reliably demonstrate aneurysms larger than 3 mm. A meta-analysis reviewing the accuracy of MRA for aneurysm detection reported an overall sensitivity of 87% and a specificity of 95% for MRA examinations performed at field strengths less than 3.0T. Sensitivity was much greater for aneurysms larger than 3 mm (94%) compared with aneurysms measuring 3 mm and smaller (only 38%).[52] In the years since those initial studies were performed, technological advances have improved the quality of MRA to the point where aneurysms less than 2 mm in size can now be reliably detected at 1.5T.[53] In spite of this, MRA at 1.5T remains inferior to DSA in a number of areas which are important for pretreatment aneurysm assessment.

Early studies of 3.0T MRA have shown that aneurysms as small as 1 mm in diameter can be detected using 3D TOF MRA. Furthermore, good anatomic correlation with DSA in characterizing the size and morphology of aneurysms has also been described.[54] The question of whether imaging at 3.0T truly improves sensitivity for aneurysm detection remains unanswered. To date, a single study encompassing 28 aneurysms has compared 3.0T TOF MRA with 1.5T TOF MRA in the evaluation of aneurysms.[55] In this study, image quality was deemed significantly better at 3.0T, but no aneurysms were detected at 3.0T which were not also visible at 1.5T (**Fig. 4**).

Investigators have also compared 3D TOF MRA and CE MRA at 3.0T for evaluation of unruptured aneurysms,[17,56] without having arrived at a consensus as to which technique is superior. In one study, TOF MRA demonstrated better overall

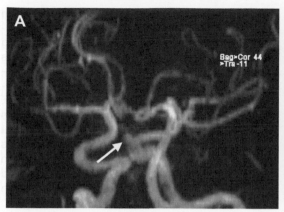 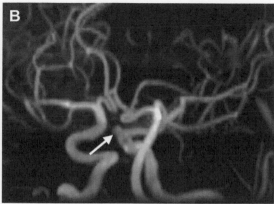

Fig. 4. Comparison of intracranial 3D TOF MRA at 1.5T (*A*) and 3.0T (*B*) for depiction of a 3 mm left ophthalmic segment internal carotid artery aneurysm. The 3.0T examination (*B*) demonstrates noticeably improved resolution and vessel sharpness compared with the 1.5T examination (*A*), but at both field strengths, the aneurysm can be easily seen (*arrow*). For the 1.5T study, the imaging parameters were: TR 37 milliseconds, TE 7.15 milliseconds, FA 25°, FOV 200 × 162 mm², matrix 512 × 192, acquisition time 7:12. For the 3.0T study, the imaging parameters were: TR 32 milliseconds, TE 3.69 milliseconds, FA 25°, FOV 200 × 200 mm², matrix 576 × 256, acquisition time 6:23.

image quality than CE MRA and detected more aneurysms than CE MRA (100% versus 92.9%).[17] Another study found no significant difference in the image quality of the two techniques, and found that CE MRA was able to detect all aneurysms which were identified on TOF MRA.[56] These two studies differed substantially in their imaging protocols and reported spatial resolutions, making it difficult to directly compare them. Of note, both studies reported that CE MRA was better in the depiction of giant aneurysms and aneurysms with slow flow, presumably because of greater susceptibility of TOF MRA to flow saturation.

MR Angiography for Follow-up of Coil-Treated Aneurysms

Endovascular treatment of intracranial aneurysms has become an accepted alternative to surgical clip ligation, but there is a 0.2% reported risk of rebleeding per patient year following embolization of ruptured aneurysms;[57] furthermore, aneurysm recanalization following coiling has been estimated to occur in anywhere from 10% to 40% of patients, because of continual expansion of the aneurysm sac or coil compaction.[58] As a result, aneurysms treated by endovascular means require prolonged imaging follow-up. At a number of institutions, including our own, a 3 to 6 month follow-up DSA is mandatory following coil embolization, and many institutions perform serial surveillance angiograms out to 3 years or longer.[59] Unfortunately, conventional angiography carries

a small but measurable risk of significant morbidity, which is compounded in cases of coiling by the need for multiple angiograms. Furthermore, the necessary duration of follow-up remains unknown. Because of the potential morbidity and added cost associated with performing surveillance DSA, a number of investigators have turned their attention toward MRA (which is safe for coiled aneurysms at static field strengths up to 3.0T)[60,61] as a potential replacement for DSA for posttreatment surveillance,[62–69] and some institutions now use MRA almost exclusively for follow-up of coiled aneurysms.[58]

Kwee and Kwee[62] performed a meta-analysis of 16 studies on the use of MRA after coiling. Fourteen of these studies evaluated TOF MRA, and seven evaluated CE MRA. For the studies examining TOF MRA, the sensitivity for detecting residual flow within the neck of a coiled aneurysm ranged from 29.4% to 100% with a pooled sensitivity estimate of 81%. Specificity for TOF MRA ranged from 50% to 100% with a pooled estimate of 90.6%. For CE MRA, sensitivity was 72% to 100% (pooled sensitivity = 86.8%), and specificity was 73.7% to 100% (pooled specificity = 91.9%). A few studies directly compared CE MRA with 3D TOF MRA for evaluating coiled aneurysms. While the overall trend seems to suggest that CE MRA may be slightly more sensitive for aneurysm remnants and recurrences, there does not appear to be a true consensus on the matter, and some have suggested that the optimal strategy for postembolization MRA follow-up may be to perform both techniques in a complementary fashion.[58]

Some investigators have suggested that administration of intravenous contrast with 3D TOF MRA may improve signal intensity in residual pouches and, therefore, improve detection.[70,71] However, a study by Cottier and colleagues[65] found that the addition of contrast did not improve the ability of TOF MRA to detect residual or recurrent aneurysms. The major limitation of TOF MRA for evaluation of coiled aneurysms is susceptibility to changes in the local magnetic field caused by the coil masses themselves. Susceptibility effects tend to be more pronounced at a higher TE, and it has been shown that MRA techniques using a TE greater than 5 milliseconds will demonstrate an artifact of approximately 1 to 2 mm in the vicinity of a coil mass.[58] At 1.5T, the use of short TEs (<2.5 millisecond) reduces signal dropout associated with coils, thereby improving visualization nearby vessels and, in some cases, small aneurysm remnants.[72]

With the exception of the report by Majoie and colleagues,[66] the studies included in the meta-analysis by Kwee and Kwee[62] were all performed at MR field strengths of 1.5T or less. To date, the authors are aware of five published clinical studies assessing MRA at 3.0T in the follow-up of coiled aneurysms.[38,66–68,73] Three of these reports compared 3D TOF MRA at 3.0T with DSA,[66–68] and found that MRA agreed with DSA on the presence of residual aneurysm flow in 86% to 94% of cases. In all three reports, there were a number of cases in which MRA demonstrated aneurysm patency while DSA showed complete occlusion, presumably due to the limited number of projections obtained at DSA. In these cases, the patent aneurysms were confirmed on repeat angiography and retreated successfully either endovascularly or surgically. In addition, there were several instances in these reports in which the morphology of unoccluded aneurysm compartments could be more easily assessed on MRA, primarily as a result of obscuration of the aneurysm by the coil mass on DSA.[68]

A direct comparison between 1.5T and 3.0T MRA for follow-up of coiled aneurysms has thus far been reported in only one study—which found that for 3D TOF MRA, imaging at 3.0T conferred no benefit in detection of aneurysm remnants or recurrences.[67] This may be due to more pronounced susceptibility artifacts at 3.0T, resulting in greater perianeurysmal vessel obscuration compared with 1.5T. In ex vivo experiments, Walker and colleagues[74] demonstrated that the volume of susceptibility-induced signal loss caused by the coil packs on TOF MRA was significantly higher at 3.0T than at 1.5T, and more tightly packed coils also caused larger artifacts. At both field strengths, artifact was more pronounced in the frequency encoding direction, and susceptibility artifacts could be reduced by minimizing the TE. Based on these findings, the investigators concluded that 1.5T is superior to 3.0T for assessment of coiled aneurysms when 3D TOF techniques are being used.[74] Much to the contrary, Majoie and colleagues[66] found in their series comparing TOF MRA at 3.0T with DSA that susceptibility artifacts caused by coil masses was minimal and did not interfere with evaluation of aneurysm occlusion, but it should be noted that this analysis did not include a comparison with MRA performed at 1.5T.

CE MRA has been shown to be less susceptible to coil induced artifacts at 3.0T.[38,74] Recently, Anzalone and colleagues[38] found that CE MRA was equal to TOF MRA in 79.6% of cases and better than TOF MRA in 20.4% of cases for visualization of aneurysm patency after coiling (**Fig. 5**). Furthermore, there were no instances in which TOF MRA was better than CE MRA. These results suggest that high-resolution CE MRA may be the preferred MRA technique for embolization follow-up at 3.0T.

Arteriovenous Malformations and Fistulas

For diagnosis and characterization of AVMs and dural AVFs, conventional DSA, which boasts a spatial resolution on the order of 0.1×0.1 mm^2 and frame rates of 10 per seconds and higher,[36] continues to be the gold standard. However, MRA techniques have proven reasonably effective for AVM imaging, particularly in preoperative planning for stereotactic radiosurgery.[75–77] High spatial resolution is essential for assessment of the angioarchitecture of AVMs, including feeding arteries, nidus size, and draining veins. Furthermore, good temporal resolution allows differentiation of small feeding arteries from veins, assessment of retrograde and cortical venous drainage, and detection of early draining veins (which may be the only sign of residual shunting in treated AVMs and AVFs).

Duran and colleagues[78] compared conventional 3D TOF MRA with an ultrafast CE-MRA sequence at 1.5T in the assessment of intracranial AVMs. Spatial resolution was better for the TOF technique than the CE technique, but CE MRA was found to be superior to TOF MRA with regards to the ability to identify arterial feeders, number of venous drainers, and the pattern of venous drainage. The superiority of CE MRA was due largely to its improved ability to depict venous structures (which would be considered a drawback in most other applications which require suppression of signal from venous structures). Nonetheless,

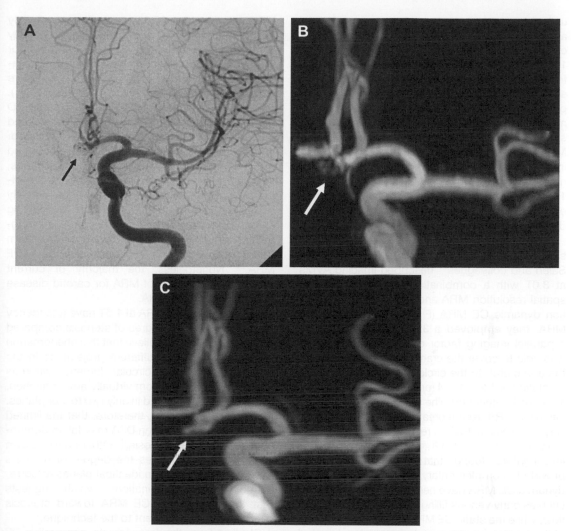

Fig. 5. (A) Left internal carotid artery digital subtraction angiogram performed following embolization of an anterior communicating artery aneurysm demonstrates complete occlusion. (B, C) MIP reconstructions from a 3D TOF MRA (B) and CE MRA (C) performed for follow-up 3 months after embolization. The TOF MRA (B) demonstrates some high signal intensity inhomogeneity in the region of the aneurysm neck (*arrow*) but does not clearly demonstrate a remnant. The CE MRA (C) clearly demonstrates the presence of a small remnant (*arrow*). (*From* Anzalone N, Scomazzoni F, Cirillo M, et al. Follow-up of coiled cerebral aneurysms at 3.0T: comparison of 3D time-of-flight MRA and contrast-enhanced MRA. AJNR Am J Neuroradiol 2008;29:1530; with permission. Copyright © 2008 by American Society of Neuroradiology.)

neither MRA technique was as good as DSA for evaluating AVMs.

Heidenreich and colleagues[79] compared 3D TOF MRA at 1.5T and 3.0T for AVM evaluation. MRA at 3.0T was superior to 1.5T in detection of feeding arteries, superficial veins, and deep veins. Overall, over 20% more feeding arteries were detected at 3.0T compared with 1.5T (73% versus 52%, respectively). In evaluating deep and superficial draining veins, 3.0T MRA identified 72% and 58% of deep and superficial draining veins respectively, while 1.5T MRA only identified 59% and 25% respectively. Neither MRA at 3.0T nor 1.5T was

comparable to DSA, and none of the MRAs performed at either field strength were able to visualize angioarchitecture of AVMs in a manner appropriate to determine embolization therapy. Furthermore, at both field strengths, there was a tendency to overestimate nidus size in small AVMs and to underestimate nidus size in larger AVMs.

Dynamic time-resolved CE MRA is now being used to investigate AVMs, as it is able to provide hemodynamic information and has the ability to capture transient processes, such as early venous filling which characterizes AVMs and AVFs. At 1.5T, dynamic CE-MRA techniques with frame rates of up to 1 frame per second and temporal resolutions as low as 900 milliseconds have been described.[80–84] Time-resolved CE-MRA techniques at 1.5T have demonstrated a sensitivities ranging from 95% to 100% for detecting arteriovenous shunting due to AVMs or AVFs, and have been reported to show high agreement with DSA in determining the type of venous drainage (deep versus superficial).[39,80–83] Furthermore, dynamic CE MRA has been shown to be superior to TOF MRA in its ability to detect AVMs[80] and AVFs.[82] Unfortunately, high temporal resolution MRA techniques at 1.5T all suffer from limited spatial resolution, which can hinder detection of small feeding arteries and draining veins.[82,84]

Time-resolved CE-MRA techniques benefit substantially from SNR gains at 3.0T. Recently, Saleh and colleagues[85] described imaging AVMs at 3.0T with a combination of both static high spatial resolution MRA and high temporal resolution dynamic CE MRA (Fig. 6). For dynamic CE MRA, they employed a 3D GRE sequence with a parallel imaging factor of three (iPAT-3) which was able to cover the craniocervical vessels from the aortic arch to the circle of Willis with a spatial resolution of $1.2 \times 1 \times 4$ mm^3 and a temporal resolution of 1.5 seconds. The static high spatial resolution CE MRA used a breath-hold spoiled 3D GRE sequence with a iPAT-4, resulting in near isotropic voxel dimensions of $0.8 \times 0.7 \times 0.8$ mm^3.[7] The investigators found that the two techniques provided complementary information, as the dynamic CE MRA gave hemodynamic information such as early venous filling and retrograde venous flow, while the static CE MRA demonstrated 100% of the feeding arteries and draining veins detected by DSA and also accurately measured nidus size.

Extracranial Carotid Stenosis

Carotid MRA is now used as a first-line noninvasive imaging tool for the evaluation of carotid stenosis at a number of institutions, including our own. The optimal MRA technique for this purpose remains controversial. A recent meta-analysis of the diagnostic accuracy of MRA for internal carotid artery (ICA) disease reported an overall sensitivity of TOF MRA (2D and 3D) for 70% to 99% stenoses to be 91.2% (95% CI: 88.9% to 93.1%) with a specificity of 88.3% (86.7% to 89.7%); whereas the overall sensitivity of CE MRA was 94.6% (92.4% to 96.4%) with a specificity of 91.9% (90.3% to 93.4%).[86] The sensitivity of CE MRA for detection of ICA occlusions was slightly better (99.4% sensitivity versus 94.5% for TOF MRA). For less severe stenoses, neither TOF MRA or CE MRA were particularly sensitive, but again CE

MRA was superior (65.9% sensitivity versus only 37.9% for TOF MRA). Analysis of reports directly comparing TOF MRA and CE MRA found that for high grade stenoses, the techniques had equivalent specificities, but that CE MRA was more sensitive than TOF MRA (96.2% versus 89.6%). This review included studies using 2D and 3D techniques for their analysis of TOF MRA, and studies dating as far back as 1991 were included. With the significant advances that have occurred with MR technology over the last two decades, there are those who believe that current state-of-the-art 3D TOF MRA techniques are now actually more accurate than CE MRA for quantifying carotid disease severity,[87,88] and some have suggested that optimal strategy may be to perform both high-resolution CE MRA and 3D TOF MRA.[33] Nonetheless, the majority of current research on the topic of MRA for carotid disease has focused on CE MRA.

Both TOF and CE MRA at 1.5T have a tendency to overestimate the degree of stenosis compared with DSA.[89,90] Some believe that this phenomenon is due to the use of different projections in the measurement of noncircular lumens—whereas MRA can be viewed from virtually any projection, DSA is typically acquired in only two to four planes. It has been suggested, therefore, that the limited number of projections on DSA may fail to demonstrate the tightest stenosis.[91] Others have shown that MRA overestimates the degree of stenosis even when viewed from identical planes to corresponding DSA examinations, which suggests that the tendency of CE MRA toward stenosis overestimation is inherent to the technique.[89]

Studies from the last decade comparing CE MRA at 1.5T with DSA[30,34,88,89,92–96] have reported sensitivities for MRA ranging from 92% to 100% and specificities of 80.6% to 99.3% for stenoses of 70% or higher. Of note, the specific imaging parameters reported in these studies vary considerably, with wide ranges in reported spatial resolutions and scan times. Interestingly, the imaging protocol with the best combination of sensitivity and specificity (100% and 99.3% respectively)[34] happened to have the longest imaging time (58 seconds) and among the smallest voxel sizes (0.66 mm^3). Based on the collective experience with high-resolution CE MRA, it has been suggested that longer scan times (and consequently higher resolution scans) result in more accurate examinations. Some investigators have proposed using double doses of contrast to provide improved SNR and contrast-to-noise (CNR) which can support higher resolution imaging.[15]

Due in large part to the lack, until recently, of commercially available multichannel neurovascular

Time Resolved CEMRA

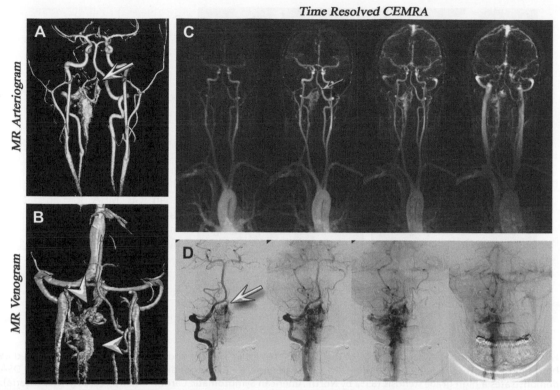

Fig. 6. Coronal volume-rendered projections from CE MRA in a 22-year-old woman with a history of intraspinal hemorrhage and cervical laminectomy. Arterial (*A*) and venous (*B*) phase images show a diffuse serpiginous cervical AVM. Note the feeding vessel is derived from the right vertebral artery (*arrows*). Venous drainage was through the paravertebral venous plexus and the occipital sinus (*arrowheads*). (*C*) Time-resolved CE MRA images with 1.5-second temporal resolution and 1.2 × 1 mm in-plane resolution show enhancement of the AVM via the right vertebral artery (*arrows*) and subsequent venous drainage. (*D*) A phase-by-phase comparison with DSA is presented. MRA and DSA examinations were performed on the same day, before surgery. (*From* Saleh RS, Lohan DG, Villablanca JP, et al. Assessment of craniospinal arteriovenous malformations at 3.0T with highly temporally and highly spatially resolved contrast-enhanced MRA. AJNR Am J Neuroradiol 2008;29:1026; with permission. Copyright © 2008 by American Society of Neuroradiology.)

coils, there is a relative paucity of literature on 3.0T MRA for the evaluation of carotid stenosis. Currently, all major manufacturers now market dedicated neurovascular coils with eight or more channels. Existing publications on cervical carotid MRA at 3.0T have all reported improved image quality over 1.5T (**Fig. 7**).[7,15,33,37] Standard commercially available sequences for CE MRA at 3.0T are still inferior to DSA for carotid stenosis measurement, however. Some investigators have performed small FOV (14 to 16 cm) high-resolution CE MRA focusing on the carotid bifurcation using dedicated surface coils,[15,33] with exquisite spatial resolution on the order of 0.27 mm³ (further improved to 0.03 mm³ after zero fill interpolation), and preliminary results have shown excellent correlation of the technique with DSA for stenosis measurement. It stands to reason that the improved spatial resolution of MRA at 3.0T will translate into improved ability to diagnose and to

quantify carotid stenoses compared with 1.5T scans and may one day rival DSA, but studies designed to confirm this assertion have yet to be performed.

Brief mention should be made of the potential for improved carotid plaque characterization at 3.0T. A great deal of interest has been directed toward high spatial resolution MR imaging of carotid plaque, and in vivo studies performed at 1.5T have shown that carotid plaque morphology and composition can be accurately described with MR imaging.[97–99] Unlike luminal techniques such as MRA and DSA, high-resolution carotid plaque MR imaging can demonstrate findings indicative of plaque instability (eg, plaque rupture, large lipid core, and intraplaque hemorrhage), which may eventually turn out to be a better predictor of stroke risk than simple percent stenosis measurements. Early work on carotid plaque imaging at 3.0T has shown that criteria for

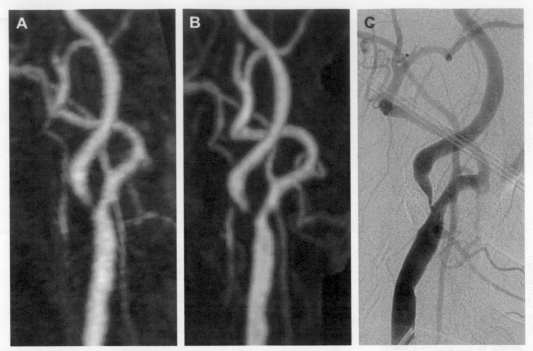

Fig. 7. MIP reconstructions from CE MRA of the carotid arteries at 1.5T (*A*) and 3.0T (*B*). The MRAs performed at both field strengths suggest a high grade (70%–99%) stenosis. (*C*) Corresponding oblique projection from a DSA demonstrates a high grade stenosis (85% by North American Symptomatic Carotid Endarterectomy Trial criteria). The 3.0T MRA (TR 2.43 milliseconds, TE 1.12 milliseconds, FA 17°, FOV 280 × 184 mm^2, matrix 320 × 144, acquisition time 7 seconds) demonstrates substantially improved resolution compared with the 1.5T scan (TR 3.06 milliseconds, TE 1.17 milliseconds, FA 25°, FOV 280 × 210 mm^2, matrix 256 × 154, acquisition time 7.45 seconds), but does not match the resolution of the DSA and, may overestimate the degree of stenosis in this case.

interpretation of carotid plaque findings 1.5T are applicable to 3.0T and that overall image quality, manifested by better carotid wall SNR, improved lumen/wall CNR, and better spatial resolution, is improved at 3.0T compared with 1.5T.[15,100,101] Recently, however, Underhill and colleagues[101] found that although there was generally good agreement in characterization of plaque composition at 1.5T and 3.0T, images at 1.5T were in fact better in the assessment of certain plaque components. Specifically, detection of hemorrhage was better at 1.5T; in addition, calcifications measured significantly larger at 3.0T, presumably because of more pronounced susceptibility effects at higher field strength. It remains to be seen whether improvements in image quality at 3.0T will actually result in improvements in risk stratification and treatment follow-up over existing 1.5T techniques.

SUMMARY

The field of neurovascular MR imaging has seen dramatic improvements over the last 2 decades, both with innovations initially developed on 1.5T systems (eg, parallel imaging, elliptic centric imaging, and view sharing) and, more recently,

with the introduction of 3.0T MR imaging systems for clinical use. The combination of higher SNR and improved background suppression at 3.0T has led to higher resolution and overall image quality for existing TOF MRA techniques, and CE MRA has also seen substantial gains both in spatial and temporal resolution as a result of higher SNR. In addition, marked reductions in scan time made possible at 3.0T enable the performance of highly temporally resolved CE MRA, which provides hemodynamic information previously unavailable with existing static MRA techniques. These advances have led to improved MR depiction of neurovascular anatomy and pathology, including aneurysms, carotid stenoses, and AVMs, but it remains be seen whether the leap from 1.5T to 3.0T will equate to better diagnostic performance in the future.

REFERENCES

1. Frayne R, Goodyear BG, Dickhoff P, et al. Magnetic resonance imaging at 3.0 Tesla: challenges and advantages in clinical neurological imaging. Invest Radiol 2003;38:385–402.

2. Campeau NG, Huston J 3rd, Bernstein MA, et al. Magnetic resonance angiography at 3.0 Tesla: initial clinical experience. Top Magn Reson Imaging 2001;12:183–204.

3. Wilson GJ, Hoogeveen RM, Willinek WA, et al. Parallel imaging in MR angiography. Top Magn Reson Imaging 2004;15:169–85.

4. Sodickson D, Manning W. Simultaneous acquisition of spatial harmonics (SMASH): fast imaging with radiofrequency coil arrays. Magn Reson Med 1997;38:591–603.

5. Griswold MA, Jakob PM, Heidemann RM, et al. Generalized autocalibrating partially parallel acquisitions (GRAPPA). Magn Reson Med 2002;47:1202–10.

6. Pruessman KP, Weiger M, Scheidegger MB, et al. SENSE: sensitivity encoding for fast MRI. Magn Reson Med 1999;42:952–62.

7. Nael K, Ruehm SG, Michaely HJ, et al. High spatial-resolution CE-MRA of the carotid circulation with parallel imaging: comparison of image quality between 2 different acceleration factors at 3.0 Tesla. Invest Radiol 2006;41:391–9.

8. Ethofer T, Mader I, Seeger U, et al. Comparison of longitudinal metabolite relaxation times in different regions of the human brain at 1.5 and 3 Tesla. Magn Reson Med 2003;50:1296–301.

9. Bernstein MA, Huston J 3rd, Lin C, et al. High-resolution intracranial and cervical MRA at 3.0T: technical considerations and initial experience. Magn Reson Med 2001;46:955–62.

10. Al-Kwifi O, Emery DJ, Wilman AH. Vessel contrast at three Tesla in time-of-flight magnetic resonance angiography of the intracranial and carotid arteries. Magn Reson Imaging 2002;20:181–7.

11. Ross JS. The high-field strength curmudgeon. AJNR Am J Neuroradiol 2004;25:168–9.

12. Hu X, Norris DG. Advances in high-field magnetic resonance imaging. Annu Rev Biomed Eng 2004;6:157–84.

13. Thomas SD, Al-Kwifi O, Emery DJ, et al. Application of magnetization transfer at 3.0 T in three-dimensional time-of-flight magnetic resonance angiography of the intracranial arteries. J Magn Reson Imaging 2002;15:479–83.

14. Schmitz BL, Aschoff AJ, Hoffmann MHK, et al. Advantages and pitfalls in 3T MR brain imaging: a pictorial review. AJNR Am J Neuroradiol 2005;26:2229–37.

15. DeLano MC, DeMarco JK. 3.0 T versus 1.5 T MR angiography of the head and neck. Neuroimaging Clin N Am 2006;16:321–41.

16. Willinek WA, Born M, Simon B, et al. Time-of-flight MR angiography: comparison of 3.0-T imaging and 1.5-T imaging—initial experience. Radiology 2003;229:913–20.

17. Gibbs GF, Huston J 3rd, Bernstein MA, et al. 3.0-Tesla MR angiography of intracranial aneurysms: comparison of time-of-flight and contrast-enhanced techniques. J Magn Reson Imaging 2005;21:97–102.

18. Gaa J, Weidauer S, Requardt M, et al. Comparison of intracranial 3D-ToF-MRA with and without parallel acquisition techniques at 1.5T and 3.0T: preliminary results. Acta Radiol 2004;45:327–32.

19. Wolff SD, Balaban RS. Magnetization transfer contrast (MTC) and tissue water proton relaxation in vivo. Magn Reson Med 1988;10:135–44.

20. Edelman RR, Ahn SS, Chien D, et al. Improved time-of-flight MR angiography of the brain with magnetization transfer contrast. Radiology 1992;184:395–9.

21. Haacke EM, Masaryk TJ, Wielopolski P, et al. Optimizing blood vessel contrast in fast three-dimensional magnetic resonance imaging. Magn Reson Med 1990;14:202–21.

22. Parker DL, Yuan C, Blatter DD. MR angiography by multiple thin slab 3D acquisition. Magn Reson Med 1991;17:434–51.

23. Blatter DD, Parker DL, Robison RO. Cerebral MR angiography with multiple overlapping thin slab acquisition: part 1. Quantitative analysis of vessel visibility. Radiology 1991;179:805–11.

24. Ding X, Tkach JA, Ruggieri PR, et al. Sequential three-dimensional time-of-flight angiography of the carotid arteries: value of variable excitation and postprocessing in reducing venetian blind artifact. AJR Am J Roentgenol 1994;163:683–8.

25. Laub G. Principles of contrast-enhanced MR angiography. Basic and clinical applications. Magn Reson Imaging Clin N Am 1999;7:783–95.

26. Fain SB, Riederer SJ, Bernstein MA, et al. Theoretical limits of spatial resolution in elliptical-centric contrast-enhanced 3D-MRA. Magn Reson Med 1999;42:1106–16.

27. Carroll TJ, Korosec FR, Petermann GM, et al. Carotid bifurcation: evaluation of time-resolved three-dimensional contrast-enhanced MR angiography. Radiology 2001;220:525–32.

28. Levy RA, Maki JH. Three-dimensional contrast-enhanced MR angiography of the extracranial carotid arteries: two techniques. AJNR Am J Neuroradiol 1998;19:688–90.

29. Huston J 3rd, Fain SB, Riederer SJ, et al. Carotid arteries: maximizing arterial to venous contrast in fluoroscopically triggered contrast-enhanced MR angiography with elliptic centric view ordering. Radiology 1999;211:265–73.

30. Huston J 3rd, Fain SB, Wald JT, et al. Carotid artery: elliptic centric contrast-enhanced MR angiography compared with conventional angiography. Radiology 2001;218:138–43.

31. Foo TK, Saranathan M, Prince MR, et al. Automated detection of bolus arrival and initiation of data acquisition in fast, three-dimensional,

gadolinium-enhanced MR angiography. Radiology 1997;203:275–80.

32. Wilman AH, Riederer SJ, King BF, et al. Fluoroscopically triggered contrast-enhanced three-dimensional MR angiography with elliptical centric view order: application to the renal arteries. Radiology 1997; 205:137–46.

33. DeMarco JK, Huston J 3rd, Nash AK. Extracranial carotid MR imaging at 3T. Magn Reson Imaging Clin N Am 2006;14:109–21.

34. Willinek WA, von Falkenhausen M, Born M, et al. Noninvasive detection of steno-occlusive disease of the supra-aortic arteries with three-dimensional contrast-enhanced magnetic resonance angiography: a prospective, intra-individual comparative analysis with digital subtraction angiography. Stroke 2005;36:38–43.

35. Villablanca JP, Nael K, Habibi R, et al. 3 T contrast-enhanced magnetic resonance angiography for evaluation of the intracranial arteries: comparison with time-of-flight magnetic resonance angiography and multislice computed tomography angiography. Invest Radiol 2006;41:799–805.

36. Cashen TA, Carr JC, Shin W, et al. Intracranial time-resolved contrast-enhanced MR angiography at 3T. AJNR Am J Neuroradiol 2006;27:822–9.

37. Markl M, Uhl M, Wieben O, et al. High resolution 3T MRI for assessment of cervical and superficial cranial arteries in giant cell arteritis. J Magn Reson Imaging 2006;24:423–7.

38. Anzalone N, Scomazzoni F, Cirillo M, et al. Follow-up of coiled cerebral aneurysms at 3T: comparison of 3D time-of-flight MR angiography and contrast-enhanced MR angiography. AJNR Am J Neuroradiol 2008;29:1530–6.

39. Gauvrit JY, Leclerc X, Oppenheim C, et al. Three-dimensional dynamic MR digital subtraction angiography using sensitivity encoding for the evaluation of intracranial arteriovenous malformations: a preliminary study. AJNR Am J Neuroradiol 2005;26:1525–31.

40. Wu Y, Goodrich KC, Buswell HR, et al. High-resolution time-resolved contrast-enhanced 3D MRA by combining SENSE with keyhole and SLAM strategies. Magn Reson Imaging 2004; 22:1161–8.

41. van Vaals JJ, Brummer ME, Dixon WT, et al. "Keyhole" method for accelerating imaging of contrast agent uptake. J Magn Reson Imaging 1993;3:671–5.

42. Fink C, Ley S, Kroeker R, et al. Time-resolved contrast-enhanced three-dimensional magnetic resonance angiography of the chest: combination of parallel imaging with view sharing (TREAT). Invest Radiol 2005;40:40–8.

43. Frydrychowicz A, Bley TA, Winterer JT, et al. Accelerated time-resolved 3D contrast-enhanced MR

angiography at 3T: clinical experience in 31 patients. MAGMA 2006;19:187–95.

44. Nael K, Michaely HJ, Villablanca P, et al. Time-resolved contrast enhanced magnetic resonance angiography of the head and neck at 3.0 Tesla: initial results. Invest Radiol 2006;41:116–24.

45. Ziyeh S, Strecker R, Berlis A, et al. Dynamic 3D MR angiography of intra- and extracranial vascular malformations at 3T: a technical note. AJNR Am J Neuroradiol 2005;26:630–4.

46. Willinek WA, Hadizadeh DR, von Falkenhausen M, et al. 4D time-resolved MR angiography with keyhole (4D-TRAK): more than 60 times accelerated MRA using a combination of CENTRA, keyhole, and SENSE at 3.0T. J Magn Reson Imaging 2008;27:1455–60.

47. Gu T, Korosec FR, Block WF, et al. PC VIPR: a high-speed 3D phase-contrast method for flow quantification and high resolution angiography. AJNR Am J Neuroradiol 2005;26:743–9.

48. Barger AV, Block WF, Toropov Y, et al. Time-resolved contrast-enhanced imaging with isotropic resolution and broad coverage using a undersampling 3D projection trajectory. Magn Reson Med 2002;48:297–305.

49. Turk AS, Johnson KM, Lum D, et al. Physiologic and anatomic assessment of a canine carotid artery stenosis model utilizing phase contrast with vastly undersampled isotropic projection imaging. AJNR Am J Neuroradiol 2007;28:111–5.

50. Moftakhar R, Aagaard-Kienitz B, Johnson K, et al. Noninvasive measurement of intra-aneurysmal pressure and flow pattern using phase contrast with vastly undersampled isotropic projection imaging. AJNR Am J Neuroradiol 2007;38:1710–4.

51. Lotz J, Doker R, Noeske R, et al. In vitro validation of phase-contrast flow measurements at 3T in comparison to 1.5T: precision, accuracy, and signal-to-noise ratios. J Magn Reson Imaging 2005;21:604–10.

52. White PM, Wardlaw JM, Easton V. Can noninvasive imaging accurately depict intracranial aneurysms? A systematic review. Radiology 2000;217:361–70.

53. Chung TS, Joo JY, Lee SK, et al. Evaluation of cerebral aneurysms with high-resolution MR angiography using a section-interpolation technique: correlation with digital subtraction angiography. AJNR Am J Neuroradiol 1999;20:229–35.

54. Tang PH, Hui F, Sitoh YY. Intracranial aneurysm detection with 3T magnetic resonance angiography. Ann Acad Med Singap 2007;36:388–93.

55. Gibbs GF, Huston J 3rd, Bernstein MA, et al. Improved image quality of intracranial aneurysms: 3.0-T versus 1.5-T time-of-flight angiography. AJNR Am J Neuroradiol 2004;25:84–7.

56. Nael K, Villablanca JP, Saleh R, et al. Contrast-enhanced MR angiography at 3T in the evaluation of intracranial aneurysms: a comparison

with time-of-flight angiography. AJNR Am J Neuroradiol 2006;27:2118–21.

57. Molyneux AJ, Kerr RS, Yu LM, et al. International subarachnoid aneurysm trial (ISAT) of neurosurgical clipping versus endovascular coiling in 2143 patients with ruptured intracranial aneurysms: a randomised comparison of effects on survival, dependency, seizures, rebleeding, subgroups, and aneurysm occlusion. Lancet 2005;366:809–17.

58. Wallace RC, Karis JP, Partovi S, et al. Noninvasive imaging of treated cerebral aneurysms, part I: MR angiographic follow-up of coiled aneurysms. AJNR Am J Neuroradiol 2007;28:1001–8.

59. Cognard C, Weill A, Spelle L, et al. Long-term angiographic follow-up of 169 intracranial berry aneurysms occluded with detachable coils. Radiology 1999;212:348–56.

60. Shellock FG. Biomedical implants and devices: assessment of magnetic field interactions with a 3.0-Tesla MR system. J Magn Reson Imaging 2002;16:721–32.

61. Hennemeyer CT, Wicklow K, Feinberg DA, et al. In vitro evaluation of platinum Guglielmi detachable coils at 3 T with a porcine model: safety issues and artifacts. Radiology 2001;219:732–7.

62. Kwee TC, Kwee RM. MR angiography in the follow-up of intracranial aneurysms treated with Guglielmi detachable coils: systematic review and meta-analysis. Neuroradiology 2007;49:703–13.

63. Weber W, Yousry TA, Felber SR, et al. Noninvasive follow-up of GDC-treated saccular aneurysms by MR angiography. Eur Radiol 2001;11:1792–7.

64. Pierot L, Delcourt C, Bouquigny F, et al. Follow-up of intracranial aneurysms selectively treated with coils: prospective evaluation of contrast-enhanced MR angiography. AJNR Am J Neuroradiol 2006;27: 744–9.

65. Cottier JP, Bleuzen-Couthon A, Gallas S, et al. Intracranial aneurysms treated with Guglielmi detachable coils: is contrast material necessary in the follow-up with 3D time-of-flight MR angiography? AJNR Am J Neuroradiol 2003;24:1797–803.

66. Majoie CB, Sprengers ME, van Rooij WJ, et al. MR angiography at 3T versus digital subtraction angiography in the follow-up of intracranial aneurysms treated with detachable coils. AJNR Am J Neuroradiol 2005;26:1349–56.

67. Buhk JH, Kallenberg K, Mohr A, et al. No advantage of time-of-flight magnetic resonance angiography at 3 Tesla compared to 1.5 Tesla in the follow-up after endovascular treatment of cerebral aneurysms. Neuroradiology 2008;50:855–61.

68. Urbach H, Dorenbeck U, von Falkenhausen M, et al. Three-dimensional time-of-flight MR angiography at 3T compared to digital subtraction angiography in the follow-up of ruptured and coiled intracranial aneurysms: a prospective study. Neuroradiology 2008;50:383–9.

69. Okahara M, Kiyosue H, Hori Y, et al. Three-dimensional time-of-flight MR angiography for evaluation of intracranial aneurysms after endosaccular packing with Guglielmi detachable coils: comparison with 3D digital subtraction angiography. Eur Radiol 2004;14:1162–8.

70. Boulin A, Pierot L. Follow-up of intracranial aneurysms treated with detachable coils: comparison of gadolinium enhanced 3D time-of-flight MR angiography and digital subtraction angiography. Radiology 2001;219:108–13.

71. Anzalone N, Righi C, Simionato F, et al. Three-dimensional time-of-flight MR angiography in the evaluation of intracranial aneurysms treated with Guglielmi detachable coils. AJNR Am J Neuroradiol 2000;21:746–52.

72. Gonner F, Heid O, Remonda L, et al. MR angiography with ultrashort echo time in cerebral aneurysms treated with Guglielmi detachable coils. AJNR Am J Neuroradiol 1998;19:1324–8.

73. Sprengers ME, Schaafsma J, von Rooij WJ, et al. Stability of intracranial aneurysms adequately occluded 6 months after coiling: a 3T MR angiography multicenter long-term follow-up study. AJNR Am J Neuroradiol 2008;29:1768–74.

74. Walker MT, Tsai J, Parish T, et al. MR angiographic evaluation of platinum coil packs at 1.5T and 3T: an in vitro assessment of artifact production: technical note. AJNR Am J Neuroradiol 2005;26: 848–53.

75. Ehricke HH, Schad LR, Gademann G, et al. Use of MR angiography for stereotactic planning. J Comput Assist Tomogr 1992;16:35–40.

76. Schad LR, Bock M, Baudendistel K, et al. Improved target volume definition in radiosurgery of arteriovenous malformations by stereotactic correlation of MRA, MRI, blood bolus tagging, and functional MRI. Eur Radiol 1996;6:38–45.

77. Bednaz G, Downes B, Werner-Wasik M, et al. Combining steriotactic angiograpy and 3D time-of-flight magnetic resonance angiography in treatment planning for arteriovenous malformation radiosurgery. Int J Radiat Oncol Biol Phys 2000; 46:1149–54.

78. Duran M, Schoenberg SO, Yuh WT, et al. Cerebral arteriovenous malformations: morphologic evaluation by ultrashort 3D gadolinium-enhanced MR angiography. Eur Radiol 2002;12:2957–64.

79. Heidenreich JO, Schilling AM, Unterharnscheidt F, et al. Assessment of 3D-TOF-MRA at 3.0 Tesla in the characterization of the angioarchitecture of cerebral arteriovenous malformations: a preliminary study. Acta Radiol 2007;48:678–86.

80. Aoki S, Yoshikawa T, Hori M, et al. MR digital subtraction angiography for the assessment of

cranial arteriovenous malformations and fistulas. AJR Am J Roentgenol 2000;175:451–3.

81. Warren DJ, Hoggard N, Walton L, et al. Cerebral arteriovenous malformations: comparison of novel magnetic resonance angiographic techniques and conventional catheter angiography. Neurosurgery 2001;48:973–82.

82. Meckel S, Maier M, Ruiz DS, et al. MR angiography of dural arteriovenous fistulas: diagnosis and follow-up after treatment using a time-resolved 3D contrast-enhanced technique. AJNR Am J Neuroradiol 2007;28:877–84.

83. Griffiths PD, Hoggard W, Warren DJ, et al. Brain arteriovenous malformations: assessment with dynamic MR digital subtraction angiography. AJNR Am J Neuroradiol 2000;21:1892–9.

84. Wetzel SG, Bilecan D, Lyrer P, et al. Cerebral dural arteriovenous fistulas: detection by dynamic MR projection angiography. AJR Am J Roentgenol 2000;174:1293–5.

85. Saleh RS, Lohan DG, Villablanca JP, et al. Assessment of craniospinal arteriovenous malformations at 3T with highly temporally and highly spatially resolved contrast-enhanced MRA angiography. AJNR Am J Neuroradiol 2008;20:1024–31.

86. Debrey SM, Yu H, Lynch JK, et al. Diagnostic accuracy of magnetic resonance angiography for internal carotid artery disease: a systematic review and meta-analysis. Stroke 2008;39:2237–48.

87. Townsend TC, Saloner D, Pan XM, et al. Contrast material enhanced MRA overestimates severity of carotid stenosis, compared with 3D time-of-flight MRA. J Vasc Surg 2003;38:36–40.

88. Fellner C, Lang W, Janka R, et al. Magnetic resonance angiography of the carotid arteries using three different techniques: accuracy compared with intraarterial x-ray angiography and endarterectomy specimens. J Magn Reson Imaging 2005; 21:424–31.

89. U-King-Im JM, Trivedi RA, Graves MJ, et al. Contrast-enhanced MR angiography for carotid disease: diagnostic and potential clinical impact. Neurology 2004;62:1282–90.

90. Nederkoorn PJ, Elgersma OE, Mali WP, et al. Overestimation of carotid artery stenosis with magnetic resonance angiography compared with digital subtraction angiography. J Vasc Surg 2002;36:806–13.

91. Porsche C, Walker L, Mendelow D, et al. Evaluation of cross-sectional luminal morphology in carotid atherosclerotic disease by use of spiral CT angiography. J Vasc Surg 2002;36:806–13.

92. Anzalone N, Scomazzoni F, Castellano R, et al. Carotid artery stenosis: intraindividual correlations of 3D time-of-flight MR angiography, contrast enhanced MR angiography, conventional DSA, and rotational angiography for detection and grading. Radiology 2005;236:204–13.

93. Alvarez-Linera J, Benito-Leon J, Escribano J, et al. Prospective evaluation of carotid artery stenosis: elliptic centric contrast-enhanced MR angiography and spiral CT angiography compared with digital subtraction angiography. AJNR Am J Neuroradiol 2003;24:1012–9.

94. Cossottini M, Pingitore A, Puglioli M, et al. Contrast-enhanced three-dimensional magnetic resonance angiography of atherosclerotic internal carotid stenosis as the noninvasive imaging modality in revascularization decision making. Stroke 2003; 34:660–4.

95. Wutke R, Lang W, Fellner C, et al. High-resolution, contrast-enhanced magnetic resonance angiography with elliptical centric k-space ordering of supra-aortic arteries compared with selective x-ray angiography. Stroke 2002;33:1522–9.

96. Lenhart M, Framme N, Volk M, et al. Time-resolved contrast-enhanced magnetic resonance angiography of the carotid arteries: diagnostic accuracy and inter-observer variability with selective catheter angiography. Invest Radiol 2002;37:535–41.

97. Yuan C, Beach KW, Smith LH Jr, et al. Measurement of atherosclerotic carotid plaque size in vivo using high resolution magnetic resonance imaging. Circulation 1998;98:2666–71.

98. Cai J, Hatsukami TS, Ferguson MS, et al. In vivo quantitative measurement of intact fibrous cap and lipid-rich necrotic core size in atherosclerotic carotid plaque: comparison of high-resolution, contrast-enhanced magnetic resonance imaging and histology. Circulation 2005; 112:3437–44.

99. Toussaint JF, LaMuraglia GM, Southern JF, et al. Magnetic resonance images lipid, fibrous, calcified, hemorrhagic, and thrombotic components of human atherosclerosis in vivo. Circulation 1996;94:932–8.

100. Yarnykh VL, Terashima M, Hayes CE, et al. Multicontrast black-blood MRI of carotid arteries: comparison between 1.5 and 3 Tesla magnetic field strengths. J Magn Reson Imaging 2006;23:691–8.

101. Underhill HR, Yarnykh VL, Hatsukami TS, et al. Carotid plaque morphology and composition: initial comparison between 1.5- and 3.0T magnetic field strength. Radiology 2008;248:550–60.

Susceptibility-Weighted Imaging: Clinical Angiographic Applications

Samuel R.S. Barnes, MS[a], E. Mark Haacke, PhD[b,c],*

KEYWORDS

- Susceptibility • Susceptibility-weighted imaging
- BOLD • Phase • Venography

Susceptibility-weighted imaging (SWI) provides a new means to enhance contrast in MR imaging.[1] Conventional imaging relies on the magnitude information to generate the image; the phase information, however, has typically been discarded except for a few applications in flow imaging. Historically, phase images have been difficult to interpret, because the valuable information about susceptibility changes between tissues was hidden by background field inhomogeneities caused by air-tissue interfaces and main magnetic field effects. It has been shown, however, that by using a special high pass filter it is possible to remove most of these unwanted effects, leaving behind only the valuable information about susceptibility changes between tissues.[2] The contrast in the phase image is complimentary to the magnitude contrast and the two can be combined to create what is now referred to as "susceptibility-weighted" images. This triplet of images (magnitude, phase, and susceptibility-weighted images) has now become part of the standard clinical neuroimaging protocol in at least one manufacturer's product.

SWI represents a new type of contrast[3–28] that is complementary to conventional spin-density, T1-, and T2-weighted imaging methods. SWI is particularly suited for imaging venous blood because it is very sensitive to deoxyhemoglobin, making it useful in imaging hemorrhages from trauma, visualizing blood products and the vascularization of tumors, and high-resolution MR venography. It has also proved useful in other applications relating to iron, such as measuring iron content in multiple sclerosis lesions, and aging.[8]

GRADIENT ECHO IMAGING

SWI is collected with a long TE, fully flow-compensated gradient echo scan; this can be in the form of a single-echo, multiple-echo, or echo-planar scan. Imaging with long echoes at 1.5 T became possible by using three-dimensional gradient echo imaging.[29] This allowed for thinner slices (1–2 mm), which reduced dephasing across the slice and improved image quality. In general, imaging at high resolution (approximately 1 mm^3) reduces dephasing across the voxel and allows for longer echo times, from 40 to 80 milliseconds at 1.5T.[30]

Flow compensation in all directions is useful at 1.5 T because of the long echo times required and because phase is being used as a measure

This work was supported by National Institutes of Health grant No. 2R01 HL062983-04A2 and by Siemens Medical Solutions USA.
[a] Department of Radiology, Loma Linda University Medical Center, 11234 Anderson Street, Room B623, Loma Linda, CA 92350, USA
[b] Department of Radiology, Wayne State University, 3990 John R, Detroit, MI 48201, USA
[c] Department of Biomedical Engineering, Wayne State University, MRI Institute for Biomedical Engineering, 440 East Ferry Street, Unit 2, Detroit, MI 48202, USA
* Corresponding author. Department of Biomedical Engineering, Wayne State University, MRI Institute for Biomedical Engineering, 440 East Ferry Street, Unit 2, Detroit, MI 48202, USA.
E-mail address: nmrimaging@aol.com (E.M. Haacke).

of susceptibility. This reduces flow-related signal loss in the magnitude image, and flow-induced phase changes in the phase image. Changes in the phase image are generated according to the formula (for a right-handed system):

$$\Delta\phi = -\gamma \cdot \Delta B \cdot TE \qquad (1)$$

$$\Delta\phi = -\gamma \cdot (\Delta\chi B_0 G + \Delta B_{CS} + \Delta B_{geometry} + \Delta B_{main\ field}) \cdot TE \qquad (2)$$

where γ is the gyromagnetic ratio, G represents a constant dependent on the geometry of the object, CS refers to chemical shift, and $B_{geometry}$ refers to the geometry of the brain and air-tissue interfaces. The last two terms represent unwanted field effects. The first two terms are of particular interest and are meant to represent the local changes in field, such as those that might be caused by iron in tissue. In equation (2), $\Delta\chi$ represents the local susceptibility change between tissues. The last two terms tend to be slowly varying spatial terms and can be, to a large degree, removed using a high-pass spatial frequency filter. Ideally, one can isolate the first two terms, $-\gamma G \Delta\chi B_0 TE$ and $-\gamma \Delta B_{CS} TE$. Both of them lead to similar phase results inside the object of interest. A paramagnetic object causes a local increase in field and a negative phase change relative to surrounding tissues.

CREATING A SUSCEPTIBILITY-WEIGHTED IMAGING DATASET

The unwanted background field effects are usually removed from the phase image with a high-pass ho-modyne filter. To do this, a low-pass or smoothed version of the original image is created using an appropriate filter size (ranging from 32 × 32 up to 128 × 128, depending on the dataset). This is then divided into the original complex image, effectively removing the low spatial frequencies and generating a high-pass filtered phase image. When severe aliasing occurs, it is possible to get better results by first applying a phase unwrapping algorithm before the high-pass filter is applied. This removes much of the phase aliasing that could not be removed by the high-pass filter alone and helps improve results in areas of rapid phase change (near air-tissue interfaces, such as the sinuses).[31] This filtered phase image is used in all subsequent steps and is referred to as the SWI "filtered-phase" image.

The contrast in the SWI filtered-phase image is complimentary to that in the magnitude image. The goal is to take advantage of features in both the magnitude and phase images, so the final step is to combine these features together to generate a susceptibility-weighted image. The phase image

is used to create a mask that is applied to the magnitude image. This mask focuses on certain phase values that enhance the contrast of the original magnitude image. For example, if areas with increased iron are the subject of interest, then the mask is designed to enhance information related to negative phase as follows:

$$f(x) = \begin{cases} \frac{\pi + \varphi(x)}{\pi} & for -\pi < \varphi(x) < 0 \\ 1 & otherwise \end{cases} \qquad (3)$$

where the phase values can range from $-\pi$ to π, $\varphi(x)$ is the phase at location x, and f(x) is the phase mask. This phase mask can be multiplied by an integer m number of times into the original magnitude image $(\rho(x))$ to create the susceptibility-weighted image:

$$\rho'(x) = f^m(x) \cdot \rho(x) \qquad (4)$$

The number of times the mask is applied changes the contrast in the susceptibility-weighted image. It has been shown that four multiplications produces good contrast-to-noise for a wide range of phase values.[32]

In each individual slice, the veins now appear dark and look like a set of circles or vessel cross-sections. To get a good SWI venogram, it is best to take a minimum intensity projection (mIP) over a number of slices (Fig. 1); this is similar to the maximum intensity projection used in angiography. A disadvantage of using mIPs is that the dark background surrounding the brain masks out the brain if it is included in the projection. The slice included in the mIP having the smallest visible brain area dictates how much of the brain is visible in the final projection. This can be problematic at the top and bottom of the brain where the size changes very rapidly. This problem can be partly overcome by using a brain extraction algorithm, such as a complex threshold approach,[33] to set the noise values outside the brain to a value much higher than the brain during the mIP processing and then back to zero afterward. Clinically, mIPs are usually limited to projections over 4 to 8 mm, although it is certainly possible to project over more slices near the center of the brain or if the background has been removed.

VENOGRAPHIC CONTRAST

The iron in deoxyhemoglobin in venous blood acts as an intrinsic contrast agent, causing T2*-related losses in the magnitude image and a shift in the phase relative to surrounding tissues in the phase image caused by susceptibility differences. The oxygen in oxyhemoglobin shields the iron so the T2* and susceptibility effects are only seen in venous blood. This provides a natural separation of venous and arterial blood, and allows for

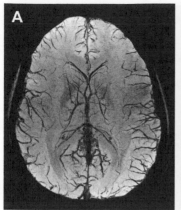 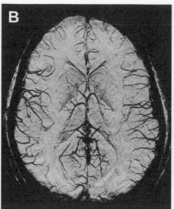 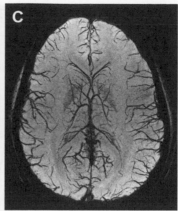

Fig. 1. SWI data at 4 T showing a mIP over 26 mm of the magnitude (A), phase (B), and susceptibility-weighted (C) images. The susceptibility-weighted images combine the contrast of the magnitude and phase images. Note the magnitude and the susceptibility-weighted processed data both have spatial inhomogeneities from radiofrequency penetration effects, whereas the phase image (B) is remarkably uniform.

venographic images without any arterial contamination.

The iron in deoxyhemoglobin induces changes to the local magnetic field, both inside and outside the veins. The changes to the local field depend on the shape of the structure of interest. If blood vessels are modeled as infinitely long cylinders, the field inside and outside the vessels can be analytically calculated. The field inside is given by:

$$\Delta B_{in} = \Delta \chi \cdot B_0 \left(3 \cdot \cos^2(\theta) - 1\right)\frac{1}{6} \qquad (5)$$

where θ is the angle the cylinder makes to the main magnetic field and $\Delta \chi$ is the change in susceptibility between the cylinder and the surrounding substance. The field outside the cylinder is more complicated, and is given by:

$$\Delta B_{out} = \frac{\Delta \chi \cdot B_0 \cdot \sin^2(\theta) \cdot \cos(2\Phi) \cdot a^2}{2 \cdot r^2} \qquad (6)$$

where r is the distance to the axis of the cylinder, a is the radius of the cylinder, and Φ is the angle the vector r makes to the projection of the main field direction onto a plane perpendicular to the axis of the vessel.

The changes in local field (which generate the contrast in the phase image, see equation [1]) depend on both the shape (modeled here as a cylinder) and the orientation of the blood vessels. This could potentially cause problems, because the field change inside the vessel disappears at the so-called "magic angle" ($\Delta B_{in} = 0$ when $\theta = 54.7$ degrees) and vessels parallel to the field have a negative phase shift (caused by a positive local field change), whereas vessels perpendicular to the field have a positive phase shift (caused by a negative local field). Practically, this is overcome by collecting data with anisotropic resolution.

Data are usually collected with anywhere from a 2:1 to a 5:1 aspect ratio, meaning the voxels are two to five times larger in the direction of B_0 than in the other two directions. The thicker slices allow the phase from outside the vessels (in the direction of B_0) to average with the phase inside the vessel. This makes the average phase in a voxel negative for veins that are perpendicular to the field and at the magic angle even though the phase inside goes to zero or is positive. It has been shown that the optimal aspect ratio for maximum contrast in the phase image is generally 4:1, although it does depend on the resolution, the size of the vessels of interest, and even the field strength.[34]

Because the phase shift is directly proportional to field strength and echo time (see equation [2]), scanning at higher fields allows the echo time to be shortened proportionally while maintaining the same contrast in the phase image. This fact, and the increased signal-to-noise ratio available at higher fields, makes SWI well suited for high-field and ultra-high-field MR imaging because the shorter echo times make it possible to scan much faster (Fig. 2). Because SWI uses small flip angles, there is little problem with specific absorption rate. Increases in field strength allow increased resolution and generally improved image quality,[5,35] although 1.5 T can still produce very nice SWI venographic images. Table 1 shows acceptable parameters for optimal venous contrast at different field strengths.

SIMULTANEOUS MR VENOGRAPHY AND MR ANGIOGRAPHY
Single-Echo Approach

SWI provides a natural separation of arteries and veins, making it possible to image both

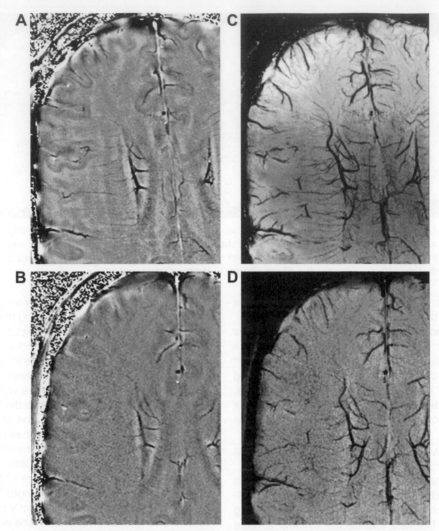

Fig. 2. Filtered phase images (*A* and *B*) and mIPS of susceptibility-weighted images over 8 mm (*C* and *D*) at 3 T (*B, D*) and 7 T (*A, C*) at identical resolutions on the same volunteer. This shows the improved visualization of veins at higher fields caused by the higher signal-to-noise ratio and increased susceptibility even at the same resolution. Imaging parameters are TR/TE/FA = 45 ms/28 ms/15 degrees at 3 T and 35 ms/16 ms/15 degrees at 7 T with identical resolutions of 0.44 × 0.44 × 2 mm^3. (*Courtesy of* Yulin Ge, New York, NY.)

simultaneously and have them be easily evaluated separately. Veins are dark because of T2* losses and SWI processing with the phase image, whereas arteries are bright from time-of-flight inflow enhancement. It is possible to increase the contrast in the arteries without overly degrading the venography by using a slightly higher flip angle, short TR, and a thin slab. This is particularly effective at high and ultra-high field because shorter echoes can be used to reduce flow dephasing in the arteries without affecting the venous contrast; this technique is unsuitable for 1.5 T and lower fields.

By imaging both the arteries and the veins, a more complete picture of the vasculature can

be created. The advantage of collecting both angiographic and venographic data in a single acquisition is that there are no registration artifacts and that their relationship to each other and to the overall brain tissue structure can be carefully reviewed.

In conventional imaging, a contrast agent is often used to enhance the arterial signal, but a longstanding problem has been the veins' tendency also to get bright in the steady state. That is much less a difficulty with SWI because the veins may actually get darker in the presence of a contrast agent (while the arteries brighten), making it possible to do an even better job imaging both parts of the vascular system simultaneously.

Table 1			
Suggested parameters for susceptibility-weighted imaging as a function of field strength			
Field	**FA in Degrees**	**TR in Milliseconds**	**TE in Milliseconds**
1.5 T	20	50	40
3 T	12	30	20
4 T	12	25	15
7 T	10–15	25	10–15

Recommended susceptibility-weighted imaging venography parameters. Usually a bandwidth of 100 Hz/pixel is used but lower bandwidths are possible at the expense of more distortion near air-tissue interfaces and loss of rapidly flowing blood signal in the center of the arteries.

The shortened T1 boosts the signal in the arteries and veins but the increased venous signal leads to increased T2* or signal cancellation effects; this is referred to as a "T1 to T2* coupling effect." The question then arises, "How are the data processed to arrive at both an MR angiography and MR venography projection?"

The arteries can be visualized using a standard maximum intensity projection and veins can be visualized with a mIP after SWI processing. The choice of flip angle and echo time are particularly important in determining image quality. Although a higher flip angle helps increase the time-of-flight effect and enhance contrast in the arteries, it also starts to degrade the venography by oversuppressing the cerebrospinal fluid. Likewise, the choice of echo time is also a compromise, because a longer echo time increases venous contrast, but leads to flow-related losses in rapidly flowing arteries. This is caused by the fact that higher-order flow effects for the low-bandwidth gradients being used, and the flow through local field inhomogeneities (which disrupt the flow compensation) are not flow-compensated. Generally, a slightly shorter echo time than is normally run (15 milliseconds instead of 20 milliseconds at 3 T), higher bandwidth (120–140 Hz/pixel), and very thin slices (0.5 mm, to reduce dephasing) give good results, especially with the use of a contrast agent. There can be problems, however, visualizing the faster-flowing blood (eg, in the middle cerebral arteries). Some examples of this approach are given in **Fig. 3**.

The thin slices improve the angiography by reducing through-plane dephasing, but SWI processing suffers because the data are not collected with the optimal 4:1 aspect ratio. This can be overcome by combining four slices together to generate a new dataset with a resolution of 0.5 × 0.5 × 2 mm, which has the 4:1 aspect ratio. These new data can then be used to do the SWI processing, resulting in improving the quality of the venography (**Fig. 4**).

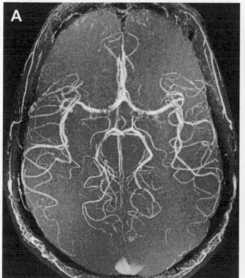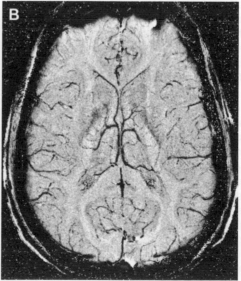

Fig. 3. Both the MR angiography (MRA) maximum intensity projection over 128 slices (*A*) and the mIP over 32 SWI filtered phase slices (*B*) are acquired from a single-echo SWI data set. The data were acquired at 3 T with TR = 35 ms, TE = 15 ms, FA = 15 degrees, 0.5-mm isotropic resolution, and 128 partitions. These high-resolution scans depict the usual M4 arteries with excellent edge definition. There are some flow-related losses in the MCA. The venous network is seen to be quite different than the arterial network in its distribution of vessels.

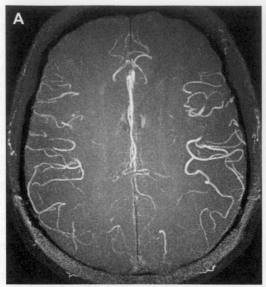
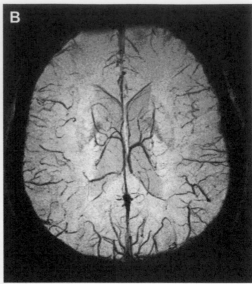

Fig. 4. Both the MRA maximum intensity projection (*A*) and the mIP over SWI processed data (*B*) are acquired from a single-echo SWI data set with 0.5-mm isotropic resolution. The data were acquired at 4 T with TR = 26 ms, TE = 15 ms, FA = 11 degrees, and 80 partitions. These high-resolution scans depict the usual M4 arteries with excellent edge definition. Again, the venous anatomy is seen to be quite different than the arterial pattern. The 4 T image shows the capability of higher fields to produce better MR angiography and venography images.

Double-Echo Approach

An alternate approach is to use a double-echo scan with the short echo used to generate the angiography and the long echo for the venography.[36] This is particularly useful at 1.5 T because the long echo times required for SWI give ample time to insert a short echo, and are too long to generate a useful angiography. This becomes less effective or necessary at higher field strengths because of the need for higher bandwidth. Further, the shorter optimal echo times for SWI no longer suffer from the same arterial dephasing problems.

The approach taken by Du and Zin[36] added an extra echo to the flow-compensated gradient echo imaging used for SWI. Flow compensation was applied in both phase-encoding directions. Asymmetric echoes were used to save time and achieve a shorter echo time for the first echo. Flyback gradients were also added between the two echoes to maintain the flow compensation on both echoes. In this way, a short echo time-of-flight MR angiography dataset and a long echo SWI MR venography dataset are obtained in the same amount of time as collecting either of them separately.

CLINICAL APPLICATIONS
Traumatic Brain Injury

Shown here are some new results related to venous involvement in traumatic brain injury.

This is an area of interest throughout the world and particularly in the United States. Traumatic brain injury is a major cause of morbidity, mortality, disability, and lost years of productive life. Tong and colleagues[4,25,26] have shown that SWI was three to six times more sensitive than conventional T2*-weighted gradient echo sequences in detecting the size, number, volume, and distribution of hemorrhagic lesions in diffuse axonal injury. From this work it is clear that SWI shows an increase in the number and size of lesions compared with other sequences. The studies of Tong and coworkers[4,25,26] also show that most patients had lesions in frontal white matter or parieto-temporo-occipital gray or white matter. SWI could play a very meaningful role in establishing the degree of injury more accurately, providing valuable prognostic information, and guiding the management and rehabilitation of patients with head injury.

Fig. 5 shows a case of a motorcycle accident where conventional MR imaging methods were unable to locate the many bleeds present. The gradient echo image shows evidence of a single microbleed. SWI, however, shows a number of damaged veins, from the confluence at the large septal vein to several smaller veins at the periphery of the brain. The smaller microbleeds are likely caused by shearing of the venules. The postcontrast T1-weighted image shows no evidence of vascular damage (**Fig. 5**). A more dramatic

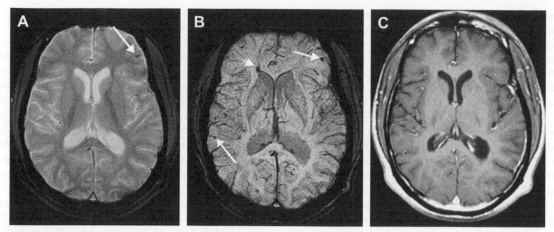

Fig. 5. Traumatic brain injury is often occult to conventional imaging methods in CT or MR imaging. Here is shown a case of a motorcycle accident where conventional MR imaging methods were unable to locate the many bleeds present. (*A*) The gradient echo image shows some sign of a microbleed (*arrow*). (*B*) SWI shows a number of venous confluences (particularly striking is the junction of the medullary veins with the septal vein) that have shearing injury (*arrows*). The smaller microbleeds are likely caused by shearing of the venules (see Fig. 12). (*C*) The postcontrast T1-weighted image shows no evidence of vascular damage.

example is shown in **Fig. 6**, where damage can be clearly seen in the corpus callosum.

Vascular Malformations and Venous Disease

Cerebral vascular malformations result from localized defects during vascular development. Most malformations are present at birth and may or may not grow with time. Cerebral cavernous malformations, developmental venous angiomas, and capillary telangiectasias have attenuated flow and can be less conspicuous or entirely missed by conventional neuroimaging techniques. Although lesions that have previously bled can be detected by conventional MR imaging, those that

have not bled tend to show as faint enhancements after contrast administration. Because SWI measures the presence of deoxyhemoglobin, there is no dependence on flow to visualize this blood and so these lesions are easily seen.[28]

Similar arguments on behalf of SWI hold for studying Sturge-Weber syndrome. This is a rare neurocutaneous disorder, typically manifested in children and characterized by cutaneous angioma, glaucoma, and leptomeningeal venous angiomatosis. It has been shown that T1-weighted gadolinium postcontrast MR imaging can demonstrate focal cortical atrophy, contrast-enhancing leptomeningeal angiomatosis, and abnormal cerebral veins. T1-weighted gadolinium postcontrast

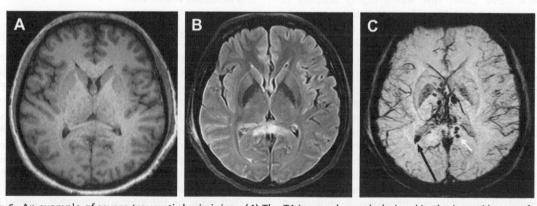

Fig. 6. An example of severe traumatic brain injury. (*A*) The T1 image shows dark signal in the lateral horns of the ventricles and some suspicious low signal intensity in the corpus callosum. (*B*) The FLAIR image shows some edema in the corpus callosum. (*C*) The SWI data clearly shows blood inside the posterior horn of the right lateral ventricle (*black arrow*) and a hemorrhage in the corpus callosum (*white arrow*). (*Courtesy of* Lei Jing, Tianjin Huan Hospital, China.)

imaging is currently an imaging standard for clinical Sturge-Weber syndrome diagnosis.[12] SWI complements conventional MR imaging by demonstrating numerous deep medullary veins that are not well visualized by any other MR imaging sequence, particularly in the early mild cases of Sturge-Weber syndrome.

Cerebral venous thrombosis is an infrequent neurologic condition but one that is notoriously difficult to diagnose because of its nonspecific clinical presentation.[37] Direct evidence of sinus thrombosis, such as "triangle sign" and "empty delta" on CT and loss of the normal flow voids on MR imaging, can be easily missed unless clinical suspicion is high and direct signs are actively sought.[38] Indirect signs of venous thrombosis vary, including cerebral edema, infarction, and hemorrhage. Cerebral venous thrombosis can be potentially deadly if it is not diagnosed and thrombolytic treatment is not started in time.[39,40] SWI has become a useful method to evaluate cerebral venous thrombosis by demonstrating venous stasis and collateral slow flow. Dural sinus thrombosis causes the concentration of deoxyhemoglobin to increase in the involved veins, which appears as a prominent hypointense signal in the SWI data. If treated successfully, this effect disappears in the SWI data.

Atherosclerosis

Outside of imaging atherosclerosis in the carotid artery, another potential application of MR imaging is in imaging peripheral arterial occlusive disease. Similar to atherosclerosis, peripheral arterial occlusive disease is also a major clinical problem affecting 8 to 10 million Americans.[41] To date, there have been few MR imaging studies of peripheral arterial occlusive disease[42–46] and most have used the black blood spin echo T2 approach. These techniques have had some success with imaging the wall of the femoral artery but have some difficulty suppressing the venous blood signal.

Calcification plays a significant role in atherosclerosis. Calcification scores have been associated with the stage of the disease and may be a better marker than the traditional risk factors in identifying people who are at high risk for amputation.[47] The presence or absence of atherosclerosis also plays a key role in deciding whether treatment should consist of percutaneous transluminal angioplasty or surgery.[48,49] It is possible to image the vessel wall and calcifications with SWI without the need to suppress the signal from the blood. It is also possible to use the phase as a complement to the magnitude SWI MR angiography data as a means to discriminate calcium from hemorrhage.

A high-resolution SWI scan was performed at 3 T using an eight-channel transmit-receive knee coil with an echo time of 15.6 milliseconds and a low bandwidth of 80 Hz/pixel. The data were collected sagittally with an in-plane resolution of 0.5 × 0.5 mm and a slice thickness of 1 mm. A flip angle of 10 degrees was used to maximize inflow effects and minimize saturation effects. The MR imaging data were compared with multidetector CT data using a 64-detector CT scanner. The scan protocol was as follows: 64 × 0.625 mm collimation, interval 0.625 mm, 120 kv, 420 mA, pitch 1.375, tablefeed 110 mm, with a 512 × 512 matrix size. The multidetector CT scanning ranged from the upper pole of the patella to the fibular head.

The magnitude SWI data are similar to low-flip angle time-of-flight MR angiography imaging. The phase images show that the vessel walls are slightly diamagnetic compared with surrounding tissue (**Fig. 7**). The vessel walls shown in **Fig. 7** are for a healthy volunteer; show no disease; and are straight (as one might expect). For patients with calcifications, comparisons between SWI and multidetector CT have been very encouraging. Both the size of the calcification and its distance to other structures appears the same in the SWI and multidetector CT data. The magnitude images clearly show the vessel lumen from the bright blood and the calcifications in the darker vessel wall (**Fig. 8**). The SWI filtered-phase images show the walls as being diamagnetic and the calcification as being much more diamagnetic. One advantage of SWI is that there is little dependence on blood flow for either patent or stenosed vessels. SWI offers an entirely new way to study and visualize both the healthy and diseased vessel wall.

Deep Venous Thrombosis and Blood Settling

Deep venous thrombosis (DVT) is a common occurrence. A recent study showed that for 2000 DVT patients with age-matched spouses, the probability of developing DVT after being stationary in a plane, train, or car for more than 4 hours was increased more than twofold.[50] DVT is known to occur when there is blood stasis and where there is damage to the vessel wall.[51] Blood stasis is known to occur when someone is seated or lying still for a long period.[52,53]

SWI relies on the susceptibility shift caused by deoxyhemoglobin in the venous blood to generate contrast. SWI is only sensitive to the deoxyhemoglobin in blood, so an increased concentration of red blood cells causes increased contrast; this

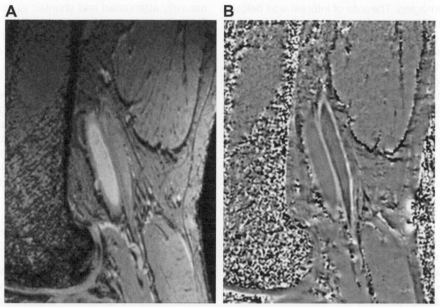

Fig. 7. Delineation of femoral artery wall in a normal subject. (*A*) Magnitude image shows the lumen bright, which serves as a good marker between the inside wall and blood. Note the vessel wall is straight with no indication of wall thickening. (*B*) The phase image shows the vessel wall with a brighter than background signal indicating that the vessel wall is diamagnetic. The phase of the venous wall seems to be brighter than that of the arterial wall indicating it is even more diamagnetic than the arterial wall.

makes it ideal for imaging blood settling or the early formation of potential clots. SWI has been used to image the veins of the leg and to determine if the red blood cells settle during rest. Perhaps blood settling will prove to be a potential risk factor for DVT formation. As an initial investigation, the authors have investigated blood settling with SWI as described next.

A total of nine subjects (18–58 years old) were scanned on a 1.5-T system with a single-channel knee coil. A three-dimensional SWI sequence with the following image parameters was used: TR = 21 milliseconds; TE = 9.95 milliseconds; FA = 20 degrees; BW = 190 Hz/pixel; a matrix of 384 × 512 × 64; a resolution of 0.39 × 0.39 × 1.6 mm^3; an acquisition time of 8 minutes; and

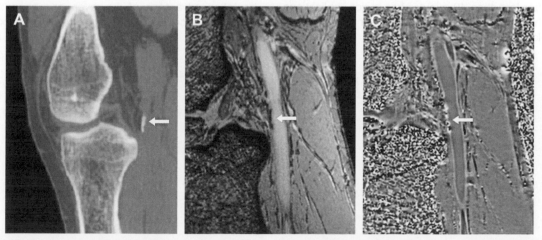

Fig. 8. (*A*) CT scan showing calcification at the edge of the popliteal artery just behind the knee (*arrow*). (*B*) Magnitude gradient echo image showing the signal loss from the calcification in the same area (*arrow*). (*C*) SWI filtered phase image showing the diamagnetic effect from the calcification (*arrow*). Note the similar shape and extent of the calcification in both the CT and MR imaging results.

no parallel imaging. The area of interest was below the knee at the level of the popliteal trifurcation with the region of interest centered 12 cm below the tibial plateau. The knee was positioned to be slightly bent within the coil.

A layering effect in the veins was observed, with the bottom of the vein (defined according to the direction of gravity) accumulating much more phase than the top layer. The layering was also observed to increase with time spent stationary in the magnet. Two scans were performed on each subject, the early scan (approximately 10 minutes stationary) showed very little or no layering, whereas the late scan (approximately 40 minutes stationary) showed increased layering (**Fig. 9**). The larger vessels showed an increase in size of the dark layer at the later time points, filling up to roughly 70% of the vessel, whereas some of the smaller vessels became completely dark in the later scans as if the flow to them had completely stopped and all the oxygen had been used up.

The layering effect was more prominent in the older subjects; younger subjects (including two father-son matched pairs) showed less layering in fewer veins, whereas older subjects showed much more pronounced layering in a greater number of veins. The younger subjects tended to have smaller veins with faster flow, whereas the veins of the older subjects were much larger (up to twice the diameter) with slower flow. Layering was seen to some extent in all subjects except the 18 year old. One other subject (female, 49) did not initially show layering, but after being kept in the magnet an additional 20 minutes (60 minutes total) and rescanned some minor layering in the smaller veins was observed.

The separation of the blood into different layers after less than 40 minutes has major implications. The denser red blood cells appear to sink as the blood flow from certain vessels seems to be naturally attenuated and shunted to other vessels. Deoxyhemoglobin in red blood cells is responsible for the phase shift in venous blood and as the cells settle out, the increased concentration of deoxyhemoglobin causes an increased phase shift in the lower layer.

This method could potentially be used as a screening procedure to determine a patient's risk factor for developing a DVT. The increased concentration of red blood cells could increase the likelihood of a clot forming and the layering seems to be correlated with age, which is a well-known risk factor for DVT.[51] These remain unproved postulates, however, at this time.

IMAGING OXYGEN SATURATION WITH SUSCEPTIBILITY-WEIGHTED IMAGING

Measuring oxygen saturation in the brain is very important for monitoring the oxygen extraction fraction and the amount of oxygen getting to the tissue. This is important for stroke and venous thrombosis. SWI offers the potential to investigate oxygen saturation by measuring the phase in three dimensions throughout a large field-of-view. In addition to neuroimaging, such a method could also be useful for measuring the oxygen saturation in the vena cava and in other parts of the body noninvasively. This section discusses the ability to use phase information as a means to monitor oxygen saturation in vessels. This was first done in 1997 to monitor changes in oxygen saturation during an fMR imaging motor task experiment.[54] Similar to the SWI approach taken today, a fully velocity-compensated flow sequence was used to make it possible to look at the susceptibility in the veins. Before the results of equation (5) can be taken advantage of, however, one needs to know the susceptibility difference between deoxygenated and oxygenated blood (referred to as

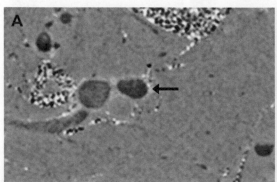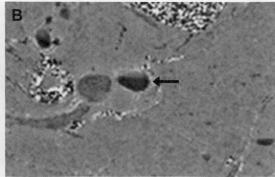

Fig. 9. Early scan (approximately 10 minutes) (*A*) and late scan (approximately 40 minutes) (*B*) of a 54-year-old man. Notice in the late scan the dark layers on the bottom (*arrows* in *B*) are more prominent than in the early scan (*arrows* in *A*).

χ_{do}). Two distinct values have been quoted in the last 20 years, but only one can be correct. Weisskoff and Kiihne[55] quoted $\chi_{do} = 0.18$ ppm in cgs units, whereas Spees and colleagues[56] quoted $\chi_{do} = 0.27$ ppm in cgs units. The authors' work demonstrates that using the phase information from an SWI sequence, it is the latter value that seems to make the MR imaging data agree with the known physiologic data. For veins, one can write

$$\varphi = -\gamma \cdot \chi_{do} \cdot TE \cdot B_0 \cdot Hct \cdot (1 - Y)$$
$$(3\cos^2 \theta - 1)\frac{1}{6} \tag{7}$$

If a specific substitution for χ_{do} is made (eg, 0.18 ppm), then a certain value for Y (the oxygen saturation) can be found once the other variables (Hct [hematocrit], B_0 [the main field], and TE [the echo time]) are known. If, however, Y also is known, then χ_{do} can be determined. Because χ_{do} is usually assumed to be 0.18 ppm, one can look instead for the deviation of χ_{do} from this value.

In this work, the phase difference between arterial and venous blood is used to determine oxygen saturation. Substituting χ_{do} with $A\chi_{do}$, setting $B_0 = 1.5$ and using

$$k = 2\pi \cdot 42.58 \cdot 4\pi \cdot 0.18 \cdot 1.5 \cdot \frac{1}{6} \tag{8}$$

A (and hence χ_{do}) can be found from:

$$A = -\frac{\varphi(vein) - \varphi(art)}{k \cdot Hct \cdot (1 - Y) \cdot TE \cdot (3\cos^2 \theta - 1)} \tag{9}$$

All data were acquired using a 1.5-T MR imager with a flexible four-channel surface array coil in the thigh region of the leg. The goal was to obtain high-resolution cross-sectional images of the femoral vein. Each subject was positioned inside the magnet feet first in a supine posture. A localizer scan was run to obtain a set of scout (or reference) images. The scout images were used to determine the imaging volume over which a two-dimensional time-of-flight MR venographic sequence was run transversely with a saturation band to reduce signal from the inflowing arterial blood so as to obtain just the venous blood signal from the imaging volume. The imaging parameters were TR = 30 milliseconds; TE = 6 milliseconds; FOV = 240 mm × 240 mm; $N_x = N_y = 256$; FA = 20 degrees; BW = 400 Hz/pixel; $N_z = 64$; and phase encoding direction laterally (left to right). Using these venous images, three-dimensional projection images were generated to determine how best to acquire the next set of three-dimensional gradient echo images so that the vein is perpendicular to the imaging slab in the center of the imaging volume. Shimming was then performed in the imaging volume to optimize the static field homogeneity. Transverse images were acquired typically using a flow-compensated, strongly T2*-weighted, high-bandwidth, four- or five-echo gradient echo SWI sequence. This sequence was designed with a symmetric echo for each echo. From these data, the arterial-venous phase difference was found for four volunteers.

To extract the phase, the authors used either the high-pass filter approach or a parabolic fitting procedure excluding the vessels to remove the local background field variations.[57–59] The latter method was found to give more consistent results between subjects than using high-pass filtering (**Figs. 10** and **11**). The real challenge comes in obtaining the actual oxygen saturation for the peripheral veins. The authors were not allowed to extract blood from this part of the body because of the need for the subjects to walk out of the scanner and leave afterward (weight bearing on this part of the body meant a higher potential for the puncture not to heal or lead to bleeding). They turned to two other approaches. One was to measure T2* (because previous research claimed to correlate T2* with oxygen saturation from in vitro measurements).[60] The problem with this approach was that the T2* measurements were very inconsistent. It is now understood why this was the case; based on the results in the previous section (where it was seen that the venous blood can develop an inhomogeneous signal from blood separation), an accurate T2* measurement in vivo is very difficult.

The second approach was to go to the literature to see what invasive measures showed for oxygen saturation. Disappointingly, the results in the field have a very high error leading to results for the in vivo oxygen saturation measurements, which can vary from 50% to 80%, a range that encompasses the values of 55% (A = 1) or 70% (A = 1.5) that the authors are interested in finding. Almost all clinically invasive studies using infrared sensors show, however, that if the femoral artery blood flow was greater than 200 mL/min, the femoral venous oxygen saturation was 70% or greater.[61–65] If this is taken at face value for young, normal volunteers, then the data suggest that A = 1.5 is the correct choice.

The correct choice of χ_{do} is critically important for predicting the forward problem: measuring the oxygen saturation from the phase of blood vessels once χ_{do} is known with certainty. In principle, the SWI sequence can be used as a means to measure oxygen saturation throughout the body

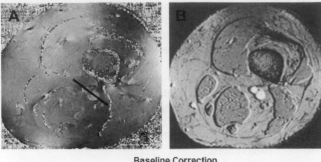

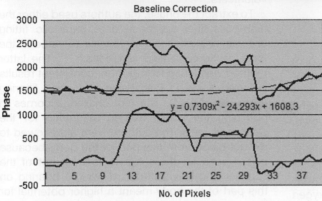

Baseline Correction

$y = 0.7309x^2 - 24.293x + 1608.3$

No. of Pixels

Fig. 10. (A) Associated phase image. (B) Magnitude image from a TE = 25 ms scan The fitted line shows the profile through the phase of the background, artery, and vein. The phase values along the profile (black line starting from bottom right moving to top left of the line) in A runs through the background tissue, artery, and vein, which are measured. The phase values from the background are then fitted to a parabola and subtracted from the phases along the profile (black line) to create a background-corrected phase of the artery (larger vessel) and vein (smaller vessel).

once the geometry of the vessel is taken into account. In the case of changes in blood oxygen saturation, a relative value can be found even without knowing the geometric correction factors.[66] The correct choice of χ_{do} determines the physiologic value of the oxygen saturation. For example, Haacke and colleagues[54] quoted 55% oxygenation in the pial veins in the brain during the resting state and 70% oxygenation during activation. If A = 1.5 (ie, χ_{do} = 0.27 ppm),

these numbers change to 70% during resting and 80% during activation.

Assuming for now that A = 1.5 and B_0 = 1.5, one can rewrite equation (9) as

$$1 - Y = -\frac{\varphi(vein) - \varphi(art)}{k \cdot Hct \cdot TE \cdot 1.5 \cdot (3\cos^2\theta - 1)} \quad (10)$$

where B_0 is given in Tesla. From equation (10), one can find Y, the oxygen saturation in any given vein.

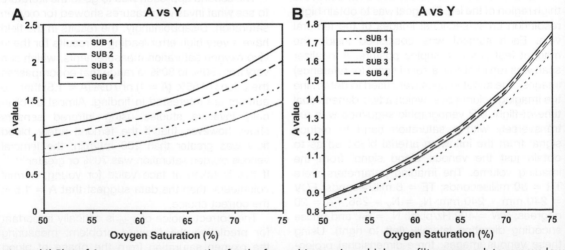

Fig. 11. (A) Plot of A versus oxygen saturation for the four subjects using a high-pass filter approach to remove low spatial frequency background. (B) Plot of A versus oxygen saturation for the four subjects using a least squares fit to a two-dimensional quadratic function to remove the phase. If the oxygen saturation is known to be 70%, that suggests that A = 1.5.

SUMMARY

By combining filtered phase and magnitude information to create a novel and intrinsic source of contrast, SWI has shown great promise in clinical angiography and venography. SWI has contributed to new insights into traumatic brain injury, the role of calcification in atherosclerosis, and the possible relationship between blood settling and DVT. A further contribution from SWI to DVT research (and also stroke) involves its application to the noninvasive measurement of oxygen saturation in the brain and in other tissues. Altogether, SWI offers manifold and diverse avenues for further research using angiographic and venographic techniques.

REFERENCES

1. Reichenbach JR, Venkatesan R, Schillinger DJ, et al. Small vessels in the human brain: MR venography with deoxyhemoglobin as an intrinsic contrast agent. Radiology 1997;204(1):272–7.

2. Haacke EM, Dmitriy SL, Yablonskiy A, et al. In vivo validation of the bold mechanism: a review of signal changes in gradient echo functional MRI in the presence of flow. Int J Imaging Systems Technology 1995;6(2–3):153–63.

3. Ashwal S, Babikian T, Gardner-Nichols J, et al. Susceptibility weighted imaging and proton magnetic resonance spectroscopy in assessment of outcome after pediatric traumatic brain injury. Arch Phys Med Rehabil 2006;87(12 Suppl 2):S50–8.

4. Babikian T, Freier MC, Tong KA, et al. Susceptibility weighted imaging: neuropsychologic outcome and pediatric head injury. Pediatr Neurol 2005;33(3):184–94.

5. Barth M, Nobauer-Huhmann IM, Reichenbach JR, et al. High-resolution three-dimensional contrast-enhanced blood oxygenation level-dependent magnetic resonance venography of brain tumors at 3 Tesla: first clinical experience and comparison with 1.5 Tesla. Invest Radiol 2003;38(7):409–14.

6. de Souza JM, Domingues RC, Cruz LC Jr, et al. Susceptibility-weighted imaging for the evaluation of patients with familial cerebral cavernous malformations: a comparison with t2-weighted fast spin-echo and gradient-echo sequences. AJNR Am J Neuroradiol 2008;29(1):154–8.

7. Essig M, Reichenbach JR, Schad L, et al [High resolution MR-venography of cerebral arteriovenous malformations]. Radiologe 2001;41(3):288–95 [in German].

8. Haacke EM, Cheng NY, House MJ, et al. Imaging iron stores in the brain using magnetic resonance imaging. Magn Reson Imaging 2005;23(1):1–25.

9. Haacke EM, DelProposto ZS, Chaturvedi S, et al. Imaging cerebral amyloid angiopathy with susceptibility-weighted imaging. AJNR Am J Neuroradiol 2007;28(2):316–7.

10. Harder SL, Hopp KM, Ward H, et al. Mineralization of the deep gray matter with age: a retrospective review with susceptibility-weighted MR imaging. AJNR Am J Neuroradiol 2008;29(1):176–83.

11. Hermier M, Nighoghossian N. Contribution of susceptibility-weighted imaging to acute stroke assessment. Stroke 2004;35(8):1989–94.

12. Hu J, Yu Y, Juhasz C, et al. MR susceptibility weighted imaging (SWI) complements conventional contrast enhanced T1 weighted MRI in characterizing brain abnormalities of Sturge-Weber Syndrome. J Magn Reson Imaging 2008;28(2):300–7.

13. Liang L, Korogi Y, Sugahara T, et al. Detection of intracranial hemorrhage with susceptibility-weighted MR sequences. AJNR Am J Neuroradiol 1999;20(8): 1527–34.

14. Matsushita T, Anami D, Arioka T, et al. Basic study of susceptibility-weighted imaging at 1.5T. Acta Med Okayama 2008;62(3):159–68.

15. Mentzel HJ, Dieckmann A, Fitzek C, et al. Early diagnosis of cerebral involvement in Sturge-Weber syndrome using high-resolution BOLD MR venography. Pediatr Radiol 2005;35(1):85–90.

16. Pinker K, Noebauer-Huhmann IM, Stavrou I, et al. High-resolution contrast-enhanced, susceptibility-weighted MR imaging at 3T in patients with brain tumors: correlation with positron-emission tomography and histopathologic findings. AJNR Am J Neuroradiol 2007;28(7):1280–6.

17. Rauscher A, Sedlacik J, Barth M, et al. Non-invasive assessment of vascular architecture and function during modulated blood oxygenation using susceptibility weighted magnetic resonance imaging. Magn Reson Med 2005;54(1):87–95.

18. Schad LR. Improved target volume characterization in stereotactic treatment planning of brain lesions by using high-resolution BOLD MR-venography. NMR Biomed 2001;14(7–8):478–83.

19. Sedlacik J, Rauscher A, Reichenbach JR. Obtaining blood oxygenation levels from MR signal behavior in the presence of single venous vessels. Magn Reson Med 2007;58(5):1035–44.

20. Sehgal V, Delproposto Z, Haacke EM, et al. Clinical applications of neuroimaging with susceptibility-weighted imaging. J Magn Reson Imaging 2005;22(4): 439–50.

21. Sehgal V, Delproposto Z, Haddar D, et al. Susceptibility-weighted imaging to visualize blood products and improve tumor contrast in the study of brain masses. J Magn Reson Imaging 2006; 24(1):41–51.

22. Somasundaram S, Kesavadas C, Thomas B. Susceptibility weighted imaging in holohemispheric venous angioma with cerebral hemiatrophy. Neurol India 2008;56(1):104–5.

23. Tan IL, van Schijndel RA, Pouwels PJ, et al. MR venography of multiple sclerosis. AJNR Am J Neuroradiol 2000;21(6):1039–42.

24. Thomas B, Somasundaram S, Thamburaj K, et al. Clinical applications of susceptibility weighted MR imaging of the brain: a pictorial review. Neuroradiology 2008;50(2):105–16.

25. Tong KA, Ashwal S, Holshouser BA, et al. Diffuse axonal injury in children: clinical correlation with hemorrhagic lesions. Ann Neurol 2004;56(1):36–50.

26. Tong KA, Ashwal S, Holshouser BA, et al. Hemorrhagic shearing lesions in children and adolescents with posttraumatic diffuse axonal injury: improved detection and initial results. Radiology 2003;227(2):332–9.

27. Warmuth C, Gunther M, Zimmer C. Quantification of blood flow in brain tumors: comparison of arterial spin labeling and dynamic susceptibility-weighted contrast-enhanced MR imaging. Radiology 2003;228(2):523–32.

28. Wycliffe ND, Choe J, Holshouser B, et al. Reliability in detection of hemorrhage in acute stroke by a new three-dimensional gradient recalled echo susceptibility-weighted imaging technique compared to computed tomography: a retrospective study. J Magn Reson Imaging 2004;20(3):372–7.

29. Reichenbach JR, Venkatesan R, Yablonskiy DA, et al. Theory and application of static field inhomogeneity effects in gradient-echo imaging. J Magn Reson Imaging 1997;7(2):266–79.

30. Akbudak E, Norberg RE, Conturo TE. Contrast-agent phase effects: an experimental system for analysis of susceptibility, concentration, and bolus input function kinetics. Magn Reson Med 1997;38(6):990–1002.

31. Rauscher A, Barth M, Reichenbach JR, et al. Automated unwrapping of MR phase images applied to BOLD MR-venography at 3 Tesla. J Magn Reson Imaging 2003;18(2):175–80.

32. Haacke EM, Xu Y, Cheng YC, et al. Susceptibility weighted imaging (SWI). Magn Reson Med 2004;52(3):612–8.

33. Pandian DSJ, Ciulla C, Haacke EM. Complex threshold method for identifying pixels that contain predominantly noise in magnetic resonance images. J Magn Reson Imaging 2008;28(3):727–35.

34. Xu Y, Haacke EM. The role of voxel aspect ratio in determining apparent vascular phase behavior in susceptibility weighted imaging. Magn Reson Imaging 2006;24(2):155–60.

35. Koopmans PJ, Manniesing R, Niessen WJ, et al. MR venography of the human brain using susceptibility weighted imaging at very high field strength. MAGMA 2008;21(1–2):149–58.

36. Du YP, Jin Z. Simultaneous acquisition of MR angiography and venography (MRAV). Magn Reson Med 2008;59(5):954–8.

37. Ameri A, Bousser MG. Cerebral venous thrombosis. Neurol Clin 1992;10(1):87–111.

38. Tang PH, Chai J, Chan YH, et al. Superior sagittal sinus thrombosis: subtle signs on neuroimaging. Ann Acad Med Singap 2008;37(5):397–401.

39. Hinman JM, Provenzale JM. Hypointense thrombus on T2-weighted MR imaging: a potential pitfall in the diagnosis of dural sinus thrombosis. Eur J Radiol 2002;41(2):147–52.

40. Preter M, Tzourio C, Ameri A, et al. Long-term prognosis in cerebral venous thrombosis: follow-up of 77 patients. Stroke 1996;27(2):243–6.

41. Criqui MH, Fronek A, Barrett-Connor E, et al. The prevalence of peripheral arterial disease in a defined population. Circulation 1985;71(3):510–5.

42. Boos M, Böttcher U, Laup G, et al. Clinical value of high resolution MRI of vessel wall lesions in peripheral atherosclerosis disease: first in vivo experience before and after PTA. Prague: Proceedings of the 13th Annual Scientific Meeting of the European Society for Magnetic Resonance in Medicine and Biology; 1996. p. 127.

43. Zimmermann GG, Erhart P, Schneider J, et al. Intravascular MR imaging of atherosclerotic plaque: ex vivo analysis of human femoral arteries with histologic correlation. Radiology 1997;204(3):769–74.

44. Vink A, Schoneveld AH, Borst C, et al. The contribution of plaque and arterial remodeling to de novo atherosclerotic luminal narrowing in the femoral artery. J Vasc Surg 2002;36(6):1194–8.

45. Wyttenbach R, Gallino A, Alerci M, et al. Effects of percutaneous transluminal angioplasty and endovascular brachytherapy on vascular remodeling of human femoropopliteal artery by noninvasive magnetic resonance imaging. Circulation 2004;110(9):1156–61.

46. Isbell DC, Meyer CH, Rogers WJ, et al. Reproducibility and reliability of atherosclerotic plaque volume measurements in peripheral arterial disease with cardiovascular magnetic resonance. J Cardiovasc Magn Reson 2007;9(1):71–6.

47. Guzman RJ, Brinkley DM, Schumacher PM, et al. Tibial artery calcification as a marker of amputation risk in patients with peripheral arterial disease. J Am Coll Cardiol 2008;51(20):1967–74.

48. Pentecost MJ, Criqui MH, Dorros G, et al. Guidelines for peripheral percutaneous transluminal angioplasty of the abdominal aorta and lower extremity vessels: a statement for health professionals from a special writing group of the Councils on Cardiovascular Radiology, Arteriosclerosis, Cardio-Thoracic and Vascular Surgery, Clinical Cardiology, and Epidemiology and Prevention, the American Heart Association. Circulation 1994;89(1):511–31.

49. Wright LB, Matchett WJ, Cruz CP, et al. Popliteal artery disease: diagnosis and treatment. Radiographics 2004;24(2):467–79.

50. Cannegieter SC, Doggen CJ, van Houwelingen HC, et al. Travel-related venous thrombosis: results from a large population-based case control study (MEGA study). PLoS Med 2006;3(8):e307.

51. Mammen EF. Pathogenesis of venous thrombosis. Chest 1992;102(6 Suppl):640S–4S.

52. Aldington S, Pritchard A, Perrin K, et al. Prolonged seated immobility at work is a common risk factor for venous thromboembolism leading to hospital admission. Intern Med J 2008;38(2):133–5.

53. Shvartz E, Gaume JG, White RT, et al. Hemodynamic responses during prolonged sitting. J Appl Phys 1983;54(6):1673–80.

54. Haacke EM, Lai S, Reichenbach JR, et al. In vivo measurement of blood oxygen saturation using magnetic resonance imaging: a direct validation of the blood oxygen level-dependent concept in functional brain imaging. Hum Brain Mapp 1997;5(5):341–6.

55. Weisskoff RM, Kiihne S. MRI susceptometry: image-based measurement of absolute susceptibility of MR contrast agents and human blood. Magn Reson Med 1992;24(2):375–83.

56. Spees WM, Yablonskiy DA, Oswood MC, et al. Water proton MR properties of human blood at 1.5 Tesla: magnetic susceptibility, $T(1)$, $T(2)$, $T^*(2)$, and non-Lorentzian signal behavior. Magn Reson Med 2001;45(4):533–42.

57. Elangovan IR. Verification of magnetic susceptibility value of deoxyhemoglobin of blood using susceptibility weighted imaging. Detroit (MI): Biomedical Engineering, Wayne State University; 2006.

58. Fernandez-Seara MA, Techawiboonwong A, Detre JA, et al. MR susceptometry for measuring global brain oxygen extraction. Magn Reson Med 2006;55(5):967–73.

59. Haacke EM, Prabhakaran KP, Elangovan IR, et al. Verification of the susceptibility value of deoxyhemoglobin in the blood using susceptibility weighted imaging (SWI) [abstract 1557]. In: Proc of the 13th Annual Meeting of ISMRM; 2005. p. 13.

60. Li D, Wang Y, Waight DJ. Blood oxygen saturation assessment in vivo using T2* estimation. Magn Reson Med 1998;39(5):685–90.

61. Brismar B, Cronestrand R, Jorfeldt L, et al. Estimation of femoral arterial blood flow from femoral venous oxygen saturation. Acta Chir Scand 1978;144(3):125–8.

62. Costes F, Barthelemy JC, Feasson L, et al. Comparison of muscle near-infrared spectroscopy and femoral blood gases during steady-state exercise in humans. J Appl Phys 1996;80(4):1345–50.

63. Esaki K, Hamaoka T, Radegran G, et al. Association between regional quadriceps oxygenation and blood oxygen saturation during normoxic one-legged dynamic knee extension. Eur J Appl Phys 2005;95(4):361–70.

64. MacDonald MJ, Tarnopolsky MA, Green HJ, et al. Comparison of femoral blood gases and muscle near-infrared spectroscopy at exercise onset in humans. J Appl Phys 1999;86(2):687–93.

65. Sonnenfeld T, Nowak J, Cronestrand R, et al. Leg venous oxygen saturation in the evaluation of intraoperative blood flow during arterial reconstructive surgery. Scand J Clin Lab Invest 1979;39(6):577–84.

66. Shen Y, Kou Z, Kreipke CW, et al. In vivo measurement of tissue damage, oxygen saturation changes and blood flow changes after experimental traumatic brain injury in rats using susceptibility weighted imaging. Magn Reson Imaging 2007;25(2):219–27.

Neuroradiologic Applications of Dynamic MR Angiography at 3 T

Hemant Parmar, MD[a],*, Marko K. Ivancevic, PhD[a,b],
Nancy Dudek, BS[a], Dheeraj Gandhi, MD[a,d], Liesbeth Geerts, PhD[c],
R. Hoogeveen, PhD[c], S.K. Mukherji, MD[a],
Thomas L. Chenevert, PhD[a]

KEYWORDS

- Time-resolved MR angiography • 4D-MR angiography
- 3 Tesla • Head and neck

Four-dimensional time-resolved MR angiography (4D-MRA) using keyhole imaging techniques is a new method of performing contrast-enhanced vascular imaging. By combining parallel imaging (sensitivity encoding, SENSE)[1,2] and keyhole imaging techniques, it is possible to obtain dynamic MRA scans up to 60 times faster, thereby achieving subsecond sampling of the contrast hemodynamics. Furthermore, imaging at 3 T gives higher signal intensity and thus affords higher spatial resolution, allowing dynamic three-dimensional (3D) MRA to approach a diagnostic performance similar to that of conventional digital subtraction angiography (DSA).

This article presents the authors' clinical experience using time-resolved 4D-MRA in the evaluation of various vascular abnormalities in the brain, spine, orbits, and neck at 3 T, demonstrates the imaging findings of this novel technique, and discusses its advantages and use in current neuroradiology practice.

Catheter DSA is the standard technique for imaging craniocervical vessels. High temporal resolution is obtained, and 3D reformats of multiple rotational datasets are possible. Because of the risk of arterial catheterization, the need to use ionizing radiation, and the costs of such procedures, however, safer angiographic procedures are being developed.

MRA has gained wide clinical acceptance for evaluating arterial and venous anatomy in the head, neck, and spine. The two-dimensional and 3D flow-sensitive sequences predominantly used in the past[3-5] are widely being replaced with gadolinium contrast-enhanced technique. High-flow intracranial arteriovenous malformations (AVM) and arteriovenous fistulae (AVF) require the highest spatial and temporal resolution and are demanding for any imaging system. Flow-sensitive techniques such as time-of-flight (TOF) MRA have limitations because of the large number of flow-related artifacts, the low spatial resolution (compared with DSA), and the essential absence of temporal resolution.

Contrast-enhanced MRA produces high-resolution 3D volume acquisitions, but exact timing is critical to obtain optimal image quality and accurate depiction of vasculature.

Centric elliptic k-space ordering has been used traditionally to acquire the peak of arterial contrast and to avoid edge-enhancement artifacts.[3] Later, contrast-enhanced timing-robust angiography (CENTRA) was introduced, in which the first 4 seconds of the central k-space was sampled randomly to lessen the need for precise timing of the peak arterial phase.[6] Routine 3D contrast-enhanced sequences reduce some of the flow-related artifacts of the TOF technique but are

[a] Department of Radiology, University of Michigan Health System, 1500 East Medical Center Drive, Ann Arbor, MI 48109-5030, USA
[b] Philips Healthcare, MR Clinical Science, 595 Miner Road, Cleveland, OH 44143, USA
[c] Philips Healthcare, MR Clinical Science, 5680 DA, Veenpluis 4–6, Best, The Netherlands
[d] Johns Hopkins Hospital, 600 N Wolfe Street, Baltimore, MD, USA
* Corresponding author.
E-mail address: hparmar@umich.edu (H. Parmar).

Magn Reson Imaging Clin N Am 17 (2009) 63–75
doi:10.1016/j.mric.2009.01.004

unable to provide high temporal resolution in depicting complex lesions.[7] The scan duration of a traditional contrast-enhanced MRA acquisition is too long to acquire dynamic information. Limitations of a single-time-point acquisition include lack of dynamic information, and occasionally a mistimed bolus results in suboptimal arterial signal or venous contamination. To image dynamic contrast kinetics, techniques based on undersampling k-space profiles, such as temporal interpolation of k-space views[8] and keyhole,[9] initially were proposed. As discussed in the article in this issue by Ivancevic and colleagues, the contrast features of an image are determined by the center of k-space, whereas the periphery of k-space determines high-resolution details. Keyhole acquisition dynamically updates only the center of k-space at a high temporal rate and reuses peripheral k-space (updated at a slower rate) to achieve a compromise between spatial and temporal information content.

More recently, 4D time-resolved angiography using keyhole acquisition (4D-TRAK) has been introduced by combining CENTRA with parallel imaging (SENSE),[1,2] partial Fourier, and keyhole techniques (**Fig. 1**). With 4D-TRAK it is possible to accelerate dynamic MRA scans up to 60 times to achieve a subsecond temporal sampling rate and to follow contrast hemodynamics with a nearly isotropic spatial resolution of 1 to 1.5 mm. Furthermore, 3-T field strength gives a higher signal-to-noise ratio, which can be used to obtain images with high spatial resolution. This technique allows dynamic high-resolution 3D MRA to attain a temporal performance closer to that of DSA, faster than that achieved with conventional MRA techniques.

This article reviews the authors' experiences in clinical practice in using 4D-TRAK at 3T for time-resolved MRA evaluation of various vascular abnormalities in arterial, capillary, and venous phases in the head and neck. The purpose of the examination is to evaluate time-resolved hemodynamic characteristics of these abnormalities while maintaining adequate spatial resolution.

TECHNIQUES

For the clinical examples presented in this article, contrast-enhanced MRA was performed on a 16-channel 3.0-T system equipped with a commercially available eight-channel SENSE-capable head coil. The dual gradient system allows gradient amplitude of 80 mT/m at 100 mT/m/ms or 40 mT/m at 200 mT/m/ms slew rate. Patients were positioned with a 20-gauge intravenous catheter inserted into the antecubital vein. An automated power injector was used for a biphasic injection protocol comprised of 20 cm^2 of gadobenate dimeglumine followed by a saline flush of 25 cm^2, all at a flow rate of 2 cm^2/s. The 4D-MRA sequence was started immediately after the contrast injection.

4D-TRAK data were acquired using the keyhole method,[6,9,10] partial Fourier, parallel imaging (SENSE). Individually, these techniques accelerate scan acquisition. Keyhole imaging with 20% of the full 3D k-space actually acquired yields an acceleration factor (AF) of 5 compared with a non-keyhole acquisition. Partial Fourier typically acquires only 80% of full k-space, which is an incremental AF of 1.25. In addition, parallel imaging using a SENSE factor of 3 in the in-plane phase encode direction and a SENSE factor of 1.8 in the slice direction yields an incremental AF of 3 × 1.8. In total, the combined AF = (5 × 1.25 × 3 × 1.8) = 33.75. That is, if a conventional 3D MRA requires 33.75 seconds at the specified spatial resolution, it can be acquired dynamically every 1 second by this technique. Each of the individual acceleration parameters can be adjusted to achieve up to AF = 60 using this system. In the clinical examples presented in this article, the AF ranged from 28 to 36. The periphery of k-space was collected in the reference dataset at the end of the acquisition in an elliptical order. The resulting data were used for reconstruction of each of the dynamic phases as described in the keyhole approach. Image processing included mask subtraction to suppress the background signal of the stationary tissue. For this purpose, one of three dynamic volumes acquired before administration of the contrast agent with the same time-resolved MR angiographic sequence was used. Default sequence parameters are listed in **Table 1**. Depending on the field of view, resolution, and coverage

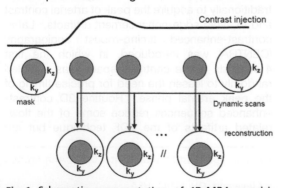

Fig. 1. Schematic representation of 4D-MRA acquisition and reconstruction. The last dynamic is fully sampled, and the peripheral part of k-space is used to reconstruct the CENTRA keyhole dynamics. A precontrast fully sampled mask can be used for postprocessing subtractions.

Table 1
Summary of default sequence parameters

Parameter	Brain	Carotids
TR/TE/flip angle	3/1.9/25°	4.6/1.41/25°
Field-of-view, matrix	240 mm, 288 × 288	300 mm, 254 × 332
Slice thickness (overcontiguous)	2 mm (1 mm)'	1.2 mm (0.6 mm)
SENSE factor	5.75 (3.2 × 1.8)	5.4 (3 × 1.8)
Voxel size (mm³, acquired/ reconstructed)	0.83 × 0.83 × 2 (0.71 × 0.71 × 1)	0.9 × 0.9 × 1.2 (0.9 × 0.9 × 0.6)
Keyhole%, dynamic time, reference dynamic time (reference last)	24%, 2.6 s, 10.9s	20%, 2.3s, 11.5s
Total scan time	80 s	44 s

adjustments in individual cases, the temporal resolution range was 1.6 to 3 seconds in the brain and 1.9 to 4.8 seconds in the carotids. The in-plane acquired resolution range was 0.6 to 1 mm.

Dynamic contrast-enhanced MRA/MR venography (MRV) using 4D-MRA has been performed in more than 150 patients at the University of Michigan Health System. Various vascular abnormalities evaluated with this technique include intracranial lesions such as intracranial AVM, AVF, cervical vascular diseases (eg, carotid artery stenosis, carotid artery pseudoaneurysm, and carotid body tumor), and intraorbital vascular malformations.

Case Examples

Dynamic MRA and MRV of the head and neck using 4D-MRA allowed the visualization of arterial, intermediate, and venous phases of vessel

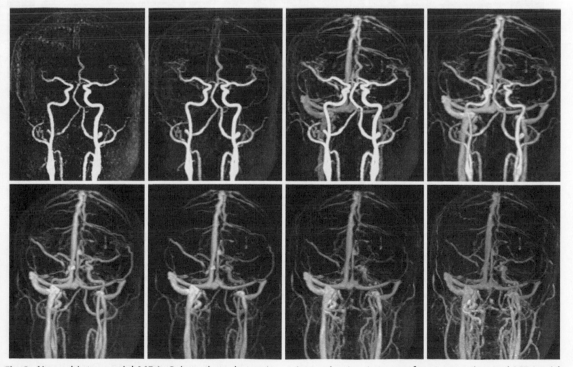

Fig. 2. Normal intracranial MRA. Selected maximum-intensity projection images of contrast-enhanced MRA with 4D-MRA of the head in coronal view showing excellent demonstration of early arterial, late arterial, and venous phases.

enhancement (**Figs. 2** and **3**). Both anatomic detail and temporal information were obtained. Representative examples are illustrated in **Figs. 2–10**.

INTRACRANIAL APPLICATIONS
Arteriovenous Malformations and Arteriovenous Fistula

Using 4D-MRA at 3 T, it is possible to identify correctly normal vasculature, enlarged arterial pedicles, lesion nidus, and the venous drainage pattern of an AVM and to resolve arterial and venous structures separately (**Fig. 4**). Similarly, in patients who have AVF (**Fig. 5**A, B), medium- and large-sized arterial pedicles are visualized

readily, and synchronous opacification of the diseased sinus or vein indicates an arteriovenous shunt. Sometimes in AVF the direct arterial feeders or the fistula may be too small to visualize with MR technique, but visualization of early filling of the corresponding vein or dural sinus should point toward this abnormality, prompting a DSA.

Cerebral Venous Thrombosis

At the University of Michigan Health System, dynamic contrast-enhanced MRV is used for all patients suspected of having dural venous thrombosis (**Fig. 6**). Although this technique provides the same information as single-phase contrast-enhanced MRV, the authors believe the added

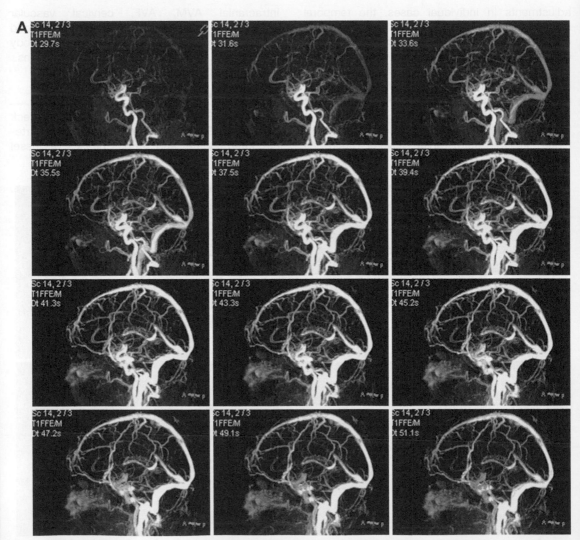

Fig. 3. Normal intracranial MRV: contrast-enhanced MRA of the head including delayed venous phase. (*A*) Sagittal maximum-intensity projection of acquired image series. (*B*) Sagittal maximum-intensity projection after subtraction of early arterial phase to display venous kinetics preferentially.

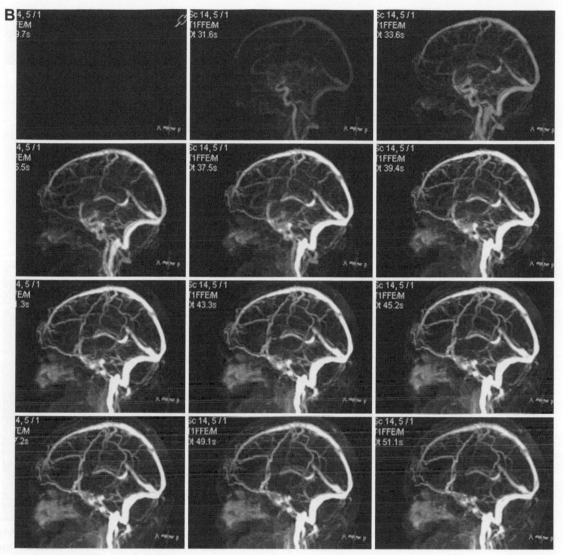

Fig. 3. (*continued*)

information about venous flow pattern, collateral circulation, and intracranial circulation times in diseased states is helpful in better evaluating this disease.[11]

APPLICATION IN ORBITS AND HEAD AND NECK
Vascular Malformations

As in intracranial AVM, dynamic contrast-enhanced MRA is helpful in identifying correctly normal vasculature, enlarged arterial pedicles, lesion nidus, and the venous drainage pattern. MRI has the added advantage of visualizing the rest of the soft tissues around the AVM. The authors increasingly are using dynamic

MRA for follow-up posttreatment head and neck AVM (**Fig. 7**A and B), reserving DSA for cases in which there is an abnormality of the dynamic MRA.

CAROTIDS ARTERIES
Carotid Body Tumor

Diseases involving the carotid space can include vascular tumors such as carotid body tumors, lymphoma, and nerve sheath tumors. In such patients visualization of contrast enhancement within the tumor in the early arterial phase is important for a correct diagnosis, because other tumors do not show such early enhancement

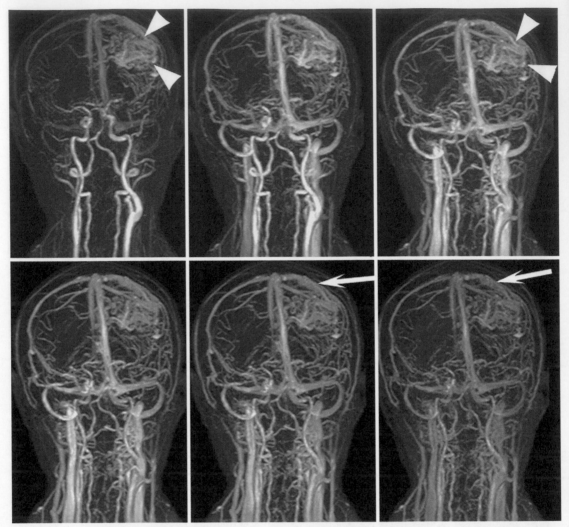

Fig. 4. Intracranial AVM. A 48-year-old woman had headaches and seizures. CT scan (not shown) showed an AVM in the left frontal lobe. Coronal maximum-intensity projection images of dynamic MRA (*above*) shows a large AVM nidus in the left frontal lobe (*arrowheads*) with feeders from left MCA and a large draining vein (*arrow*) emptying into superior sagittal sinus.

(**Fig. 8**). Although, after contrast enhancement, routine MRI can show this lesion, the authors believe that the MR imaging sometimes may not show the early arterial phase as well as dynamic MRA. Dynamic MRA also can show the arterial feeders and venous drainage patterns in such tumors, helping the surgeon or guiding preoperative embolization.

Carotid Artery Stenosis/Fibromuscular Dysplasia

By using an extended field of view, the arch of aorta, cervical, and cerebral vessels can be demonstrated simultaneously in a single image. In patients who have advanced atherosclerosis (**Fig. 9**) or fibromuscular dysplasia (**Fig. 10**), delayed filling of the cerebral vessels sometimes is observed on the side of the stenotic or occluded carotid vessel.[12,13] It is possible to demonstrate the patency of the distal vasculature and assess the compensatory collateral circulation. Although the information from this study is analogous to that obtained with catheter angiography, the degree of stenosis still is difficult to estimate accurately, and other techniques such as single-phase contrast-enhanced MRA or CT angiography need to be coupled with dynamic MRA.

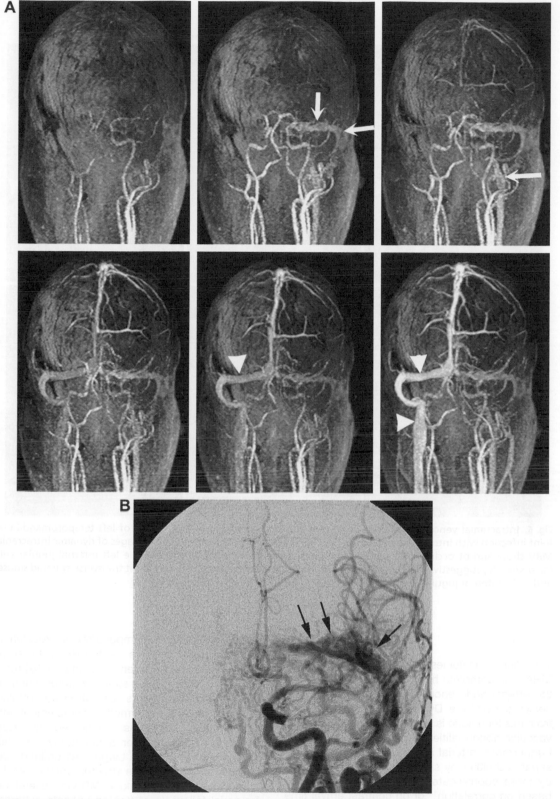

Fig. 5. Intracranial AVF. A 42-year-old man presented with chronic headaches. (*A*) Coronal maximum-intensity projection images of dynamic MRA show early opacification of the left transverse sinus and left internal jugular vein (*arrows*), suggestive of abnormal arteriovenous connection. Compare this image with the normal and late opacification of the right transverse sinus and internal jugular vein (*arrowheads*). (*B*) Anteroposterior image of left common carotid DSA reveals extensive AVFs (*arrows*) between the left internal and external carotid branches and between the left transverse sinus and left internal jugular vein.

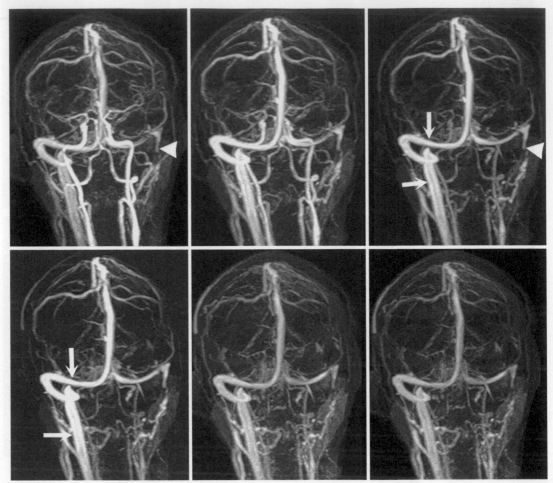

Fig. 6. Intracranial venous thrombosis. A 40-year-old man presented with a history of left temporomandibular joint infection with intracranial extension. Coronal maximum-intensity projection images of dynamic intracranial MRV show abrupt occlusion of the left sigmoid sinus with non-opacification of the left internal jugular vein (*arrowheads*), suggestive of venous thrombosis. Note the normal opacification of right transverse-sigmoid sinuses and right internal jugular vein (*arrows*).

DISCUSSION

The clinical usefulness of 4D-MRA for dynamic MRA with complete hemodynamic information of the arterial and venous system in the head and neck is shown here. Dynamic information obtained from this technique is useful in evaluating complex vascular abnormalities, such as AVF and AVM. Furthermore, arterial and venous phases can be separated either by simple subtraction (**Fig. 3**) or by more sophisticated postprocessing methods based on correlation[14] or on contrast arrival time maps.[15]

It was necessary, however, to compromise high spatial resolution to achieve high temporal resolution. The higher signal gained from 3-T field strength therefore is particularly important in achieving adequate temporal/spatial resolution. Time-resolved MRA is performed with some compromise between temporal and spatial resolution. To study more subtle features such as flow-related aneurysms or intranidal fistulae, dynamic MRA is performed in complement with single-phase MRA (as suggested by Nael et al[16]) or with catheter angiography for initial assessment of patients. Large, well-defined malformations with a simple structure may be evaluated by dynamic MRA alone. MRA is a useful tool for serial follow-up of treated patients, whereas catheter angiography is reserved for complex cases or cases in which MRA findings are unclear. In addition, 4D-MRA allows the full 3D volume coverage with adequate spatial and

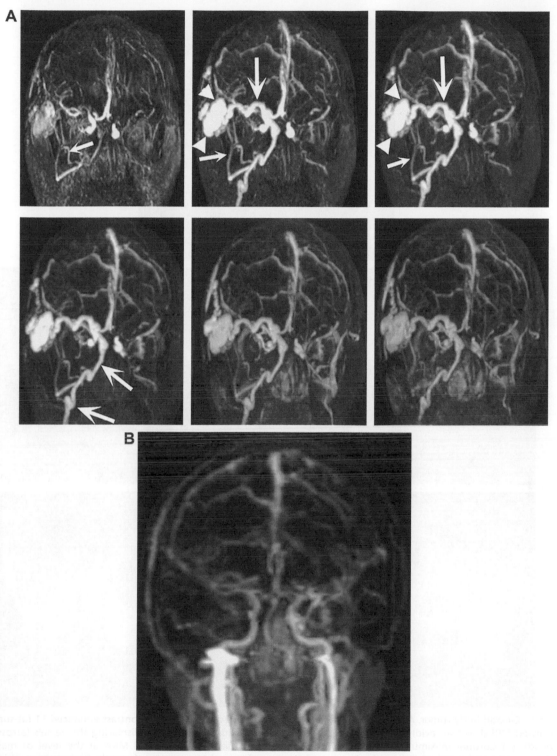

Fig. 7. Orbital AVM. A 12- year-old girl presented with enlarging right periorbital AVM. (*A*) Coronal maximum-intensity projection images show a large AVM (*arrowheads*) in the right peri-orbital region that was fed by the branches of the right external carotid artery (*small arrows*). A large draining vein extends over the supraorbital ridge and empties into the angular facial vein (*large arrows*). (*B*) Postembolization MRA showed complete resolution of the AVM.

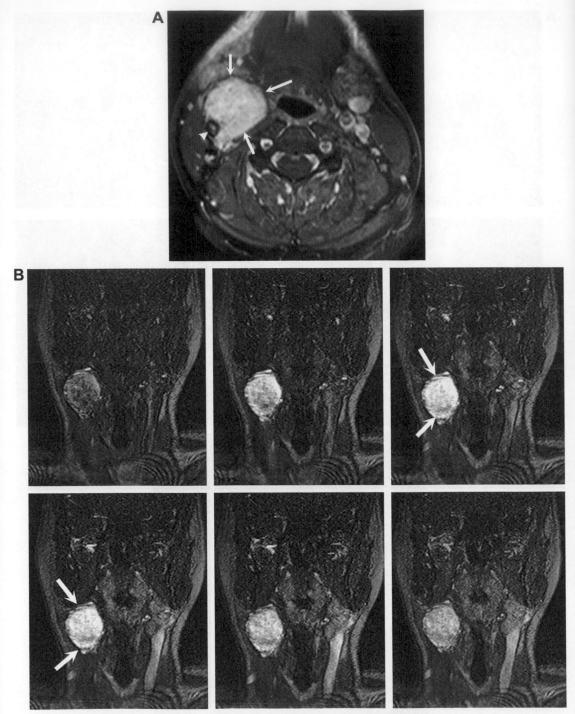

Fig. 8. Carotid body tumor. A 27-year-old man with right-sided neck swelling. (*A*) Contrast-enhanced T1 fat-suppressed MRI shows an avidly enhancing mass in the right carotid space (*arrows*) displacing the vessels (*arrowhead*). (*B*) Coronal maximum-intensity projection images of the dynamic carotid MRA at the level of mass shows early and rapid contrast enhancement of the mass (*arrows*), suggestive of carotid body tumor, which was proven at surgery.

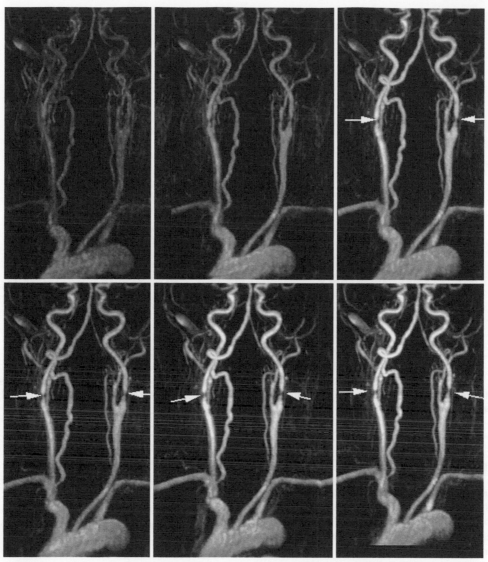

Fig. 9. Carotid artery stenosis. Coronal maximum-intensity projection images of the carotid arteries show severe stenosis of proximal segments of bilateral internal carotid arteries in a 65-year-old man who has advanced atherosclerosis (*arrows*).

temporal resolution with no risk of ionizing radiation exposure, iodizing contrast agent, or catheterization. In the future this technique can be extended to other indications (eg, to image the surgical shunt in carotid surgery bypass without the risk of arterial damage from direct catheterization or to demonstrate the delayed opacification of the vertebral artery in subclavian steal syndrome).[11]

This technique, although promising, has limitations. A dedicated team, including a neuroradiologist, is needed to define the temporal/spatial strategy and anatomic coverage, and a skilled MR technologist is needed to adjust scanning parameters accordingly. The most significant drawback of this approach is that one must decide prospectively to favor spatial or temporal features at the expense of the other.

In conclusion, multichannel RF technology with parallel imaging, shared k-space technique, and signal gain from a 3-T magnetic field allows high-performance time-resolved 4D-MRA angiography. This technique provides a useful clinical tool for evaluating the arterial and venous phases of complex vascular diseases, providing spatial and temporal information in a noninvasive manner.

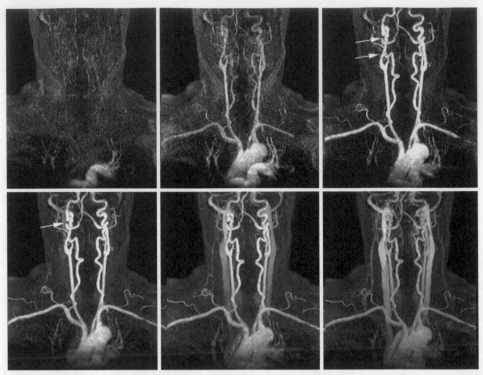

Fig. 10. Fibromuscular dysplasia. Coronal maximum-intensity projection images of the carotid arteries show multiple areas of narrowing and dilatations giving rise to a "beaded" appearance (*arrow*) of the internal carotid and vertebral arteries.

REFERENCES

1. Pruessmann KP, Weiger M, Scheidegger MB, et al. SENSE: sensitivity encoding for fast MRI. Magn Reson Med 1999;42:952–62.
2. Weiger M, Pruessmann KP, Kassner A, et al. Contrast-enhanced 3D MRA using SENSE. J Magn Reson Imaging 2000;12:671–7.
3. Lanzer P, Gross GM, Keller FS, et al. Sequential 2D inflow venography: initial clinical observations. Magn Reson Med 1991;19:470–6.
4. Holtz DJ, Debatin JF, McKinnon GC, et al. MR venography of the calf: value of flow-enhanced time-of-flight echoplanar imaging. AJR Am J Roentgenol 1996;166:663–8.
5. Huston J, Fain SB, Wald JT, et al. Carotid artery: elliptic centric contrast enhanced MR angiography compared with conventional angiography. Radiology 2001;218:138–43.
6. Willinek WA, Gieseke J, Conrad R, et al. Randomly segmented central k-space ordering in high-spatial resolution contrast-enhanced MR angiography of the supraaortic arteries: initial experience. Radiology 2002;225:583–8.
7. Farb RI, McGregor C, Kim JK, et al. Intracranial arteriovenous malformations: real-time, auto triggered elliptic centric-ordered 3D gadolinium-enhanced MR angiography: initial assessment. Radiology 2001;220:244–51.
8. Korosec FR, Frayne R, Grist TM, et al. Time-resolved contrast enhanced 3D MR angiography. Magn Reson Med 1996;36:345–51.
9. van Vaals JJ, Brummer ME, Dixon WT, et al. "Keyhole" method for accelerating imaging of contrast agent uptake. J Magn Reson Imaging 1993;3:671–5.
10. Jones RA, Haraldseth O, Muller TB, et al. K-space substitution: a novel dynamic imaging technique. Magn Reson Med 1993;29:830–4.
11. Coley SC, Wild JM, Wilkinson ID, et al. Neurovascular MRI with dynamic contrast-enhanced subtraction angiography. Neuroradiology 2002;45:843–50.
12. Aoki S, Yoshikawa T, Hori M, et al. Two-dimensional thick-slice MR digital subtraction angiography for assessment of cerebrovascular occlusive diseases. Eur Radiol 2000;10:1858–64.
13. Wetzel SG, Haselhurst R, Bilecen, et al. Preliminary experience with dynamic MR projection angiography in the evaluation of cervico-cranial steno-occlusive disease. Eur Radiol 2001;11:295–302.

14. Bock M, Schoenberg SO, Floemer F, et al. Separation of arteries and veins in 3D MR angiography using correlation analysis. Magn Reson Med 2000;43:481–7.
15. Du J, Thornton FJ, Mistretta CA, et al. Dynamic MR venography: an intrinsic benefit of time-resolved MR angiography. J Magn Reson Imaging 2006;24:922–7.
16. Nael K, Michaely HJ, Villablanca P, et al. Time-resolved contrast enhanced magnetic resonance angiography of the head and neck at 3 Tesla: initial results. Invest Radiol 2006;41:116–24.

Dynamic Four-Dimensional MR Angiography of the Chest and Abdomen

Michael Griffin, PhD, Thomas M. Grist, MD, Christopher J. François, MD*

KEYWORDS
- MR angiography • Time-resolved MR angiography
- Dynamic MR angiography • MR angiography chest
- MR angiography abdomen

Conventional x-ray digital subtraction angiography (DSA) has long been considered the gold standard for the investigation of diseases of the vasculature. DSA provides high spatial and temporal resolution of the anatomy and flow dynamics of the vasculature. It suffers from several limitations and well-recognized adverse effects, however, including (1) limited information on vessel morphology and extraluminal anatomy, (2) invasiveness of arterial catheterization, (3) radiation risk, and (4) toxicity of iodinated contrast. CT angiography (CTA) has gained widespread use for vascular investigations, in part because of its noninvasiveness and near universal availability in the hospital setting. CTA has replaced DSA in several applications, particularly in applications where rapid diagnosis is necessary (trauma, acute dissection, pulmonary embolus, and so forth). Advances in CT technology, including multiple detectors and advanced postprocessing, allow for fast scan speed, high spatial resolution of entire anatomic regions, and the ability to form additional projections from the three-dimensional data set. As with DSA, however, CTA requires the use of ionizing radiation and iodinated contrast. Additionally, CTA requires accurate timing of the contrast bolus. Because of concerns with radiation exposure, it is not clinically acceptable to perform time-resolved imaging with CTA to assess vascular flow dynamics.

The use of contrast-enhanced MR angiography (CE-MRA) has circumvented many of the limitations and drawbacks of DSA and CTA. Gadolinium contrast agents have a better allergic safety profile than iodinated contrast agents. For patients at risk of nephrogenic systemic fibrosis, non–CE-MRA techniques should be considered (discussed elsewhere in this issue). In addition, CE-MRA does not require the use of ionizing radiation, which is particularly advantageous for the pediatric population. Because no ionizing radiation is involved with CE-MRA, repeated imaging can be performed without increased risk. Data can be acquired in any plane to maximize vessel coverage while minimizing the number of slices.

Advances in gradient hardware, pulse sequences, and computational power have allowed for greatly reduced scan times. By reducing the scan time to several seconds or less, it is possible to image the precontrast, arterial, parenchymal, and venous contrast phases within a single breath hold (**Fig. 1**). Digital subtraction can be used to isolate each vascular phase. Rapid sequential acquisitions also ensure that at least one acquired phase of images is obtained during the peak

Department of Radiology, University of Wisconsin, 600 Highland Avenue, Madison, WI 53792, USA
* Corresponding author.
E-mail address: cfrancois@uwhealth.org (C.J. François).

Magn Reson Imaging Clin N Am 17 (2009) 77–90
doi:10.1016/j.mric.2008.12.001

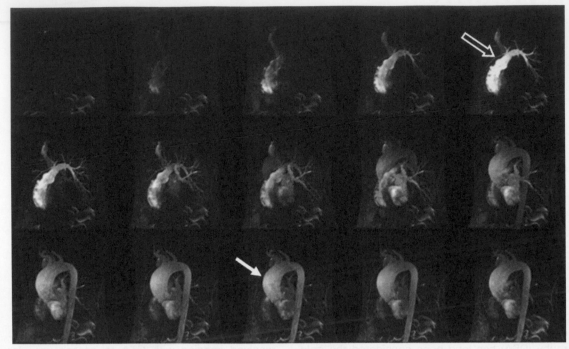

Fig. 1. Maximum intensity projection (MIP) images from a time-resolved CE-MRA of the chest. A high temporal resolution, low spatial resolution technique was used so that each image corresponds to an approximately 1.5-second time frame. There is clear distinction between the peak pulmonary artery (*open arrow*) and peak aorta (*solid arrow*) enhancement.

vascular phase of interest,[1,2] eliminating the need for contrast bolus timing. These techniques provide information on the dynamics of contrast arrival and rates of enhancement of vascular structures and organs,[3–6] often critical information in the hemodynamic assessment of stenoses and full characterization of complex vascular pathologies.[7–10]

Approaches to achieving high temporal resolution can be divided into those based on imaging with high-performance hardware, imaging based on interpolating undersampled k-space, parallel imaging, or a combination of these techniques. Regardless of the technique used, there is always a tradeoff between spatial resolution and temporal resolution. The appropriate balance between these two depends on the pathology being investigated. This article reviews the techniques used to perform time-resolved, or four-dimensional, CE-MRA and provides an overview of its clinical use for body MRA applications.

FOUR-DIMENSIONAL CONTRAST-ENHANCED MR ANGIOGRAPHY TECHNIQUES
Time-Resolved Imaging of Contrast Kinetics

Currently, the most commonly used approach to reduce acquisition time and perform time-resolved CE-MRA is to use undersampled k-space techniques. The use of time-resolved imaging of

contrast kinetics (TRICKS) allows for rapid acquisitions on moderate-performance imaging hardware while maintaining high spatial resolution.[1] In the basic form of this technique, k-space is divided into three to four sections in the slice direction. The central k-space segment, which contains low-frequency data responsible for image contrast, is alternately sampled with sections of more peripheral k-space, which contain high-frequency data responsible for image detail. To reconstruct images, each sample of central k-space is then combined with the linearly interpolated values of the remaining k-space pairs acquired most closely in time. TRICKS thereby oversamples the central k-space relative to the more peripheral regions, and because most of the data needed to create an MRA image is present within the center of k-space, high spatial resolution is maintained during short acquisition times. To reduce acquisition time further, TRICKS also uses zero-filling in the phase- and slice-encoding dimensions, with typically half of the data being acquired and half zero-filled.

The standard TRICKS technique has undergone several modifications further to increase spatial or temporal resolution. Projection reconstruction (PR)-TRICKS uses radially undersampled projection reconstruction in the kx-ky plane combined with variable-rate k-space sampling.[11,12] Cartesian encoding is then used in the slice direction. This technique provides equivalent spatial resolution to standard TRICKS with a nearly threefold increase in temporal resolution. Streak artifact from angular undersampling may occur as the number of angular samples is reduced. Blood vessels are the dominant signal source in MRA, however, and streak artifacts generally occur over background tissues.

A more recent modification of the TRICKS technique is highly constrained back-projection (HYPR)-TRICKS.[13,14] HYPR-TRICKS is a two-part technique that uses a TRICKS acquisition of low-frequency data during the first pass of the contrast bolus combined with a single high-resolution acquisition of high-frequency data obtained after venous opacification. This extended sampling improves the signal-to-noise ratio and resolution over standard TRICKS. With HYPR-TRICKS, however, the edge information is fixed and temporal information is limited to the low spatial frequencies. The amount of dynamic information in the study depends on the fraction of the total k-space acquired during the time-resolved portion of the acquisition.

This has been further modified by combining the PR and HYPR techniques in PR-HYPR-TRICKS, which combines the high in-plane spatial resolution of PR-TRICKS with a multistep acquisition analogous to HYPR-TRICKS.[12] Static high-spatial-frequency data in the slice-encoding direction are sampled after venous opacification to increase the through-plane spatial resolution. PR-HYPR-TRICKS has a twofold increase in spatial resolution over PR-TRICKS, with similar temporal resolution and signal-to-noise. The increased total acquisition time for PR-HYPR-TRICKS makes patient motion a primary concern with this technique, however, because the temporal filtering and mask subtraction used with this technique assume that tissues are stationary during the entire examination.

Spiral-TRICKS is another variant of the TRICKS algorithm that uses spiral sampling of k-space in-plane and Cartesian encoding in the slice direction, which is partitioned into multiple regions and sampled using a TRICKS sequence.[15-17] This allows more efficient data sampling of k-space with each TR, thereby allowing longer sampling intervals and increased signal-to-noise ratio over standard radial projection reconstruction. Each line of k-space that is sampled begins at the origin, so low-frequency data are inherently oversampled. With spiral-TRICKS, a 1-second temporal resolution can be achieved without undersampling the spiral trajectories.

Although PR-TRICKS uses radial undersampling of k-space in the in-plane direction and Cartesian encoding in the slice direction, the "vastly undersampled isotropic projection reconstruction" technique extends undersampling of radial trajectories to all three dimensions.[18,19] Projection angles are selected to cover three-dimensional k-space uniformly, and the maximum k-space radius sampled determines the resolution in all three spatial directions. To increase temporal resolution, the projection acquisition order is interleaved such that all spatial frequency orientations are coarsely sampled less than or equal to the desired frame rate. The k-space origin is sampled with every projection. An advantage of the vastly undersampled isotropic projection reconstruction technique is that it provides isotropic spatial resolution, which allows for equal spatial resolution in any reformatted oblique plane and facilitates volume rendering.

Parallel Imaging in Four-Dimensional Contrast-Enhanced MR Angiography

Parallel imaging techniques have been developed that use an array of radiofrequency detector coils to acquire multiple data points simultaneously with a single phase-encoding gradient strength. This allows k-space to be undersampled, which results in aliasing in traditional single-coil images. Various techniques have been developed to correct for the aliasing, including sensitivity encoding and simultaneous acquisition of spatial harmonics reconstruction techniques.[20,21] With parallel imaging, the maximum increase in speed is proportional to the number of coils. Although massively parallel acquisitions could theoretically lead to substantial acceleration factors, in practice this has been limited by reductions in the signal-to-noise. The signal-to-noise is reduced by shorter acquisition times, and it is also reduced by the amplification of noise that occurs in regions where the geometry of coil sensitivities is suboptimal. This reduction in signal-to-noise can be partially overcome by injecting the contrast bolus faster, thereby achieving higher contrast concentrations. The use of parallel imaging techniques in combination with the undersampling techniques described previously allows for even greater improvements in both spatial and temporal resolution,[16,22-27] particularly when imaging at 3 T.[5,28-30]

CLINICAL USES OF FOUR-DIMENSIONAL CONTRAST-ENHANCED MR ANGIOGRAPHY IN THE CHEST AND ABDOMEN
Aortic Dissection

Aortic dissection is a potentially catastrophic illness that results from a tear in the aortic tunica intima.[31–34] Blood passes from the true lumen, through the tear, into a second false lumen as it separates the intima from the media or adventitia. The persistent intraluminal pressure drives extension of the false lumen distally or proximally, creating an intimal flap. Dissections that involve the ascending aorta regardless of the site of origin are classified as Stanford type A and are surgical

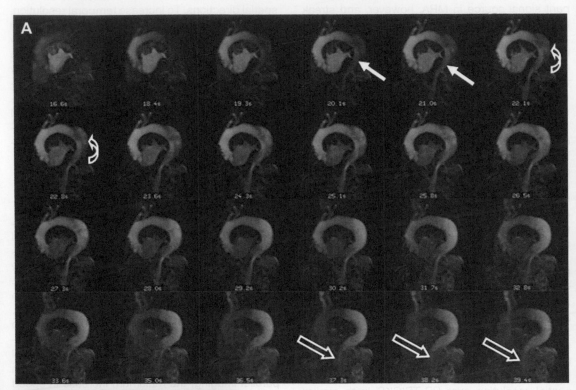

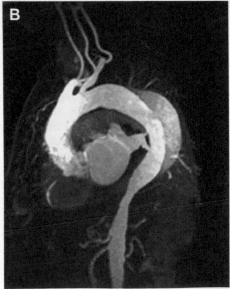

Fig. 2. MIP images from a time-resolved CE-MRA of the chest in a patient with an acute Stanford type B aortic dissection. Using a high temporal resolution, low spatial resolution technique (*A*), it is possible to demonstrate delayed filling of the false lumen (*curved arrows*) relative to the true lumen (*solid arrows*). Delayed phases show the distal extent of the false lumen (*open arrows*), which is not seen on the high spatial resolution three-dimensional CE-MRA (*B*). (*Courtesy of* J. Carr, MD, Chicago, IL.)

emergencies. Retrograde extension of the dissection to the aortic valve can lead to aortic regurgitation or pericardial tamponade. All dissections not involving the ascending aorta are classified as Stanford type B and are often treated medically, unless there are signs of malperfusion of abdominal organs. Malperfusion may occur when the branch vessel originates from the false lumen or may occur secondary to obstruction by the intimal flap.

The role of imaging in the setting of aortic dissection is to determine the following:[33,35]

1. Origin
2. Extent
3. Entry and re-entry locations
4. Branch vessel, including coronary artery involvement
5. Presence of false lumen thrombus
6. Presence of aortic regurgitation
7. Presence of pericardial effusion

Three-dimensional CE-MRA, as with CTA, has a sensitivity and specificity for detection of aortic dissection of nearly 100%. It is also useful for assessing the proximal and distal extent of the dissections, false lumen patency, and branch vessel involvement. Using multiplanar reformations it is often possible to locate the sites of intimal tears and re-entry locations. Fast, breath held, three-dimensional CE-MRA acquisitions require accurate timing of the contrast bolus either with an automatic trigger or a test bolus, which may be problematic in aortic dissection because of delayed filling of the false lumen. In addition, patients with aortic dissection are often acutely ill and unable to cooperate with breathing instructions.

Time-resolved CE-MRA is beneficial in fully characterizing an aortic dissection (**Fig. 2**) because it helps identify entry and re-entry locations, minimizes venous overlay, and minimizes pulsation artifacts in the aortic lumen that can mimic dissection.[36,37] Time-resolved CE-MRA can also be used to show whether there is a difference in flow through the true and false lumens (**Fig. 2A**). Frequently, enhancement of the false lumen is delayed relative to the true lumen and persists longer because of slower blood flow. If a non–time-resolved acquisition is used, synchronization of

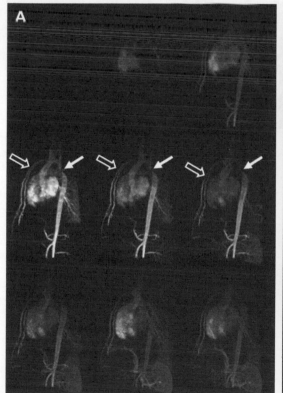
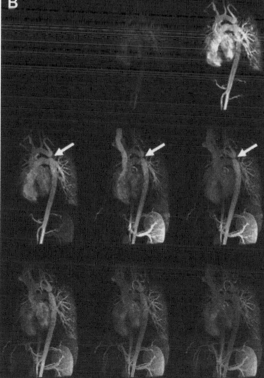

Fig. 3. MIP images from a time-resolved CE-MRA of the chest in two patients with aortic coarctation. (*A*) The patient has dilated internal mammary artery collaterals (*open arrows*), indicating a hemodynamically significant stenosis in the proximal descending aorta (*solid arrows*). (*B*) The patient does not have any dilated collateral arteries, indicating a milder stenosis in the proximal descending aorta (*arrows*).

acquisition with contrast arrival in the true lumen could make the depiction of the false lumen inadequate. If only a single CE-MRA phase is acquired, the full extent of the dissection may not be demonstrated, because the slow enhancement of the distal false lumen continues beyond the acquisition time of a single phase. The growth rate of

a dissection has been previously shown to be related to the presence of a patent false lumen.[38]

Coarctation of the Aorta

Coarctation of the aorta is most often a focal narrowing of the aorta just distal to the origin of the left subclavian artery (**Fig. 3**). Coarctation can occur

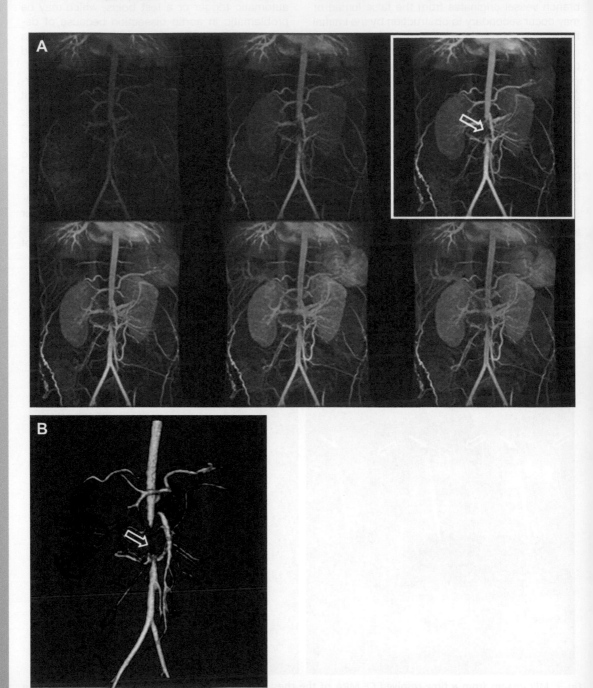

Fig. 4. (*A*) MIP images from a time-resolved CE-MRA of the abdomen in a patient with aortic occlusion (*open arrows*) related to aortitis. (*B*) The phase with the greatest arterial enhancement (*square*) can then be used to create additional multiplanar reformatted or volume-rendered images for further evaluation.

anywhere along the aorta, however, or may even be diffuse. It is generally a sporadic congenital malformation, and it is frequently associated with Turner's syndrome, bicuspid aortic valve, ventricular septal defect, patent ductus arteriosus, aortic stenosis, and intracranial aneurysms. Focal aortic coarctation is often asymptomatic unless the resulting hypertension is severe. Aortic coarctations are often found incidentally in adults. If the coarctation is severe, multiple body wall collaterals develop. The degree of collateral formation parallels the severity of aortic narrowing, often with the highest density near the site of the coarctation. Severe or diffuse coarctation typically presents in early infancy with heart failure or shock as the ductus arteriosus closes.

Single-phase CE-MRA provides an accurate overview of the vascular morphology, including the location of the coarctation site and the degree of luminal narrowing. Time-resolved CE-MRA techniques, however, are also helpful in this setting given the variable rate of contrast filling distal to the stenosis. Time-resolved techniques can also demonstrate delayed filling of the aorta distal to the coarctation site and differential flow through various body wall collaterals (see **Fig. 3**).[39]

Aortitis

There are numerous causes of inflammation of the aorta, but it most commonly occurs secondary to infection or immune disorders, such as Takayasu's arteritis, giant cell arteritis, polyarteritis nodosa, or systemic lupus erythematosus. Takayasu's arteritis is a progressive, large vessel granulomatous vasculitis of unknown etiology, although immuno-pathogenic mechanisms are suspected.[40,41] It occurs primarily in women and has a worldwide distribution with increased prevalence in Asians. It primarily affects the aorta, its major branches, and the pulmonary artery. The inflammatory process can result in either dense medial and adventitial scarring causing vessel narrowing, or disruption of the elastic lamina and media causing vessel dilation. Vascular symptoms are rare early in the disease, but with disease progression vascular insufficiency results in symptoms of end-organ ischemia. Proximal subclavian artery involvement is common and may lead to

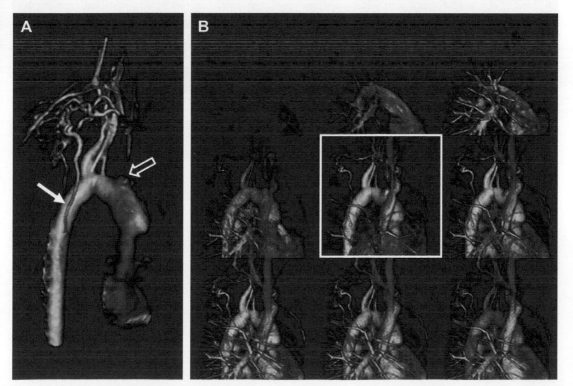

Fig. 5. (A) Volume-rendered time-resolved CE-MRA of the chest in a patient with aortitis and an occluded right innominate artery (open arrow). The right subclavian, common carotid, and vertebral arteries fill through a large intercostal artery collateral arising from the proximal descending thoracic aorta (solid arrow). (B) By selecting the phase with the greatest systemic arterial enhancement (white square), it is possible to evaluate the systemic arteries without interference from the pulmonary arteries or systemic veins.

subclavian steal. Diagnosis is established by a combination of clinical features and imaging.

Three-dimensional CE-MRA is useful for both diagnosis and monitoring of disease progression.

Luminal narrowing and dilation, mural thrombus, and collateral pathways can be assessed with CE-MRA.[42] This can be supplemented with delayed postcontrast inversion recovery images to

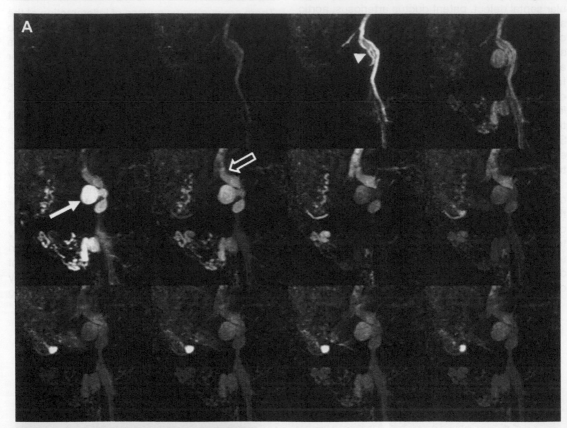

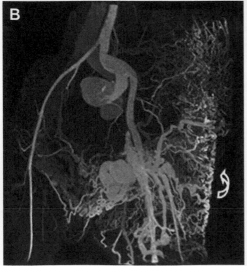

Fig. 6. MIP images from a high temporal resolution, low spatial resolution time-resolved CE-MRA (*A*) and three-dimensional high spatial resolution CE-MRA (*B*) of the pelvis in a patient with Parkes Weber syndrome. The patient has multiple arteriovenous malformations and fistulas in the left hemipelvis and left lower extremity. An arteriovenous fistula is present between the left internal iliac artery (*arrowhead*) and vein (*open arrow*) and is associated with an aneurysm (*solid arrow*). There is also filling of innumerable dilated subcutaneous veins on the left (*curved arrow*). Note the discrepancy in size of the iliac arteries between the left and right.

assess the degree of vessel wall inflammation.[43] Given the variability in the vessel filling distal to obstructions, a time-resolved approach is useful in this case to simplify the acquisition of a pure arterial phase over a large region of interest (**Figs. 4** and **5**). Time-resolved CE-MRA can also be used to show retrograde filling of vessels distal to an obstruction, such as with subclavian steal.

Pulmonary Sequestration

Pulmonary sequestration refers to a congenital pulmonary malformation consisting of a nonfunctioning mass of primitive lung tissue that does not communicate with the tracheobronchial tree. Its blood supply arises from the systemic circulation rather than the pulmonary artery. Sequestration

may be intrapulmonary, where the mass is surrounded by normal functioning lung tissue and venous drainage is commonly to the pulmonary veins; or it may be extrapulmonary, where it is surrounded by its own pleural sac and venous drainage is commonly to the systemic venous system. Intrapulmonary sequestration is often diagnosed in childhood or adolescence following multiple episodes of pneumonia, whereas extrapulmonary sequestration often presents in infancy with cough and respiratory distress. Rarely, communication with the gastrointestinal tract can occur. Other congenital anomalies appear in 10% of the cases.

DSA remains the reference standard for diagnosis, although CTA and CE-MRA are noninvasive alternatives. Time-resolved CE-MRA allows

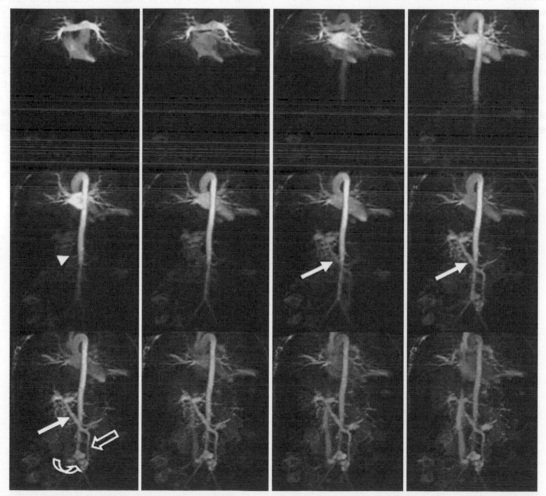

Fig. 7. MIP images from a high temporal resolution (1 second per frame), low spatial resolution time-resolved CE-MRA of the abdomen in a patient with a hepatic artery (*arrowhead*) to portal vein (*solid arrows*) fistula. Because a high temporal resolution technique was used, it is possible to confirm that there is retrograde filling of the portal vein. There is also early collateral filling of middle sacral veins (*curved arrow*) from the inferior mesenteric vein (*open arrow*). (*Courtesy of* J. Carr, MD, Chicago, IL.)

separation of the arterial and venous phases of these high-flow lesions and provides additional information on the dynamics of tissue perfusion and contrast enhancement, which can have treatment implications.[44] High temporal resolution four-dimensional CE-MRA provides accurate delineation of the arterial phase without venous overlay.

Congenital Vascular Malformations

Vascular malformations are common congenital abnormalities seen in infants and children. They are nonneoplastic and nonproliferative lesions that grow commensurate with the child. They can occur sporadically or may be associated with syndromes, such as Klippel-Trénaunay-Weber,[45–47] Parkes Weber, or Rendu-Osler-Weber.[48] They can be classified by whether the predominant anomalous vessels are arterial, capillary, venous, or lymphatic. Combinations of malformations are common. Arteriovenous malformations can occur throughout the body and are common in the extremities. As they grow, they can lead to severe disfigurement, limb hypertrophy, massive bleeding, steal phenomenon with distal ischemia and pain, and congestive heart failure. Treatment of vascular malformations depends on the location and involvement of surrounding muscles, bones, and joints and includes both surgical and minimally invasive strategies.

Comprehensive assessment of these lesions requires accurate delineation of the lesions and functional analysis of the filling and draining vessels (**Figs. 6** and **7**). Accurate differentiation between high-flow lesions (arterial and arteriovenous) and low-flow lesions (venous, capillary, and lymphatic) is essential because of the impact on treatment.[49–51] DSA and Doppler ultrasonography are well-established diagnostic modalities. MRA has become increasingly used as a noninvasive method for detection and classification of arteriovenous malformations. Although conventional CE-MRA is useful for assessing the morphology and extent of the lesion, time-resolved techniques provide functional assessment of feeding and draining vessels and aid in differentiating high- and low-flow lesions.[52]

Pelvic Congestion Syndrome

Pelvic congestion syndrome (PCS) is a common cause of chronic pelvic pain. PCS is caused by incompetent ovarian veins, which occurs in approximately 10% of women.[53] Of women with incompetent ovarian veins, approximately 60%

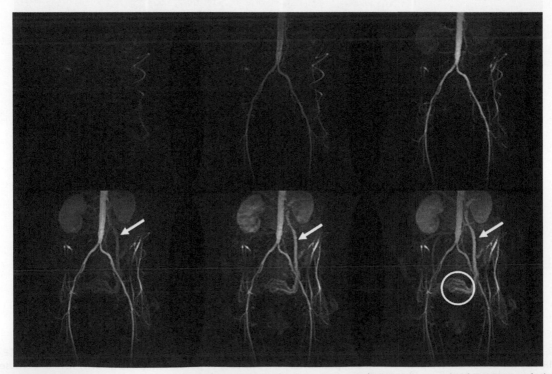

Fig. 8. MIP images from a low temporal resolution, high spatial resolution time-resolved CE-MRA of the abdomen in a patient with pelvic congestion syndrome. There is retrograde filling of the left uterine vein (*arrows*) and uterine veins (*circle*) before opacification of other veins in the pelvis.

develop PCS. As a result of incompetent ovarian veins, there is retrograde flow and dilatation of the ovarian vein, most commonly on the left. This then leads to dilatation and decreased clearance of the pelvic veins. Pelvic congestion can also be seen as a result of extrinsic compression of the left renal vein or ovarian veins by an external mass. Other, less common, causes of pelvic congestion include portal hypertension or acquired inferior vena cava syndrome. The initial imaging evaluation of patients with PCS is usually ultrasound, done to evaluate pelvic pain. MRA confirms the presence of pelvic varices which, with time-resolved CE-MRA, can be seen to fill retrograde from the ovarian vein (**Fig. 8**).

Endovascular Abdominal Aortic Aneurysm Repair

Endovascular abdominal aortic aneurysm repair is becoming a commonly performed procedure, with an estimated 40,000 procedures yearly. Following endovascular abdominal aortic aneurysm repair, patients require life-long imaging surveillance to detect graft failure caused by graft migration, endoleak, or increase in aneurysm sac size. Although postoperative assessment is commonly performed with CT, MRA is increasingly playing a role because of the growing concern of increased radiation exposure from medical imaging. This is of particular concern in this patient population because of the requirement of life-long imaging follow-up. Time-resolved CE-MRA has been shown to be a highly accurate means of correctly identifying the presence and categorizing the type of endoleak in a few small studies.[54–57] When MRA is used for follow-up, radiography is required to exclude stent fracture. In a study by van der Laan and colleagues,[56] time-resolved CE-MRA was able correctly to classify the type of endoleak in six patients who could not be classified using non–time-resolved MR images.

Spinal MR Angiography Before Thoracoabdominal Aortic Aneurysm Repair

To prevent neurologic complications during and following descending thoracic aortic aneurysm and thoracoabdominal aortic aneurysm repair, it is vital that spinal cord perfusion be maintained. An increasingly important part of the preprocedural evaluation to minimize complications from thoracic aortic aneurysm and thoracic aortic aneurysm repair is the identification of the anterior spinal artery with MRA.[58–60] Correct identification of the anterior spinal artery (**Fig. 9**) requires precise visualization of the arteries, without venous contamination.[59] At the authors' institution, this is performed

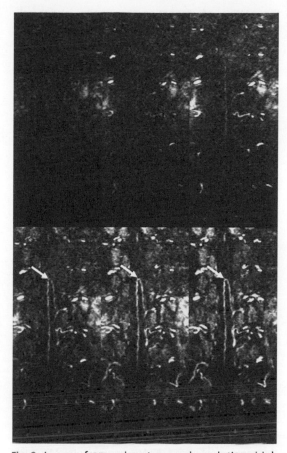

Fig. 9. Images from a low temporal resolution, high spatial resolution time-resolved CE-MRA of the spinal artery performed at 3 T in a patient before thoracoabdominal aortic aneurysm repair. Identification of the anterior spinal artery (*arrows*) before surgery assists the vascular surgeons in localizing the feeding artery that needs to be reimplanted following aneurysm repair to minimize the risk of paraplegia. To maximize spatial resolution, a very low temporal resolution (12 seconds per image) technique is used and patients are scanned at 3 T. Sublingual nitroglycerin is given to the patient before scanning to maximize vasodilation.

using a high spatial resolution, low temporal resolution time-resolved CE-MRA technique at 3 T using a spine coil and following the administration of sublingual nitroglycerin.[61]

SUMMARY

Various hardware- and software-based strategies have been developed to reduce scan times significantly for CE-MRA acquisitions allowing evaluation of the chest and abdominal vasculature with high temporal resolution. Time-resolved techniques are particularly useful in the setting of dissection, congenital abnormalities of the aorta, steno-occlusive disease, vascular malformations, PCS, and preaortic and postaortic aneurysm repair. Even in the setting of pathologically altered hemodynamics and delayed vessel filling, time-resolved techniques allow delineation of multiple vascular phases in addition to simplifying contrast administration. The balance between spatial and temporal resolution can be tailored to the pathology under investigation. High temporal resolution is essential to providing information on inflow and outflow vessels in high-flow lesions and can often identify pathologic changes in flow direction. Temporal resolution can be relaxed in favor of spatial resolution, such as for dynamic spinal MRA. With continuing advances in hardware and alternative k-space sampling techniques, this tradeoff between spatial and temporal resolution is expected to minimize. The examples presented in this article demonstrate how four-dimensional CE-MRA can be a valuable asset to the imaging armamentarium for evaluation of complex vascular pathologies of the body.

REFERENCES

1. Korosec FR, Frayne R, Grist TM, et al. Time-resolved contrast-enhanced 3D MR angiography. Magn Reson Med 1996;36:345–51.
2. Carroll TJ, Korosec FR, Swan JS, et al. Method for rapidly determining and reconstructing the peak arterial frame from a time-resolved CE-MRA exam. Magn Reson Med 2000;44:817–20.
3. Francois CJ, Shors SM, Bonow RO, et al. Analysis of cardiopulmonary transit times at contrast material-enhanced MR imaging in patients with heart disease. Radiology 2003;227:447–52.
4. Shors SM, Cotts WG, Pavlovic-Surjancev B, et al. Heart failure: evaluation of cardiopulmonary transit times with time-resolved MR angiography. Radiology 2003;229:743–8.
5. Nael K, Fenchel M, Krishnam M, et al. 3.0 Tesla high spatial resolution contrast-enhanced magnetic resonance angiography (CE-MRA) of the pulmonary circulation: initial experience with a 32-channel phased array coil using a high relaxivity contrast agent. Invest Radiol 2007;42:392–8.
6. Wang Y, Chen CZ, Chabra SG, et al. Bolus arterial-venous transit in the lower extremity and venous contamination in bolus chase three-dimensional magnetic resonance angiography. Invest Radiol 2002;37:458–63.
7. Mohrs OK, Petersen SE, Voigtlaender T, et al. Time-resolved contrast-enhanced MR angiography of the thorax in adults with congenital heart disease. AJR Am J Roentgenol 2006;187:1107–14.
8. Fenchel M, Saleh R, Dinh H, et al. Juvenile and adult congenital heart disease: time-resolved 3D contrast-enhanced MR angiography. Radiology 2007;244:399–410.
9. Goo HW, Yang DH, Park IS, et al. Time-resolved three-dimensional contrast-enhanced magnetic resonance angiography in patients who have undergone a Fontan operation or bidirectional cavopulmonary connection: initial experience. J Magn Reson Imaging 2007;25:727–36.
10. Ley S, Fink C, Zaporozhan J, et al. Value of high spatial and high temporal resolution magnetic resonance angiography for differentiation between idiopathic and thromboembolic pulmonary hypertension: initial results. Eur Radiol 2005;15:2256–63.
11. Vigen KK, Peters DC, Grist TM, et al. Undersampled projection-reconstruction imaging for time-resolved contrast-enhanced imaging. Magn Reson Med 2000;43:170–6.
12. Du J, Carroll TJ, Wagner HJ, et al. Time-resolved, undersampled projection reconstruction imaging for high-resolution CE-MRA of the distal runoff vessels. Magn Reson Med 2002;48:516–22.
13. Mazaheri Y, Carroll TJ, Du J, et al. Combined time-resolved and high-spatial-resolution 3D MRA using an extended adaptive acquisition. J Magn Reson Imaging 2002;15:291–301.
14. Huang Y, Wright GA. Time-resolved MR angiography with limited projections. Magn Reson Med 2007;58:316–25.
15. Du J, Bydder M. High-resolution time-resolved contrast-enhanced MR abdominal and pulmonary angiography using a spiral-TRICKS sequence. Magn Reson Med 2007;58:631–5.
16. Kressler B, Spincemaille P, Prince MR, et al. Reduction of reconstruction time for time-resolved spiral 3D contrast-enhanced magnetic resonance angiography using parallel computing. Magn Reson Med 2006;56:704–8.
17. Zhu H, Buck DG, Zhang Z, et al. High temporal and spatial resolution 4D MRA using spiral data sampling and sliding window reconstruction. Magn Reson Med 2004;52:14–8.
18. Barger AV, Block WF, Toropov Y, et al. Time-resolved contrast-enhanced imaging with isotropic resolution and broad coverage using an undersampled 3D projection trajectory. Magn Reson Med 2002;48:297–305.
19. Du J, Carroll TJ, Brodsky E, et al. Contrast-enhanced peripheral magnetic resonance angiography using time-resolved vastly undersampled isotropic projection reconstruction. J Magn Reson Imaging 2004;20:894–900.

20. Sodickson DK, Manning WJ. Simultaneous acquisition of spatial harmonics (SMASH): fast imaging with radiofrequency coil arrays. Magn Reson Med 1997;38:591–603.

21. Pruessmann KP, Weiger M, Scheidegger MB, et al. SENSE: sensitivity encoding for fast MRI. Magn Reson Med 1999;42:952–62.

22. Fink C, Puderbach M, Ley S, et al. Time-resolved echo-shared parallel MRA of the lung: observer preference study of image quality in comparison with non-echo-shared sequences. Eur Radiol 2005;15:2070–4.

23. Wu Y, Goodrich KC, Buswell HR, et al. High-resolution time-resolved contrast-enhanced 3D MRA by combining SENSE with keyhole and SLAM strategies. Magn Reson Imaging 2004;22:1161–8.

24. Muthupillai R, Vick GW III, Flamm SD III, et al. Time-resolved contrast-enhanced magnetic resonance angiography in pediatric patients using sensitivity encoding. J Magn Reson Imaging 2003;17:559–64.

25. Ohno Y, Kawamitsu H, Higashino T, et al. Time-resolved contrast enhanced pulmonary MR angiography using sensitivity encoding (SENSE). J Magn Reson Imaging 2003;17:330–6.

26. Brauck K, Maderwald S, Vogt FM, et al. Time-resolved contrast-enhanced magnetic resonance angiography of the hand with parallel imaging and view sharing: initial experience. Eur Radiol 2007;17:183–92.

27. Fink C, Ley S, Kroeker R, et al. Time-resolved contrast-enhanced three-dimensional magnetic resonance angiography of the chest: combination of parallel imaging with view sharing (TREAT). Invest Radiol 2005;40:40–8.

28. Frydrychowicz A, Bley TA, Winterer JT, et al. Accelerated time-resolved 3D contrast-enhanced MR angiography at 3T: clinical experience in 31 patients. MAGMA 2006;19:187–95.

29. Krishnam MS, Tomasian A, Lohan DG, et al. Low-dose, time-resolved, contrast-enhanced 3D MR angiography in cardiac and vascular diseases: correlation to high spatial resolution 3D contrast-enhanced MRA. Clin Radiol 2008;63:744–55.

30. Nael K, Michaely HJ, Lee M, et al. Dynamic pulmonary perfusion and flow quantification with MR imaging, 3.0T vs. 1.5T: initial results. J Magn Reson Imaging 2006;24:333–9.

31. DeSanctis RW, Doroghazi RM, Austen WG, et al. Aortic dissection. N Engl J Med 1987;317:1060–7.

32. Debakey ME, Henly WS, Cooley DA, et al. Surgical management of dissecting aneurysms of the aorta. J Thorac Cardiovasc Surg 1965;49:130–49.

33. Nienaber CA, Eagle KA. Aortic dissection: new frontiers in diagnosis and management: part I: from etiology to diagnostic strategies. Circulation 2003;108:628–35.

34. Nienaber CA, Eagle KA. Aortic dissection: new frontiers in diagnosis and management: part II: therapeutic management and follow-up. Circulation 2003;108:772–8.

35. Cigarroa JE, Isselbacher EM, DeSanctis RW, et al. Diagnostic imaging in the evaluation of suspected aortic dissection: old standards and new directions. N Engl J Med 1993;328:35–43.

36. Schoenberg SO, Wunsch C, Knopp MV, et al. Abdominal aortic aneurysm. Detection of multilevel vascular pathology by time-resolved multiphase 3D gadolinium MR angiography: initial report. Invest Radiol 1999;34:648–59.

37. Finn JP, Baskaran V, Carr JC, et al. Thorax: low-dose contrast-enhanced three-dimensional MR angiography with subsecond temporal resolution–initial results. Radiology 2002;224:896–904.

38. Sueyoshi E, Sakamoto I, Hayashi K, et al. Growth rate of aortic diameter in patients with type B aortic dissection during the chronic phase. Circulation 2004;110:II256–61.

39. Salanitri GC. Intercostal artery aneurysms complicating thoracic aortic coarctation: diagnosis with magnetic resonance angiography. Australas Radiol 2007;51:78–82.

40. Weyand CM, Goronzy JJ. Medium- and large-vessel vasculitis. N Engl J Med 2003;349:160–9.

41. Andrews J, Mason JC. Takayasu's arteritis: recent advances in imaging offer promise. Rheumatology (Oxford) 2007;46:6–15.

42. Yamada I, Nakagawa T, Himeno Y, et al. Takayasu arteritis: diagnosis with breath-hold contrast-enhanced three-dimensional MR angiography. J Magn Reson Imaging 2000;11:481–7.

43. Desai MY, Stone JH, Foo TK, et al. Delayed contrast-enhanced MRI of the aortic wall in Takayasu's arteritis: initial experience. AJR Am J Roentgenol 2005;184:1427–31.

44. Tuite DJ, Francois C, Dill K, et al. Diagnosis and characterization of pulmonary sequestration using dynamic time-resolved magnetic resonance angiography. Clin Radiol 2008;63:913–7.

45. Meine JG, Schwartz RA, Janniger CK, et al. Klippel-Trenaunay-Weber syndrome. Cutis 1997;60:127–32.

46. Cohen MM Jr. Klippel-Trenaunay syndrome. Am J Med Genet 2000;93:171–5.

47. Kanterman RY, Witt PD, Hsieh PS, et al. Klippel-Trenaunay syndrome: imaging findings and percutaneous intervention. AJR Am J Roentgenol 1996;167:989–95.

48. Guttmacher AE, Marchuk DA, White RI Jr, et al. Hereditary hemorrhagic telangiectasia. N Engl J Med 1995;333:918–24.

49. Jackson IT, Carreno R, Potparic Z, et al. Hemangiomas, vascular malformations, and lymphovenous malformations: classification and methods of treatment. Plast Reconstr Surg 1993;91:1216–30.

50. Goyen M, Ruehm SG, Jagenburg A, et al. Pulmonary arteriovenous malformation: characterization with time-resolved ultrafast 3D MR angiography. J Magn Reson Imaging 2001;13:458–60.

51. Herborn CU, Goyen M, Lauenstein TC, et al. Comprehensive time-resolved MRI of peripheral vascular malformations. AJR Am J Roentgenol 2003;181:729–35.

52. Ohgiya Y, Hashimoto T, Gokan T, et al. Dynamic MRI for distinguishing high-flow from low-flow peripheral vascular malformations. AJR Am J Roentgenol 2005; 185:1131–7.

53. Ganeshan A, Upponi S, Hon LQ, et al. Chronic pelvic pain due to pelvic congestion syndrome: the role of diagnostic and interventional radiology. Cardiovasc Intervent Radiol 2007;30: 1105–11.

54. Lookstein RA, Goldman J, Pukin L, et al. Time-resolved magnetic resonance angiography as a noninvasive method to characterize endoleaks: initial results compared with conventional angiography. J Vasc Surg 2004;39:27–33.

55. Cohen EI, Weinreb DB, Siegelbaum RH, et al. Time-resolved MR angiography for the classification of endoleaks after endovascular aneurysm repair. J Magn Reson Imaging 2008;27:500–3.

56. van der Laan MJ, Bakker CJ, Blankensteijn JD, et al. Dynamic CE-MRA for endoleak classification after endovascular aneurysm repair. Eur J Vasc Endovasc Surg 2006;31:130–5.

57. Haulon S, Lions C, McFadden EP, et al. Prospective evaluation of magnetic resonance imaging after endovascular treatment of infrarenal aortic aneurysms. Eur J Vasc Endovasc Surg 2001;22:62–9.

58. Backes WH, Nijenhuis RJ, Mess WH, et al. Magnetic resonance angiography of collateral blood supply to spinal cord in thoracic and thoracoabdominal aortic aneurysm patients. J Vasc Surg 2008;48:261–71.

59. Jaspers K, Nijenhuis RJ, Backes WH, et al. Differentiation of spinal cord arteries and veins by time-resolved MR angiography. J Magn Reson Imaging 2007;26:31–40.

60. Nijenhuis RJ, Mull M, Wilmink JT, et al. MR angiography of the great anterior radiculomedullary artery (Adamkiewicz artery) validated by digital subtraction angiography. AJNR Am J Neuroradiol 2006;27: 1565–72.

61. Reeder SB, Duffek C, Bley TA, et al. Presurgical localization of the artery of Adamkiewicz with time resolved MRA at 3.0T. In: 20th Annual International Conference on Magnetic Resonance Angiography. Graz, Austria, October 15th–18th, 2008.

Peripheral MR Angiography

Harald Kramer, MD*, Konstantin Nikolaou, MD,
Wieland Sommer, MD, Maximilian F. Reiser, MD,
Karin A. Herrmann, MD

KEYWORDS

- Peripheral MR angiography
- Hybrid MR angiography
- Contrast-enhanced MR angiography
- Time-resolved MR angiography • 3.0 Tesla

Imaging of the arteries of the lower extremity is most often performed in patients who have known or suspected peripheral artery occlusive disease (PAOD), which is the most common manifestation of systemic atherosclerosis other than coronary heart disease and cerebrovascular disease.[1,2] The prevalence of PAOD ranges between 3% and 10% in the general population, increasing to 10% to 15% in persons older than 70 years. If PAOD is not treated at an early stage, severe symptoms starting with intermittent claudication and progressing to rest pain and finally to potential gangrene and tissue loss may occur.[3] After family disposition, smoking is the next most severe risk factor; smokers are three times more often affected than nonsmoking individuals. Furthermore, PAOD is directly associated with arterial hypertension and diabetes mellitus.[4]

The first clinical test performed to evaluate the presence or absence of PAOD is calculation of the ankle brachial index (ABI). Here, the systolic pressure in the posterior tibial or dorsalis pedis artery is divided by the systolic blood pressure in the arms. A resting ABI of 0.90 or less correlates to a hemodynamically significant arterial stenosis and is most often used as the hemodynamic definition of PAOD. In symptomatic individuals, an ABI 0.90 or less is approximately 95% sensitive in detecting arteriogram-positive PAOD and almost 100% specific in identifying healthy individuals. Thus, this test is well suited for identifying individuals suffering from PAOD but is unspecific for the exact localization of pathologic vascular lesions.

Due to the recent advances in imaging modalities, the radiologic approach to the diagnosis of PAOD has changed substantially in the last few years.[5–9] Digital subtraction (DS) angiography is still regarded as the standard of reference; however, the well-known disadvantages of DS angiography, such as risks associated with the invasive procedure, ionizing radiation, and potentially nephrotoxic contrast agents, more and more come into account. The combination of high spatial resolution and dynamic information cannot yet be achieved by any other imaging modality. CT angiography almost meets the excellent spatial resolution of DS angiography without being invasive and with a lower amount of contrast agent but still suffers from ionizing radiation and cannot deliver any information about dynamic flow.[10–12] New generations of CT scanners allowing for time-resolved, dynamic CT angiography are rare (the techniques are under initial investigation) and may be associated with an increased radiation dose. Although Doppler ultrasonography allows for noninvasive vessel imaging without ionizing radiation or contrast agent and provides dynamic information, its disadvantage is that it is restricted to certain vessel territories and is user and patient dependent.[13,14] MR angiography, however, is a noninvasive, user-independent imaging modality. The applied contrast agents do not affect renal function when used in the recommended amount in patients who have a nonimpaired renal function (glomerular filtration rate >30 mL/min/1.73 m^2). Until now, the definite

Institute for Clinical Radiology, University Hospital Munich, Marchioninistr. 15, 81377 Munich, Germany
* Corresponding author.
E-mail address: harald.kramer@med.uni-muenchen.de (H. Kramer).

Magn Reson Imaging Clin N Am 17 (2009) 91–100
doi:10.1016/j.mric.2008.12.006

disadvantage of MR angiography compared with DS angiography and CT angiography has been the restricted spatial resolution. Recent technical developments such as the introduction of new image reconstruction algorithms and dedicated contrast agents have pushed the limits of MR angiography toward higher spatial resolution and image quality and have enabled time-resolved imaging. The combination of multichannel MR systems, high field-strength multielement angiography receiver coils, and dedicated contrast agents has helped to substantially minimize most of the traditional drawbacks of MR angiography.[15–20]

TECHNICAL CONCEPTS OF PERIPHERAL MR ANGIOGRAPHY

The main prerequisite for any diagnostic imaging modality of the arterial vasculature is to get the best possible spatial resolution in combination with sufficient vessel contrast and (if possible) dynamic information, ultimately seeking the best chance of obtaining a detailed vessel wall evaluation. An MR angiography dataset of subjectively high image quality shows excellent signal-to-noise ratio (SNR) and is free of venous enhancement. To improve these parameters, there are several technical concepts that have evolved over time. Over the past years, contrast-enhanced MR angiography has evolved as the preferred technique for MR imaging of the arterial vasculature, which relies on synchronizing maximum T1 shortening with acquisition of central k-space information. Injection of gadolinium chelate contrast media, however, leads only to transient T1 shortening of the blood pool. After having briefly enhanced the intravascular space, these contrast agents rapidly diffuse into the extracellular space. The intravascular half-life of commercially approved agents is approximately 90 seconds. Enough contrast must be injected to decrease the T1 of blood to values smaller than those of stationary background tissues. The basic principle of this technique is to acquire a luminogram during arterial first pass of contrast material. The major challenge in contrast-enhanced MR angiography is to find a balance of the desires for high spatial resolution, large anatomic coverage, and acquisition time.

Step-By-Step MR Angiography

Early techniques of peripheral MR angiography allowed for the imaging of one coronal volume only, covering approximately 40 to 50 cm of the vascular tree. Although high image quality can be achieved with gadolinium-enhanced MR angiography, in most cases, more than one field of view

(FOV; 40–50 cm) must be imaged. To accomplish imaging of the peripheral vascular tree beyond this restricted FOV, time-of-flight (TOF) techniques have been used.[21] TOF imaging, however, is time-consuming and subject to a number of typical artifacts (see later discussion). An alternative to the TOF approach is to image multiple gadolinium-enhanced volumes, with subsequent application of multiple doses of contrast agent.[22] The use of this method, however, increases the cost of the contrast material and can result in unintended effects due to an increase in intra- and extravascular levels of gadolinium. With the technique of moving-bed infusion-tracking MR angiography, only one bolus of contrast agent is used for imaging the entire peripheral vascular tree.[23,24] Depending on the MR system and the corresponding FOV, a peripheral MR angiography is performed in three to five steps, from the diaphragm to the feet. The first attempts for moving-bed peripheral MR angiography faced some technical restrictions. Without the possibility to use later-developed acquisition techniques such as parallel imaging, high–spatial resolution datasets need long acquisition times that result in severe venous enhancement in the most distal calf station when using a standard bolus-chase technique, because blood flow (and thus arrival of the contrast-agent bolus) is faster than the acquisition of the abdominal and thigh stations (**Fig. 1**). When using this technique, a defined amount of contrast agent is injected as a single bolus, and the arterial vasculature is imaged in consecutive steps. Due to long acquisition times to get high spatial resolution in every station, it is not possible to get the more distal vessels (ie, in the lower leg) in an arterial-only phase because the acquisition time of the more proximal stations together with the time for table movement is longer than the circulation time of the contrast-agent bolus from the abdominal aorta to the calf veins. This situation results in an enhancement of the calf veins, impeding diagnosis of the lower-leg arteries. Several attempts can be made to overcome this problem. First, it is important to start data acquisition in the most proximal station as early as possible to not waste any time during which imaging could be done. Second, it is possible to influence the contrast-agent bolus by using dedicated injection protocols, such as a biphasic injection, to ensure a concentrated start of the bolus and a long duration of contrast agent within the arterial vasculature.[25,26] With the introduction of dedicated coils, image acquisition techniques, and image reconstruction algorithms, acquisition times have been significantly shortened while retaining the same high spatial resolution. The implementation of

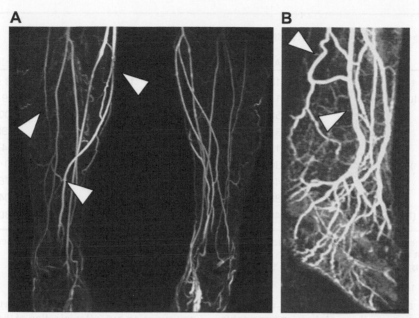

Fig. 1. Examples of venous enhancement impairing the diagnostic accuracy in the calf (*A*) and foot (*B*) station (*arrowheads*).

parallel imaging helped to reduce acquisition time by a factor of 2 or more but at the cost of reduced SNR, which again can be increased by using dedicated multielement surface coils.[27] Dedicated data-acquisition strategies such as non-Cartesian k-space readout and centric reordered readout helped to become more independent from exact bolus arrival in the most distal station, still ensuring a purely arterial contrast (**Fig. 2, Table 1**). Another

method to reduce or avoid venous contamination of the lower leg is venous compression in the thigh station. With this technique, venous return should be decelerated.[28]

Hybrid MR Angiography

As described previously, a three-dimensional (3D), contrast-enhanced MR angiography examination

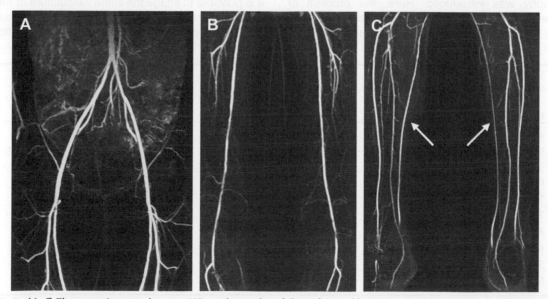

Fig. 2. (*A–C*) Three-station step-by-step MR angiography of the pelvis and lower extremities acquired with parallel imaging shows excellent image quality at high spatial resolution. There is a small amount of venous contamination of the calf station, which does not interfere with interpretation (*arrows*).

Table 1
Sequence parameters for step-by-step MR angiography with parallel imaging

Parameters	Abdomen	Thigh	Calf
Acquisition time (s)	18 s	15 s	23 s
Spatial resolution (mm³)	1.4 × 1.1 × 1.2	1 × 1 × 1	0.9 × 0.9 × 0.9
FOV (mm)	500	500	500
TR (ms)	3.31	3.51	3.98
TE (ms)	1.21	1.33	1.47
Flip angle (°)	30	30	30
Matrix	448	512	576
Slices/slab	88	88	104
Bandwidth (Hz/Px)	400	410	330

Acquisition time for each station is short enough to avoid venous enhancement in the calf station; hence, the hybrid approach is not necessary.
    Abbreviations: Hz/Px, hertz/pixel; TE, echo time; TR, repetition time.

of the pelvis and lower extremities is commonly performed using a three-station moving-table bolus-chase technique. With this technique, the timing of the bolus is optimized for the first station (abdomen/pelvis), and then imaging is performed as rapidly as possible to try to keep up with the flow of gadolinium down the peripheral vasculature. Although the MR angiography image quality is generally excellent for evaluation of the first two stations (abdomen/pelvis and thigh), it is often inadequate for assessment of the last station (calf/foot) because imaging of the lower station is often degraded by venous contamination.

To overcome this restriction, hybrid MR angiography was introduced. Here, the problem of venous enhancement in the most distal calf station is solved not by decreasing acquisition times of the more proximal stations or by the use of venous compression but (after injection of the first bolus of contrast agent) by imaging this station first and in multiple phases (**Table 2**).[29] Afterward, the more proximal abdominal and thigh stations are imaged with a second bolus of contrast agent (**Fig. 3**). For an accurate assessment of bolus arrival time, a test bolus measurement is performed at two different positions. For timing of data acquisition at the calf station, the arrival time of contrast agent is assessed at the height of the popliteal artery; for the abdominal and thigh stations, arrival time of contrast agent is measured in the abdominal aorta at the height of the diaphragm. With this protocol, it is possible to image the entire vasculature of the lower extremity from the diaphragm to the feet without any venous overlay at high spatial

Table 2
Sequence parameters for hybrid MR angiography

Parameters	Calf first	Abdomen	Thigh	Knee	Calf
Acquisition time (s)	30	19	13	18	27
Spatial resolution (mm³)	1.4 × 0.7 × 0.9	1.5 × 0.7 × 1.5	1.5 × 0.7 × 1.4	1.5 × 0.7 × 1.3	1.4 × 0.7 × 0.9
FOV (mm)	360	380	380	380	360
TR (ms)	3.51	3.01	2.48	3.42	4.30
TE (ms)	1.25	1.04	1.04	1.09	1.32
Flip angle (°)	20	20	20	20	20
Matrix	512	512	512	512	512
Slices/slab	88	60	56	52	64
Bandwidth (Hz/Px)	360	810	810	540	320

Imaging of the most distal calf station is done first, followed by consecutive imaging of the more proximal abdominal, thigh, and knee stations.
    Abbreviations: Hz/Px, hertz/pixel; TE, echo time; TR, repetition time.

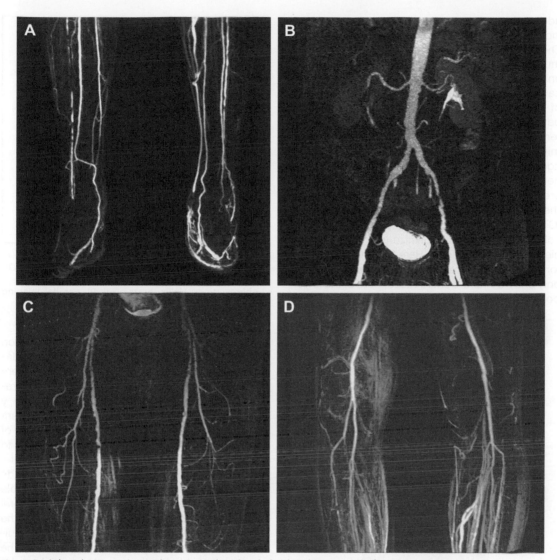

Fig. 3. Peripheral MR angiography acquired with a hybrid technique. (*A*) The most distal station is imaged first. Following a second contrast-agent bolus, the abdominal (*B*), thigh (*C*), and calf vasculature (*D*) is examined.

resolution and, at the same time, provide dynamic, time-resolved information on the contrast inflow in the lower leg. This kind of high-quality dataset is very important for treatment planning in cases with arterial occlusion when the decision stands between revascularization/bypass surgery and amputation. On the other hand, this technique may be complicated for those who do not perform peripheral MR angiography frequently, because contrast-agent timing is still somewhat complicated using the two-test-bolus approach described earlier.

Continuous Table Movement MR Angiography

To compensate for the restricted FOV for larger anatomic areas such as the lower-extremity peripheral arteries, a multistep approach as described earlier has been successfully implemented for MR angiography of the lower limb. Bolus-chase techniques with the use of multistation table motion allow the stepwise assessment of the pelvic and run-off arteries within a single examination. Although various multistation approaches have been shown to be effective, these protocols have several inherent limitations and include several disadvantages. To cover extended anatomy with high image resolution and to stay within the arterial window to prevent venous overlay, imaging time must be as short as possible. Repositioning of the table between discrete stations, however, leads to a reduction in imaging time efficiency because of the interruption of data acquisition during this process.[30] In addition, gradient nonlinearities at the edges of individual FOVs have to be taken into account. The planning and separate data acquisition of multiple steps for nonenhanced and contrast-enhanced imaging is time-consuming, complicated, and may be error ridden. Although the use of contrast agents can be classified as safe in patients who do not have substantially impaired renal function (glomerular filtration rate >30 mL/min/1.73 m^2), the issue of double-bolus contrast-agent application and the conjoint risk of inducing nephrogenic systemic fibrosis have to be considered. These limitations have been eliminated by the introduction of continuous table movement (CTM) data acquisitions that provide seamless volume coverage and optimize imaging time efficiency (**Fig. 4, Table 3**). Here, planning and performing the examination is much easier because only one FOV for the entire vasculature of the lower body part has to be positioned and only one

Table 3 Imaging parameters for continuous table movement MR angiography	
PI	2
Acquisition time (s)	64
Spatial resolution (mm^3)	1.2 × 1.2 × 1.2
FOV (mm)	1280
TR (ms)	2.36
TE (ms)	1.07
Flip angle (°)	20
Matrix	384
Slices/slab	88
Bandwidth (Hz/Px)	1000

Spatial resolution is technically limited to 1.2 mm^3. FOV in z-axis measures 1280 mm; thus, only one seamless FOV covers the entire vasculature of the lower body part.
   Abbreviations: Hz/Px, hertz/pixel; PI, parallel imaging factor; TE, echo time; TR, repetition time.

contrast-agent bolus is used.[31] Slice acquisition in the coronal plane is particularly beneficial for datasets as in peripheral MR angiography, where there is a large extension in x (left-right) and z (cranio-caudal) direction but little volume in the y (anterior-posterior) plane. Before table movement is initiated in CTM MR angiography, a number of lines are acquired without moving the table to acquire the most cranial part of the FOV. Likewise, the data acquisition is prolonged for a few seconds at the end of the imaging range (ie, after the table has stopped moving) to acquire the peripheral parts of k-space in the most distal part of the acquired volume. Table velocity during data acquisition is influenced by several parameters, the most important being the acquired spatial resolution and the applied parallel imaging factor.[32,33]

Non–Contrast-Enhanced MR Angiography

When discussing the use of contrast agents in MR imaging in patients who have impaired renal function because of new reported diseases such as nephrogenic systemic fibrosis, non–contrast-enhanced MR angiography techniques attract attention.[34–36] The first of these techniques available was the so-called "time-of-flight" MR angiography. This technique is still used for imaging of the intracranial vasculature and, in some rare cases, imaging of the feet vasculature when the decision stands between revascularization and amputation due to its very high spatial resolution achievable. TOF MR angiography relies on the differences in exposure to radiofrequency excitation between in-plane/in-slab stationary protons

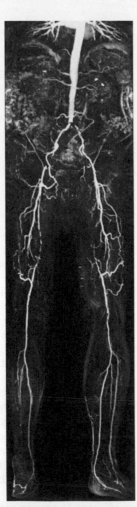

Fig. 4. Continuous table movement MR angiography displaying a seamless FOV.

and the blood protons flowing into the section/ slab. For selective imaging of arteries or veins, saturation bands can be applied on the venous or arterial side, respectively, to null the signal from the unwanted inflow of nonsaturated protons. Acquisition can be performed using two-dimensional or 3D methods, depending on the spatial resolution, extent of the imaged volume, and the available imaging time. A drawback of this imaging method remains the small imaging volume and the occurrence of artifacts due to slow, in-plane, or turbulent flow, impeding diagnosis and potentially causing false-positive results in terms of detection of significant stenoses.

Some of these limitations also apply for phase-contrast imaging; today, this technique is used for flow measurements and, only in rare cases, for angiographic imaging. This technique uses pairs of bipolar or flow-compensated and uncompensated gradient pulses to generate flow-sensitive phase images. Phase data can be used to reconstruct velocity-encoded flow-quantification images or MR angiographic images.

Upcoming techniques, especially for MR angiography of the lower extremities and the carotid arteries, are ECG-gated 3D partial-Fourier fast spin echo (FSE) sequences and balanced steady-state free precession (SSFP) sequences (**Fig. 5**).

ECG-gated 3D FSE imaging relies on different flow-patterns of arteries and veins. Slow-flowing blood, such as on the venous side of circulation, appears hyperintense bright; modulated fast-flowing arterial blood shows flow voids in the systolic phase and appears hypointense dark. Data are acquired in arterial and venous phases and later subtracted to get a pure arterial image of the examined region. This technique can be used for peripheral, thoracic, pulmonary, and (in some cases) carotid imaging.

Because balanced SSFP sequences determine their image contrast T2/T1 ratios, which produce bright blood imaging without reliance on different flow patterns (**Fig. 6**), this technique is most often used in carotid, coronary, abdominal, and renal artery imaging.

CONTRAST AGENTS FOR MR ANGIOGRAPHY

Gadolinium-based contrast agents can be subdivided into two groups: agents with no capacity to interact with intravascular proteins and those with weak or strong capacity for protein interaction. Until now, the standard contrast agent for imaging of the entire body and vasculature was a 0.5-mol/L extracellular gadolinium chelate without any protein binding. This kind of contrast agent provides good image quality for nearly all clinical indications for MR angiography. The advent of new, innovative contrast agents with properties distinct from those of the traditional extracellular gadolinium agents promises to further expand the clinical application of contrast-enhanced MRA. For some anatomic regions or indications, contrast agents with higher concentrations of gadolinium-chelates seem to be beneficial (eg, time-resolved applications or imaging of the carotid or renal arteries). In these vascular territories, already a comparably small

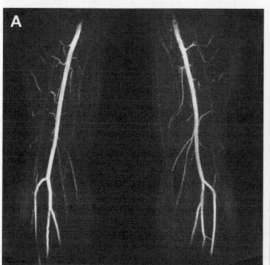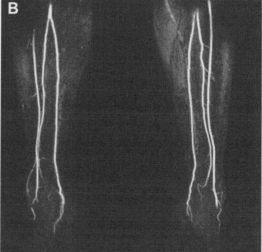

Fig. 5. Examples of MR angiography of the thigh (*A*) and calf stations (*B*) acquired without contrast agent but with a flow-sensitive sequence.

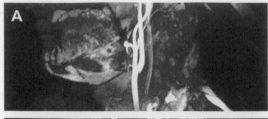

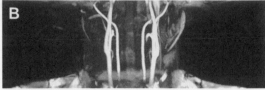

Fig. 6. (*A, B*) Maximum-intensity projection images of MR angiography of the carotid bifurcation acquired with a non–contrast-enhanced angiography technique.

volume of a highly concentrated (ie, 1.0 mol/L) contrast agent can provide a high SNR.

A completely different type of contrast agent is the intravascular or so-called "blood pool" contrast agent. These substances do not enhance in surrounding soft tissue because they do not pass the vessel wall due to their size when bound to human serum proteins such as albumin. This effect makes MR angiography independent from the short time-frame of arterial first-pass imaging and allows for high resolution at steady-state (equilibrium state), with potentially prolonged acquisition times of up to several minutes.[37–40]

SUMMARY

Recent developments in MR hardware and software have helped to significantly increase image quality of MR angiography. The introduction of high-field MR systems (ie, 3T or more) into clinical routine and the development of dedicated coils and contrast agents have made MR angiography a strong competitor of DS angiography and CT angiography. The long-lasting drawbacks of MR angiography, such as reduced spatial resolution and the absence of dynamic information, could be overcome with new coil concepts, the introduction of parallel imaging techniques, and new sequence algorithms. Several different MR angiography techniques are available for every vascular territory. Certainly, there is no single application with which every region can be examined at best-possible image quality; however, with a particular technique for a dedicated region or a combination of two or more techniques, such as the combination of a high-resolution static dataset and a dynamic examination, MR angiography

can provide complementary and complex information that cannot be provided by any other imaging method. In every contrast-enhanced MRA technique, it is recommended to acquire the data in three phases. First, a nonenhanced phase should be acquired to ensure proper anatomic coverage and precise positioning of the different FOVs of the MR angiography acquisition. The precontrast acquisition should be performed in the same fashion as the contrast-enhanced acquisitions because this familiarizes the patient with the breath-holding procedure that will likely be necessary and the expected length of the acquisition. In addition, this unenhanced mask can serve for later subtraction. After that, the arterial phase of the contrast-enhanced MR angiography is acquired for best visualization of the arterial vasculature. A delayed venous phase is the third phase acquired to identify possible late filling in dissections or distal to hemodynamically significant stenoses. This delayed phase can give information about the venous vasculature.

The combination of different acquisition techniques and strategies and different contrast agents and noncontrast MR angiography techniques makes MR angiography the diagnostic modality of choice in vascular disease. Other imaging modalities may provide for the possibility of interventional procedures or may be widely available, but every treatment decision demands optimal imaging before potential surgery or invention.

REFERENCES

1. Diehm C, Kareem S, Lawall H. Epidemiology of peripheral arterial disease. Vasa 2004;33(4):183–9.
2. Norgren L, et al. Inter-Society Consensus for the Management of Peripheral Arterial Disease (TASC II). J Vasc Surg 2007;45(Suppl S):S5–67.
3. Baumgartner I, Schainfeld R, Graziani L. Management of peripheral vascular disease. Annu Rev Med 2005;56:249–72.
4. Weckbach S. Comprehensive diabetes imaging with whole body MR imaging at 1.5 and 3.0 T in patients with longstanding diabetes. Presented at the European Congress of Radiology 2006. Vienna, March 3–6, 2006.
5. Adams MR, Celermajer DS. Detection of presymptomatic atherosclerosis: a current perspective. Clin Sci (Lond) 1999;97(5):615–24.
6. Boudewijn G, Vasbinder C, Nelemans PJ. Accuracy of computed tomographic angiography and magnetic resonance angiography for diagnosing renal artery stenosis. Perspect Vasc Surg Endovasc Ther 2005;17(2):180.

7. Cortell ED, et al. MR angiography of tibial runoff vessels: imaging with the head coil compared with conventional arteriography. AJR Am J Roentgenol 1996;167(1):147–51.

8. de Vries M, et al. Peripheral arterial disease: clinical and cost comparisons between duplex US and contrast-enhanced MR angiography—a multicenter randomized trial. Radiology 2006;240(2):401–10.

9. Ekelund L, et al. MR angiography of abdominal and peripheral arteries. Techniques and clinical applications. Acta Radiol 1996;37(1):3–13.

10. Green D, Parker D. CTA and MRA: visualization without catheterization. Semin Ultrasound CT MR 2003;24(4):185–91.

11. Prokop M. Multislice CT angiography. Eur J Radiol 2000;36(2):86–96.

12. Rankin SC. CT angiography. Eur Radiol 1999;9(2):297–310.

13. Colquhoun I, et al. The assessment of carotid and vertebral arteries: a comparison of CFM duplex ultrasound with intravenous digital subtraction angiography. Br J Radiol 1992;65(780):1069–74.

14. Koelemay MJ, et al. Diagnosis of arterial disease of the lower extremities with duplex ultrasonography. Br J Surg 1996;83(3):404–9.

15. Barkhausen J. New imaging protocols for peripheral MRA. Presented at the European Congress of Radiology 2006. Vienna, March 3–6, 2006.

16. Bilecen D, et al. MR angiography with venous compression. Radiology 2004;233(2):617–8 [author reply 618–9].

17. Kramer H. Magnetic resonance angiography (MRA) of the lower extremities with parallel imaging and a dedicated 36 element matrix-coil at 3 Tesla. Presented at the International Society of Magnetic Resonance in Medicine 2006 meeting. Seattle (WA), May 6–12, 2006.

18. Kramer H. Effects of injection rate and dose on image quality in time-resolved magnetic resonance angiography (MRA) by using a 1.0M contrast agent. Eur Radiol 2006; [online first].

19. Leiner T, et al. Contrast-enhanced peripheral MR angiography at 3.0 Tesla: initial experience with a whole-body scanner in healthy volunteers. J Magn Reson Imaging 2003;17(5):609–14.

20. Leiner T, et al. Peripheral arterial disease: comparison of color duplex US and contrast-enhanced MR angiography for diagnosis. Radiology 2005;235(2):699–708.

21. Dorweiler B, et al. Magnetic resonance angiography unmasks reliable target vessels for pedal bypass grafting in patients with diabetes mellitus. J Vasc Surg 2002;35(4):766–72.

22. Du J, et al. SNR improvement for multiinjection time-resolved high-resolution CE-MRA of the peripheral vasculature. Magn Reson Med 2003;49(5):909–17.

23. Hany TF, et al. Aorta and runoff vessels: single-injection MR angiography with automated table movement compared with multiinjection time-resolved MR angiography—initial results. Radiology 2001;221(1):266–72.

24. Huber A, et al. Moving-table MR angiography of the peripheral runoff vessels: comparison of body coil and dedicated phased array coil systems. AJR Am J Roentgenol 2003;180(5):1365–73.

25. Leiner T. Magnetic resonance angiography of abdominal and lower extremity vasculature. Top Magn Reson Imaging 2005;16(1):21–66.

26. Leiner T, et al. Use of a three-station phased array coil to improve peripheral contrast-enhanced magnetic resonance angiography. J Magn Reson Imaging 2004;20(3):417–25.

27. Kramer H, et al. High-resolution magnetic resonance angiography of the lower extremities with a dedicated 36-element matrix coil at 3 Tesla. Invest Radiol 2007;42(6):477–83.

28. Herborn CU, et al. Peripheral vasculature: whole-body MR angiography with midfemoral venous compression—initial experience. Radiology 2004;230(3):872–8.

29. Meissner OA, et al. Critical limb ischemia: hybrid MR angiography compared with DSA. Radiology 2005;235(1):308–18.

30. Vogt FM, et al. Peripheral vascular disease: comparison of continuous MR angiography and conventional MR angiography—pilot study. Radiology 2007.

31. Kramer H, et al. Peripheral magnetic resonance angiography (MRA) with continuous table movement at 3.0 T: initial experience compared with step-by-step MRA. Invest Radiol 2008;43(9):627–34.

32. Kruger DG, et al. Dual-velocity continuously moving table acquisition for contrast-enhanced peripheral magnetic resonance angiography. Magn Reson Med 2005;53(1):110–7.

33. Zenge MO, et al. High-resolution continuously acquired peripheral MR angiography featuring partial parallel imaging GRAPPA. Magn Reson Med 2006;56(4):859–65.

34. Lim RP, et al. 3D nongadolinium-enhanced ECG-gated MRA of the distal lower extremities: preliminary clinical experience. J Magn Reson Imaging 2008;28(1):181–9.

35. Miyazaki M, Lee VS. Nonenhanced MR angiography. Radiology 2008;248(1):20–43.

36. Miyazaki M, et al. Non-contrast-enhanced MR angiography using 3D ECG-synchronized half-Fourier fast spin echo. J Magn Reson Imaging 2000;12(5):776–83.

37. Knopp MV, et al. Contrast agents for MRA: future directions. J Magn Reson Imaging 1999;10(3):314–6.

38. Prokop M, Debatin JF. MRI contrast media—new developments and trends. CTA vs. MRA. Eur Radiol 1997;7(Suppl 5):299–306.

39. Tournier H, Hyacinthe R, Schneider M. Gadolinium-containing mixed micelle formulations: a new class of blood pool MRI/MRA contrast agents. Acad Radiol 2002;9(Suppl 1):S20–8.

40. van Bemmel CM, et al. Blood pool contrast-enhanced MRA: improved arterial visualization in the steady state. IEEE Trans Med Imaging 2003;22(5):645–52.

Pulmonary MR Angiography Techniques and Applications

Elizabeth M. Hecht, MD*, Andrew Rosenkrantz, MD

KEYWORDS

- Magnetic resonance angiography • Pulmonary
- Pulmonary embolism • Thoracic

The role of the pulmonary artery is to channel deoxygenated blood to the lungs where it can be replenished with oxygen at the level of the pulmonary capillaries/lung alveoli. Newly oxygenated blood returns to the heart via the pulmonary veins where it can be distributed to the heart muscle and systemic circulation. Disruption in the normal pattern of blood flow through the pulmonary artery because of arterial vasoconstriction, luminal obstruction, veno-occlusive disease, or lung disease/hypoxemia can have a devastating impact on the ability of blood to receive oxygen from the lungs. To compensate for the lack of oxygen reaching the body, the right heart chambers attempt to overcome the "obstruction" by increasing blood flow through the pulmonary artery and its branches, eventually leading to increased right heart, and in turn pulmonary artery pressure. The resulting pulmonary hypertension can lead to a variety of symptoms including shortness of breath, fatigue, syncope, peripheral edema, heart failure, and even death depending on the etiology. Rapid and accurate diagnosis of the underlying cause of pulmonary vascular compromise and quantitative evaluation of its impact on the heart and lungs is critical for triaging and managing patients. From an imaging perspective, diagnosis depends on accurate depiction of the pulmonary arterial tree from the centrally located main pulmonary artery (3-cm diameter) to the small subsegmental branches (<1 mm) in the periphery of the lung. In addition, quantitative

evaluation of pulmonary arterial pathology and its impact on lung perfusion and cardiac function is of great importance and is a role where MR imaging can be particularly valuable. Beyond just lumenography, MR can be used to assess lung perfusion, quantify pulmonary blood flow, visualize cardiac contractility, and consequently estimate function.

The purpose of this review is to discuss the well-established as well as the expanding role of MR imaging and magnetic resonance angiography (MRA) in assessment of pulmonary arterial diseases. For depiction of pulmonary arterial anatomy and morphology, MRA techniques will be compared with CTA and DSA. However, the additional benefits of MR techniques, namely perfusion, flow, and function will be emphasized, as the integrated MR examination offers a comprehensive assessment of vascular morphology and function. Nonetheless, pulmonary MRA can be challenging. Accurate depiction and interpretation of the pulmonary arterial system can be hampered by suboptimal spatial resolution and artifacts from susceptibility at air/tissue interfaces and from respiratory and cardiac motion. Advances in MR technology that improve spatial and temporal resolution and compensate for potential artifacts are required and will be discussed as they pertain to pulmonary MRA. Current and emerging gadolinium contrast-enhanced (CE) and non–contrast-enhanced (NCE) MRA techniques will be discussed. The role of pulmonary MRA, general

Department of Radiology, New York University School of Medicine, 560 First Avenue, TCH-HW202, New York, NY 10016, USA
* Corresponding author.
E-mail address: elizabeth.hecht@nyumc.org (E.M. Hecht).

Magn Reson Imaging Clin N Am 17 (2009) 101–131
doi:10.1016/j.mric.2009.01.001
1064-9689/09/$ – see front matter © 2009 Elsevier Inc. All rights reserved.

protocols, imaging findings, and interpretation pitfalls will be reviewed for many common and some not so common clinical indications including acute and chronic pulmonary embolic disease, primary pulmonary hypertension, pulmonary arteriovenous malformation, pulmonary aneurysms and dissections, congenital heart disease, pulmonary sequestration, and malignancy.

TECHNICAL ASPECTS

Before discussing the major clinical applications of MRA and related MR techniques for characterizing pathologies of the pulmonary arterial system (PAS), it is worthwhile to briefly consider the technical aspects of pulse sequence selection, artifacts, and approaches to limiting their impact on image quality and perspectives on the future evolution of these methodologies.

Pulse Sequences

Broadly speaking, there are three major potential components to the comprehensive vascular MR examination of the PAS: (1) high-resolution depiction of the pulmonary arteries themselves, (2) assessment of lung perfusion and defects thereof, and (3) quantification of blood flow in the main PA and its branches. Although not all sequences may be required for every clinical examination, a fundamental understanding of all aspects of a comprehensive pulmonary MRA examination is necessary to develop appropriate protocols for a variety of clinical indications.

High spatial-resolution contrast enhanced magnetic resonance angiography

In the past, non–contrast-enhanced time-of-flight (TOF) was the primary technique used for assessment of the pulmonary arteries; however, contrast-enhanced MRA has emerged as the current standard method. In TOF imaging, signal enhancement depends on the velocity of flowing blood and the pattern of blood flow (and is sometimes referred to as "in-flow enhancement"). Although flow sensitive, it is hampered by limited spatial resolution, insensitivity to very slow flow, and artifacts related to a number of factors including poor background tissue suppression, magnetic field inhomogeneities, motion, and saturation effects.[1] In contradistinction, the mechanism of contrast in CE-MRA is the T1 shortening of blood by an exogenous gadolinium chelate and is much less dependent on blood velocity itself. As a result, CE-MRA offers superior tissue contrast, high spatial and temporal resolution, and can be less sensitive to

motion and susceptibility artifacts compared with TOF. However, it requires accurate timing of the contrast bolus for two main reasons: (1) to ensure that the central portion (the "contrast-determining" portion) of k-space is acquired during the period of peak concentration of gadolinium within the pulmonary arteries to optimize image contrast and (2) to limit venous contamination of the MRA (ie, signal from pulmonary veins). Proper timing is achieved by either administering a test bolus (1 to 2 mL) or using an automatic triggering method timed to the main pulmonary artery, as bolus arrival timing varies depending on injection rate/volume and circulation time. A normal saline flush immediately following the contrast bolus is needed to ensure infusion of the entire contrast bolus. When using a bolus-tracking method with inversion recovery pre pulses, centric reordering of k space is warranted, as the peak arterial enhancement occurs at the beginning of the acquisition and should correspond to the central filling of k space. High-resolution CE-MRA is typically performed before and following administration of contrast using a 3-dimensional (3D) gradient-echo sequence with a very short repetition time (TR)/echo time (TE) (<5/<2 ms) such as a fast low angle single shot (FLASH) (flip angle typically 25° but may be higher or lower depending on field strength and desired background suppression) (Fig. 1). Fat suppression is not necessary and slightly lengthens scan time but may sometimes be used to reduce the conspicuity of wraparound (spatial aliasing) artifacts. In addition, fat suppression may cause artifact when using a 3D spoiled gradient-echo sequence leading to inadvertent signal loss within blood vessels.[2,3] Post processing with subtraction is useful for further reduction in background tissue and permits a more appealing display of volume-rendered (VR) and maximum intensity projection (MIP) images for referring clinicians (Fig. 1). Acquisition is usually in the coronal or coronal oblique plane to minimize scan time, as fewer partitions are required in the anterior-posterior direction when compared with other planes in human subjects. Alternatively, imaging can be performed with a dual-injection approach similar to conventional DSA using a smaller sagittal field of view over one hemithorax at a time to improved spatial resolution.[4] Resolution may vary depending on the technical capability of magnet systems but optimally, in-plane resolution should permit visualization of small (<1 mm) subsegmental vessels. Isotropic resolution is desirable to reduce stair-step artifacts in off-axis reconstructed planes. However, in patients with compromised respiratory function, breath-holding capability is

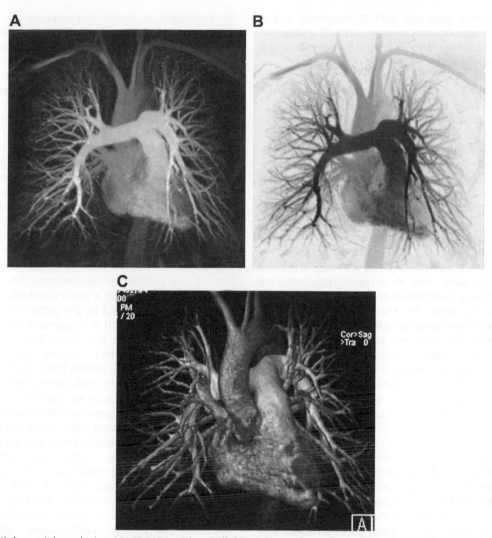

Fig. 1. High spatial resolution 3D CE MRA with parallel imaging with an acceleration factor of 2 in a 44-year-old male patient with shortness of breath and suspected pulmonary embolism. There was no evidence of filling defect or perfusional abnormality. Normal pulmonary arterial anatomy is demonstrated on the maximum intensity projection (MIP) (*A*), inverted MIP (*B*), and volume-rendered images (*C*).

limited and whereas most healthy patients can breath hold for at least 20 seconds, many patients referred for pulmonary MRA have a lower threshold. Acquisition time needs to be shortened to limit respiratory motion typically at the cost of spatial resolution. However, in such circumstances, parallel imaging (eg, sensitivity encoding [SENSE], simultaneous acquisition of spatial harmonics [SMASH], array spatial sensitivity encoding technique [ASSET]) may be implemented for improved temporal resolution.

To review, parallel imaging undersamples lines of k space data and recovers that information either before or after Fourier transform using coil sensitivity profiles of multielement coil arrays surrounding the patient.[5,6] Implementation of

parallel imaging compromises the signal-to-noise ratio (SNR) in a predictable way but it does allow for a significant increase in temporal and/or spatial resolution.[6] Parallel imaging may be used simply to accelerate the time of acquisition but can alternatively be used to increase spatial resolution without sacrificing scan time. Although parallel imaging may be used, it can lead to wraparound artifacts especially in larger patients and when used in combination with rectangular field of view. In the authors' experience, at 1.5 T, accelerations of two- to threefold may be performed for pulmonary MRA with excellent results despite the sacrifice in SNR. Other methods can be used to improve overall SNR when implementing parallel imaging such as using higher order multichannel coils (eg, with 32 elements) and/or higher magnetic field strength (>1.5 T) or high relaxivity contrast agents that are now becoming clinically available.[7,8]

Time-resolved magnetic resonance angiography–imaging of perfusion dynamics

Time-resolved MRA is a general term that refers to high temporal rate imaging performed with a modified 3D gradient-echo sequence. Data sets are acquired sequentially over time yielding a 4-dimensional (3D + time) view of the vessels of interest. This approach also permits one or more arterial-phase data sets free from venous contamination to be acquired, depending on the temporal resolution. Because multiple data sets are rapidly obtained over time, this strategy obviates the need for a timing run or bolus-tracking. The most straightforward way to achieve high temporal resolution is to reduce spatial resolution to reduce acquisition time. In recent years, additional methods have become available to permit higher temporal rates with less compromise for spatial resolution. Available methods include parallel imaging and alternative k-space filling such as keyhole and dynamic view sharing. Briefly, with view-sharing techniques such as time resolved imaging of contrast kinetics (TRICKS),[9] the center of k space (the center contributes most to image contrast) is sampled more frequently than the periphery (contributes most to edge detail). Essentially, this method improves temporal resolution by not sampling all of k space during each acquisition of data; instead, the undersampled high spatial frequency information in the periphery of k space is interpolated (ie, shared) between data sets (**Fig. 2**). Furthermore, spiral[10] or radial (eg, vastly undersampled isotropic-voxel radial projection imaging [VIPR])[11] k-space readout trajectories offer some reconstruction advantages as alternate interleaved "subscans" include both central and peripheral k-space sampling. Parallel imaging can be, in principle, combined with any of the above techniques in one or more directions to accelerate imaging and perhaps eventually match or even exceed the temporal resolution of x-ray DSA. Mask based reconstruction using a highly constrained back projection (HYPR) approach, including HYPR-VIPR[12] potentially offers dramatic temporal resolution improvement with reduced artifact and good separation of arterial and venous enhancement. This has yet to be established in time-resolved imaging of the pulmonary vasculature.

By using very high temporal-imaging methods, MRA becomes more like DSA with near "real-time" visualization of blood flow and the potential for estimation of global and regional perfusion. Although the pulmonary arteries themselves are not well depicted because spatial resolution is typically compromised for high temporal rate acquisition, the presence or absence of perfusion within a given vascular territory serves as an indirect sign of the patency or occlusion of the vessels supplying that region. In this sense, perfusion images are analogous to nuclear medicine perfusion images (using intravenous Tc-99 m–labeled macro-aggregated human albumin [MAA]), although higher spatial resolution is achievable with MR (this continues to improve with advances in parallel-imaging technology and alternative k-space sampling). The goal in MR gadolinium chelate–enhanced perfusion (MR perfusion) is not only to qualitatively assess perfusion but more importantly to demonstrate and quantify blood flow to the pulmonary parenchyma. The signal intensity changes within a given voxel reflects the T1 shortening produced by the administered gadolinium chelate, which is dependent on gadolinium concentration in the blood; thus, one can estimate regional blood volume from signal enhancement. At the present time, state-of-the-art pulmonary perfusion MRA takes advantage of high performance gradients, parallel imaging, and view sharing. First pass gadolinium pulmonary perfusion techniques have vastly improved in both temporal and spatial resolution over a very short period of time. Initially, imaging was performed using low spatial resolution 2D and 3D single and multislice techniques with relatively long acquisition times.[13–15] Soon thereafter, 3D acquisitions were explored with temporal resolution of 3 to 7 seconds using high performance gradients without parallel acquisition.[16–20] With the implementation of parallel-imaging techniques, less than 1.5-second 3D acquisitions have become achievable in the clinical setting[21,22] and, furthermore, parallel imaging may be combined with view sharing for further reduction in acquisition time or to maintain high temporal resolution of 1.5 seconds but with improved spatial resolution ($1.87 \times 3.74 \times 4$ mm^3).[23,24]

There have been many studies exploring gadolinium contrast-enhanced pulmonary perfusion MR for a variety of indications including pulmonary embolism,[15,25–27] chronic pulmonary hypertension,[28,29] pneumonia,[30] lung cancer pre[21] and post surgery,[31] lung diseases such as chronic obstructive pulmonary disease[32] and cystic fibrosis,[33] preoperative planning prior resection in cancer, pre- and postoperative assessment of congenital heart disease,[34] and post pulmonary venous ablation for atrial fibrillation to assess venous stenoses.[35] Gadolinium-based first-pass

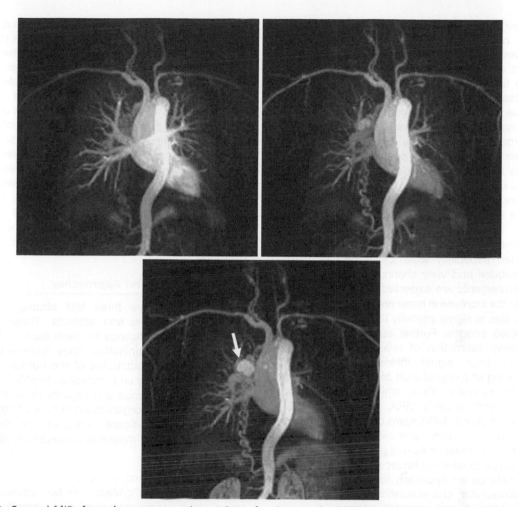

Fig. 2. Coronal MIPs from three separate time points of a time-resolved MRA performed with parallel imaging and view sharing (time resolved echo sharing angiographic technique) at 1.5 T with a temporal resolution of 3.3 seconds. Images demonstrate a right pulmonary AVM (*arrow*). Sequential imaging permits depiction of the AVM as it fills with contrast over time and demonstrates the feeding arterial branches from the mesenteric circulation distinct from the draining pulmonary veins. (*Courtesy of* Henrik J. Michaely, Mannheim, Germany.)

perfusion may be measured qualitatively, assessing for perfusion defects, semiquantitatively using signal intensity-time curves, or quantitatively using indicator-dilution theory and kinetic modeling. Quantitative analysis using indicator-dilution theory assumes there is no extravasation of contrast during the first pass of contrast through the lungs and pulmonary circulation. Quantification is based on knowledge of an arterial input function (AIF) and tissue concentration of gadolinium over time using deconvolution analysis.[36,37] Using this model, several parameters may be calculated including pulmonary blood flow (PBF), pulmonary blood volume (PBV), and the mean transit time (MTT), related by the central volume principle. There are several limitations that could lead to inherent errors in this methodology as

certain assumptions are made to implement this method of quantitative analysis. Although a complete review of perfusion is beyond the scope of this review, in brief, limitations stem from the assumption that measured signal changes correlate linearly with local gadolinium chelate concentration, which is likely of limited validity, especially at higher concentrations. In fact, low doses of gadolinium are recommended for subsequent perfusion analysis to avoid saturation effects caused by high concentrations of gadolinium at the peak of the bolus. In addition, this method assumes that gadolinium remains in the blood vessels at all times and does not leak into the interstitium, an assumption that is invalid in most of the capillaries of the body (but true, for example, in the presence of the intact blood brain barrier). Last, in this model an output function, ie, the pulmonary vein, should be measured. However, in practice to obtain regional assessment of flow, regions of interest are placed on lung tissue rather than pulmonary veins, which relates to gadolinium contrast agent remaining in tissue rather than a true output measure. It should be noted that the widespread CT perfusion approach is limited by very similar considerations.[38] Despite these potential pitfalls, an early study by Hatabu and colleagues[25] demonstrated good correlation between microsphere estimation of lung perfusion and MR perfusion measures in a pig model. Additional studies have since used this quantitative methodology in clinical patients,[29,39,40] although further validation is needed especially when using parallel imaging techniques and view sharing, as signal intensity measurements are expected to be more variable given the increase in noise and the spatial inhomogeneities in signal intensity throughout the reconstructed images. Further approaches based on dynamic estimation of relaxation rate changes (rather than signal intensity) and including modeling of extravasation are promising avenues of development. Thus, while a straightforward multiphasic dynamic MRA, or a short series of "time-resolved" MRA scans during bolus administration of a contrast agent can readily give a visual sense, or qualitative view of perfusion, it is encouraging to consider the kinetic modeling of dynamic CE data as an approach toward describing the microvascular characteristics of the pulmonary vascular system in quantitative terms.

Phase-contrast magnetic resonance angiography

In the context of pulmonary MR angiography, phase-contrast (PC)-MRA is used primarily for quantitative estimation of flow and determination of pressure gradients to complement the morphologic information provided by CE-MRA. A bipolar phase-encoding gradient is applied inducing velocity-dependent phase shifts in moving blood while stationary tissue remains unaffected.[41] Velocity images are generated by determining net phase shifts between two complex (real and imaginary) data sets with and without flow encoding gradients (or with pairs of flow encoding gradients with reversed polarity). Signal intensity on these velocity images is directly proportional to net phase shifts and, in turn, the velocity offlowing blood with the bright signal representing positive phase shifts (and by convention, positive velocities). The magnitude and duration of the velocity-encoding gradient determines the maximum

velocity that can be encoded over the phase range of $-180°$ to $+180°$. Before acquisition, the operator selects the encoding velocity (VENC), thereby determining the dynamic range of velocities that can be measured. This range should be selected to be slightly larger than the expected peak velocity of flow within the vessel of interest or aliasing will occur and lead to ambiguity of measurement. The ascending and descending aorta and the main, left, and right pulmonary arteries can be individually interrogated for assessment of flow and bronchosystemic shunting can also be calculated pre- and postintervention. This technique is most often used for congenital heart disease but could be useful for assessment of pulmonary hypertension for a number of etiologies.

Issues, Artifacts, and Approaches

Affecting the above three MR strategies are a number of issues and artifacts. These may have differing significance for each aspect of the comprehensive examination. They arise in large part from peculiar attributes of the human lung: (1) cardiac pulsatility and respiration tend to cause movement of the lungs and vessels within them, and (2) lung tissue organization includes large air spaces with significant tissue:air interfaces, leading to profound magnetic susceptibility differences and artifacts.

Respiratory and cardiac motion
Respiratory motion artifact can be reduced by using high temporal resolution breath-hold imaging. For most healthy patients, a 20-second breath-hold for a high-resolution CE pulmonary MRA is acceptable but for many patients this is exceedingly long and not tolerated. Even higher temporal resolution gadolinium chelate–enhanced imaging is certainly feasible but typically at the cost of spatial resolution, which not only may be acceptable in certain clinical scenarios but can be acceptable when assessing lung perfusion. Other technologic advances such as parallel imaging and high field imaging can be used to improve temporal resolution with reduced compromise of spatial resolution.

To compensate for cardiac motion, electrocardiogram (ECG)-gated cine gradient echo and steady state free precession techniques (SSFP) are used in daily practice for assessment of dynamic and functional flow assessment in congenital heart disease. Rapidly acquired non-ECG gated 2D and 3D SSFP non–contrast-enhanced MRA techniques can be performed for morphologic assessment and have great potential for patients who may not be candidates for

gadolinium chelate contrast agents such as pregnant patients or patients on dialysis. ECG-gated
3D gradient-echo CE-MRA is also now feasible
and may be performed in a breath hold but studies
are limited for application to pulmonary MRA
although it has been shown helpful for assessment
of mediastinal tumor invasion.[42] Depending on
patient heart rate, the resolution of ECG-gated
CE-MRA may be limited to keep scan time within
a reasonable breath hold.

Susceptibility effects

The low proton density of the lung parenchyma and
the extensive soft tissue–air interfaces at the level
of the alveoli lead to extremely rapid decay of transverse magnetization, ie, short T2*, ranging on
average from 0.86 to 2.18 ms.[43–45] Interaction
between air and tissue at the microscopic level
leads to signal loss from intravoxel phase dispersion and inhomogeneities within a static magnetic
field, which increase with increasing field strength.
The degree of oxygenation, lung expansion, and
patient positioning can dynamically accentuate
these effects.[43] Global and regional field inhomogeneities can cause signal loss within arterial
segments that have large interfaces with aerated
lung, which can lead to inaccurate depiction
and interpretation of arterial stenosis or a luminal
filling defect. Currently available gradient-echo
sequences for a high spatial-resolution 3D acquisition are performed with very short TR and TE. Short
TR (< 5 ms) permits large field of view imaging
within a breath hold and keeps background signal
to a minimum. Short TE reduces susceptibility artifacts and keeps flow-related dephasing effects to
a minimum. It should be noted that to achieve the
necessary short TE times, these fast gradient-
echo sequences rely on a high-performance
gradient system (gradient amplitude at least 30 to
45 mT/m, slew rates 120 to 200 T/m/s).

Remergence of Nongadolinium Magnetic Resonance Angiography Techniques in the Era of Nephrogenic Systemic Fibrosis

Despite the advantages of CE-MRA strategies for
depiction of the pulmonary arterial system, these
techniques still may not be suitable for some
patients. Not all patients are appropriate candidates for intravenous gadolinium chelate contrast
agents because of inadequate intravenous
access, renal dysfunction, or pregnancy. It is well
know that administration of gadolinium chelates
is not without the potential risk of renal toxicity
and has recently been implicated in the development of nephrogenic systemic fibrosis (NSF),
a potentially debilitating and fatal disease that

almost exclusively occurs in patients on dialysis
or in acute or severe renal failure.[46]

In light of such concerns, alternative non–gadolinium-enhanced (NG) contrast mechanisms need
be explored and validated. Conventional TOF
MRA, still used in head and neck imaging, offers
high spatial resolution but even with parallel
imaging is not as competitive with gadolinium
enhanced because of relatively long scan times
and the degrading impact of respiratory motion
leading to obscuration of small vessels and artifacts. Currently, true fast imaging with steady state
free precession (True FISP) holds the most
promise for clinical implementation because of
its high signal to noise and rapid acquisition time.

Arterial spin labeling, which can be combined
with SSFP and ECG-gated fast spin echo, has
been explored for pulmonary perfusion but
remains a research tool. Other sequences such
as ECG-gated fast spin echo (discussed later)
are now available but are less well established.
Of course, phase-contrast and cine MR
sequences using gradient echo or steady state
precession do not require gadolinium contrast
and are part of routine clinical protocols when
flow and functional parameters are required, suggesting the possibility of a comprehensive non–
contrast-enhanced imaging examination of the
pulmonary arterial circulation.

True fast imaging with steady state free precession

With balanced SSFP sequences, image contrast is
dependent not on blood flow or (strongly on) exogenous contrast agents but rather on the intrinsic
properties of tissue. Image contrast reflects the
T2/T1 ratio of tissues, leading to high signal for
blood without depending on TOF effects. The
impact of gadolinium-based contrast agents on
image contrast in these sequences is markedly
reduced compared with conventional gradient-
recalled echo (GRE) techniques (because gadolinium affects both T2 and T1, their ratio is not
particularly sensitive to its presence). As a result,
the loss of flow signal resulting from slow, turbulent,
or in-plane flow that challenged early attempts at
TOF MRA is less significant for this technique,
although destruction of the "steady state," which
may result from these effects in the presence of
magnetic field inhomogeneity, can lead to signal
degradation. Given that the image contrast in these
sequences is based on the intrinsic properties of
blood, high signal can be seen in both arteries
and veins making distinction between these
vessels challenging. Thus, for MRA applications,
selective preparatory pulses or saturation bands
are used to reduce venous signal. Currently, the

major applications in the chest for SSFP are 2D ECG-gated cine MR to assess cardiac contractility and valve function or 3D SSFP for anatomic imaging of the coronaries and thoracic aorta with ECG gating and diaphragmatic navigation. In addition, with SSFP sequences, entire slices can be acquired extremely rapidly to allow for real-time imaging. Finally, the high flip angle typically used for balanced SSFP contributes to a very high SNR relative to its speed; because of the high SNR, SSFP is amenable to use with parallel imaging.

Kluge and colleagues[47,48] have performed a number of clinical studies using real-time balanced SSFP (True FISP). In these studies, images were obtained in real-time with free-breathing and no respiratory or cardiac gating. To further demonstrate the robustness of the technique, acquisition began immediately after the patient was placed on the table and centered within the magnet; there was no adjustment of sequence parameters or of slice position or orientation for individual patients. Such an approach may facilitate identifying a central pulmonary embolism in a critically ill patient in as little time as possible. In an initial clinical trial of this technique in 39 patients with suspected pulmonary embolism in 2004, Kluge and colleagues[47] performed real-time 2D true FISP at 1.5 T to provide comprehensive coverage of the entire thorax by obtaining contiguous 50% overlapping slices in three orthogonal large-field-of-view planes. Individual slices with a thickness of 3 to 4 mm were acquired in 0.40 to 0.52 seconds, for a total examination time of less than 3 minutes. True FISP MRA had sensitivity and specificity of 93% and 100% per patient compared with high spatial-resolution CE-MRA, and sensitivity and specificity of 83% and 100% in a subset of 17 patients who also had perfusion scintigraphy. Overall, real-time true FISP was deemed capable of demonstrating pulmonary embolism in a fast and robust manner in critically ill patients.

Using a somewhat different technique, Hui and colleagues[49] attempted balanced SSFP for MRA using a 3D acquisition with both cardiac and respiratory navigator gating permitting higher spatial resolution. In volunteers, the free-breathing acquisition required on average 180 ± 79 seconds and produced images that were subjectively graded to be equal in image quality to 3D balanced SSFP images obtained in a 30-second breath-hold. This approach has yet to be studied for MRA in a clinical setting.

Arterial spin labeling

Arterial spin labeling (ASL) offers a method for assessing perfusion without requiring exogenous contrast agents. ASL essentially uses magnetically labeled blood as an endogenous contrast agent by applying an inversion radiofrequency pulse to selectively tag spins upstream of the vessel or organ of interest. Separate acquisitions with and without the tagging pulse are obtained and subtracted to remove background signal (**Fig. 3**). While subtraction of the two images leads to a perfusion "weighted" image, modeling of signal intensity and knowledge of T1 can allow quantitative assessment of perfusion as has been repeatedly demonstrated in the brain.[50,51] To obtain pulmonary perfusion images, cardiac blood is tagged by an inversion pulse and imaging is performed repeatedly with varying delays to demonstrate the circulation of tagged blood through the lungs. Although Mai and colleagues[52,53] have performed a number of studies that demonstrate the feasibility of ASL techniques for imaging pulmonary perfusion in healthy human subjects and in animal models of pulmonary embolism, the technique has yet to be studied in a clinical setting and is currently of indeterminate value for routine practice. ASL can be a challenging technique to perform, as it suffers from low signal to noise and is extremely vulnerable to susceptibility and motion artifacts.

CLINICAL PROTOCOL

Clinical CE-MRA should be performed on at least a 1.5-T field strength magnet with a high strength gradient system and parallel imaging capability. Before placing the patient into the bore of the magnet, a 20-g intravenous catheter is placed into an antecubital vein and connected to a power injector. A multichannel phased array coil is placed around the thorax. Two liters per minute of oxygen should be administered via nasal cannula if the patient is dyspneic or seems likely to have difficulty with breath-holding. The patient is then placed supine in the magnet, with arms raised above his or her head if possible to limit wraparound artifacts. Initial scout sequences of the thorax are obtained using an ultrafast imaging sequence such as 2D true FISP or HASTE. The scouts are used to prescribe a coronal field-of-view that is large enough to cover both lungs in their entirety and reduce wraparound artifacts but small enough to maintain adequate spatial resolution. An initial mask of a high-resolution 3D T1 GRE data set is acquired in a breath hold at end expiration and images are checked for artifact; if there are artifacts, adjustment is made and the sequence repeated. Before obtaining the CE-MRA acquisition, a timing run may be used to assess the delay between contrast

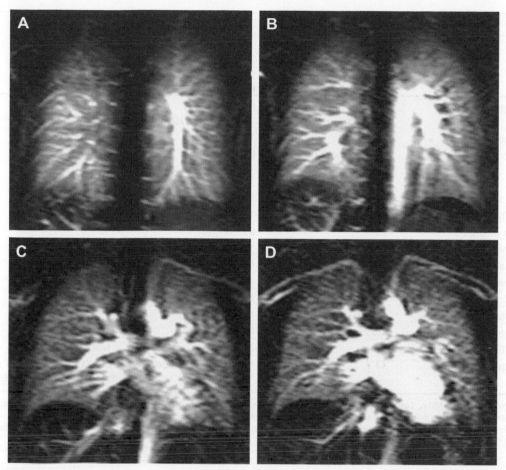

Fig. 3. (*A–D*) Arterial spin labeling (ASL) perfusion imaging in a 20-year-old pregnant patient with shortness of breath and suspected pulmonary embolism. Nonexogenous contrast-enhanced ASL demonstrates normal perfusion to both lungs without evidence of pulmonary embolism. (*Courtesy of* Quen Chen, PhD, New York, NY.)

administration and peak concentration within the main pulmonary artery or a bolus-tracking technique may be used. If time-resolved technique is used, a timing run is not necessary but the patient should be asked to suspend respiration for as long as possible to reduce motion artifact. Protocol details will vary depending on field strength, gradient strength, and performance and the availability of parallel-imaging or view-sharing techniques (**Table 1**).

CLINICAL INDICATIONS
Acute Pulmonary Embolism

Pulmonary embolism (PE) has an annual incidence of approximately 60 cases per 100,000 in the community[54] and approximately 1000 cases per 100,000 in the hospital setting.[55] PE may be associated with substantial morbidity and mortality, with one study finding a 3-month mortality of about

15%.[56] The diagnosis is often challenging to make, as the signs and symptoms may be subtle and nonspecific, often overlapping the presentation of other common cardiopulmonary disorders. Indeed, in one autopsy series of patients who died of PE, the diagnosis was not suspected before death in 70% of cases.[55] When the diagnosis is missed, the risk of a fatal recurrence has been estimated to be about 30%.[57,58]

In the past, catheter angiography was considered the gold standard for diagnosis of PE. However, a study from 1998 estimated that about one third of subsegmental emboli may be missed with angiography.[59] In addition, catheter angiography is an invasive procedure, with one study of 1111 cases reporting a mortality of 0.5% and morbidity of 6.0%.[60] More recently, multidetector-CT (MDCT) has revolutionized the diagnosis of acute PE by offering a fast, widely available, noninvasive test with high spatial

Table 1
Imaging parameters based on review of the current literature

	High-Resolution CE-MRA	Time-Resolved Perfusion MRA	Real Time Nongated Steady State Free Precession
Authors	Kluge and colleagues 2006[48]	Nikolaou and colleagues 2005[89]	Kluge and colleagues 2006[48]
Sequence	3D FLASH	3D FLASH	Real Time True FISP
IV contrast	0.125 mmol/kg @ 4 mL/sec + 20 mL saline flush	0.1 mmol/kg @ 5 mL/sec + 20 mL saline flush	None
Fat suppression	Yes	NA	No
TR/TE (in ms)	3.2/1.4	1.7/0.6	3.1/1.5
Flip angle (°)	25	25	59
Bandwidth	1500 Hz/pixel	1220 Hz/Pixel	975 Hz/Pixel
Parallel imaging	GRAPPA, R = 2	GRAPPA, R = 2	None
View sharing	None	None	None
Field of view (in mm)	350	400	340–360
Matrix	512 × 384	133 × 256	156 - 192 × 256[a]
Slice thickness (in mm)	1.5	4	3–4
Partitions	72	24	Not available
Acquisition time	14 s	1.1 s/phase; 26 s for 24 phases	0.4–0.5 s per slice; 3 min to obtain 320 slices[a]

Abbreviations: CE-MRA, contrast-enhanced magnetic resonance angiography; FISP, fast imaging with steady state free precession; FLASH, fast low angle shot; GRAPPA; TE, echo time; TR, repetition time; 3D, 3 dimensional.
[a] Three orthogonal planes were obtained (120 transverse + 100 coronal and sagittal acquired with 50% overlapping slices).

resolution that can visualize the pulmonary arteries to the subsegmental level while simultaneously assessing the remainder of the thorax for alternate diagnoses. On this basis, MDCT has replaced angiography as the primary test for the diagnosis of acute PE.[61-64]

MR imaging provides a cross-sectional depiction of the pulmonary arteries, as does CT, and may also have a role in the diagnosis of acute PE. Like CT, pulmonary MRA can be performed in conjunction with MR venography of the lower extremities. Moving table technology combined with integrated coil technology permits imaging of different sites of interest within the same examination without having to reposition the patient or the coils.

MR imaging findings
Acute pulmonary embolism may be recognized on MR images as either a partial or complete arterial occlusive filling defect similar to the features on CT and x-ray angiography.[65-68] A partially occlusive filling defect may appear as a central or marginal filling defect that forms an acute angle

with the vessel wall and is separated from the vessel well by a small amount of contrast. A completely occlusive filling defect is visualized as a concave filling defect at the point of obstruction of an enhancing vessel that represents the trailing edge of the embolus (**Figs. 4** to **7**).[65,69-71]

With perfusion imaging, pulmonary embolism is diagnosed by identifying peripheral wedge-shaped perfusion defects, analogous to the interpretation of a nuclear medicine perfusion scan. The pattern of the perfusion abnormality may be useful in distinguishing PE from other causes of altered perfusion. For instance, perfusion abnormalities resulting from chronic obstructive pulmonary disease (COPD) have been described as more coarse or heterogeneous, rather than the focal wedge-shaped defects characteristic of PE.[30,72] In addition, wedge-shaped perfusion defects related to focal areas of emphysema may be identified by the presence of a subpleural rind of preserved perfusion.[72]

However, the interpretation of MRA for acute pulmonary embolism is subject to a number of imaging pitfalls. Suboptimal timing of the contrast

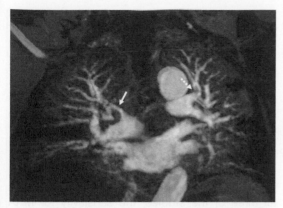

Fig. 4. Coronal MIP of a CE-MRA in a 60-year-old male with shortness of breath demonstrating an embolus at the bifurcation of the distal right pulmonary artery (*arrow*) extending into the right lobar pulmonary arteries and nonocclusive filling defects in the distal left-pulmonary artery extending into upper (*dotted arrow*) and lower lobar branches. Associated bilateral perfusion defects are demonstrated.

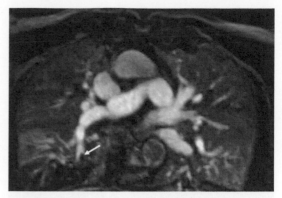

Fig. 6. Axial reconstruction of CE-MRA in an 82-year-old male with chest pain demonstrates a filling defect within a right posterior basal sub segmental branch pulmonary artery. Concave meniscus of the filling defect (*arrow*) at the point of occlusion is consistent with the trailing edge of the embolus and is associated with a perfusional defect.

bolus, poor breath holding, wraparound artifacts, and susceptibility differences at vessel-air interfaces within the lung all may degrade image quality (**Fig. 8**). As previously discussed, the latest imaging strategies using state-of-the-art equipment serve to minimize these effects. It is within this context that visualization of pulmonary arterial branches to the subsegmental level may become feasible, raising the possibility of using CE-MRA as a primary diagnostic test for acute pulmonary embolism.

Magnetic resonance angiography versus CT angiography for pulmonary embolism

Dozens of studies have demonstrated the use of MRA for evaluating the pulmonary arteries. Yet, it remains difficult to compare the sensitivity and specificity of this technique with CTA. This difficulty is in large part attributable to the continuing and rapid advances in MR technology that may

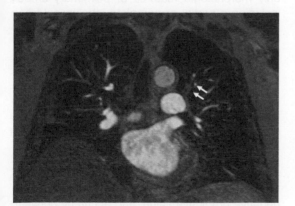

Fig. 5. Coronal image from a CE-MRA in a 49-year-old male with metastatic prostate cancer, known deep venous thrombosis, and shortness of breath demonstrates an embolus within the apical posterior segmental branch of the left upper lobar artery (*arrows*). A small amount of contrast separating the thrombus from the vessel walls creates a tram-track appearance.

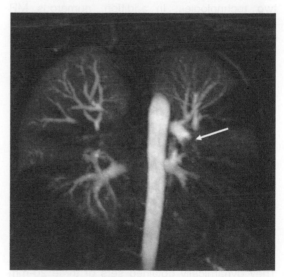

Fig. 7. Coronal MIP of a subtracted data set from a CE-MRA in a 22-year-old female with chest pain and shortness of breath demonstrates a large occlusive embolus in a left lower lobe segmental pulmonary artery (*arrow*). Numerous bilateral perfusional defects are also present and additional images revealed extensive bilateral pulmonary emboli.

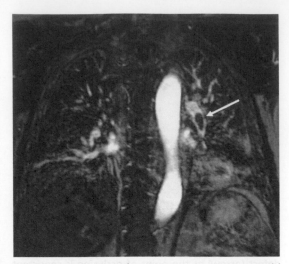

Fig. 8. Coronal MIP of a CE-MRA in a 75-year-old female with chest pain demonstrates an intravascular filling defect (*arrow*) consistent with pulmonary embolus extending from the lobar to the segmental branches of the left lower lobe pulmonary artery. The embolus is clearly visualized despite the suboptimal timing of the contrast bolus, with greater enhancement of the thoracic aorta than of the pulmonary arteries.

render the results of an earlier trial outdated. Indeed, studies of MRA that did not use a 3D acquisition, parallel imaging, or even an exogenous contrast agent, cannot be considered relevant in making an accurate comparison of the two technologies. In addition, numerous MR studies have been limited in their design, for instance lacking a definitive diagnostic test to use as a gold standard, not determining sensitivity and specificity, or studying healthy volunteers rather than actual patients. Indeed, a review of the literature in 2003 by Stein and colleagues[73] found that of 28 studies of the use of CE-MRA for diagnosing pulmonary embolism published up to that point, only 3 met strict criteria for inclusion in an analysis of the sensitivity and specificity of the modality. It is within this framework that we provide an overview of the literature comparing MRA and CTA in the setting of suspected acute pulmonary embolism.

Loubeyre and colleagues[71] published the first study that used CE-MRA to diagnose acute pulmonary embolism in a clinical setting in 1994. They dynamically obtained sets of three 20-mm thick 2D slices of the pulmonary arteries for about a minute during free breathing. Using this basic technique, the authors achieved a sensitivity of 70% and specificity of 100%, with conventional angiography as the gold standard. However, CE-MRA missed all six of the peripheral emboli in their

study sample. A large number of studies published during the ensuing decade were generally of limited clinical value for accurately assessing sensitivity and specificity. The three articles during this time to be identified by Stein and colleagues[73] as meeting their inclusion criteria were by Meaney and colleagues in 1997,[65] Gupta and colleagues in 1999,[74] and Oudkerk and colleagues in 2002.[4] The study by Oudkerk and colleagues had the largest sample size, assessing CE-MRA compared with pulmonary angiography 118 patients. These articles found respective sensitivities of 100%, 85%, and 77%, and specificities of 95%, 96%, and 98%. In all three of the studies, the sensitivity for MRA decreased for more peripheral arterial branches. Additional subsequent studies by Blum and colleagues in 2005[75] and Plezewski and colleagues in 2006[76] obtained similar results, demonstrating excellent specificity and a more limited sensitivity for MRA. Although none of these studies used parallel imaging, all used a 3D gradient-echo acquisition. This technique allowed for a reasonable spatial resolution; however, temporal resolution remained limited, requiring relatively long breath holds for a single acquisition, compared with subsequently developed approaches.

Ohno and colleagues[77] in 2004 was the first to examine pulmonary MRA with parallel imaging in a clinical cohort. Forty-eight patients with suspected pulmonary embolism underwent ventilation/perfusion scintigraphy, MDCT, conventional angiography, and time-resolved CE-MRA using an acceleration factor of 3 (SENSE) resulting in a temporal resolution of 4 seconds and a voxel size of 0.7 × 1.0 × 5 mm. Readers assessed not only morphologic features of pulmonary emboli including a partial or complete intraluminal filling defect, the railway track sign, and mural defects but also decreased areas of perfusion with or without associated filling defect. On a per-patient basis, sensitivity and specificity were 92% and 94% respectively, already considerably better sensitivity than previously reported. These improved results likely represent a combination of their use of a time-resolved technique, increased in-plane resolution, and inclusion of perfusion abnormalities in image interpretation. Interestingly, there was no significant difference in sensitivity, specificity, positive predictive value, negative predictive value, and accuracy between MR and CT on a per-patient basis. On a per-vessel basis, MR had a sensitivity of 100% for central embolus and 68% for peripheral embolus, which was in fact significantly better than the 54% sensitivity of MDCT for peripheral embolus. False positives on MR were predominantly related to perfusional defects in peripheral vascular regions and were attributed to susceptibility, motion and flow-related artifacts, and superimposition of pulmonary veins on pulmonary arteries. False negatives for perfusion resulted from incomplete peripheral vascular obstruction not associated with perfusional defects.

A more recent study by Kluge and colleagues[48] from 2006 compared the results of MR imaging and CT in 62 patients. The MR protocol consisted of three separate techniques. First, nonenhanced MRA was performed using a 2D true FISP sequence in three orthogonal planes to rule out large clot burden in critically ill patients. Contrast-enhanced high temporal rate MRA was performed without parallel imaging to allow for time-resolved imaging with a temporal resolution of 1.8 seconds compromising spatial resolution (voxel size $2.9 \times 1.6 \times 10$ mm) but permitting MR assessment of perfusion using a low dose of contrast 0.125 mmol/kg. Finally, after a second injection of similar dose of contrast material, high-spatial resolution MRA was performed using a 3D FLASH sequence with parallel imaging acceleration factor of 2, voxel size $0.7 \times 1.2 \times 1.5$ mm, and 14-second acquisition time. When all three techniques were examined in a combined fashion, MR had a sensitivity and specificity of 100% and 93% respectively, with a kappa value for interobserver agreement between MR and CT of 0.9. When comparing individual techniques, MR perfusion had a per-patient sensitivity and specificity of 100% and 91%, compared with values of 81% and 100% for high-resolution MRA. The high sensitivity of perfusion was attributable to its better performance for detecting peripheral emboli, as indicated by 93% sensitivity for subsegmental emboli compared with 55% for MRA. Although there were a few false-positive perfusional deficits because of underlying parenchymal disease, it is apparent that a split bolus combined MR protocol including perfusion and high spatial resolution MRA was as robust as MDCT, with the perfusion portion adding important value in detecting the consequence of subsegmental emboli and thereby conferring improved sensitivity.

In a more recent study, Ersoy and colleagues[78] 2007 used a time-resolved CE-MRA acquisition as a primary diagnostic test in 27 inpatients with suspected pulmonary embolism and a contraindication to iodinated contrast. MR as a primary screening test was able to confidently exclude or include pulmonary embolism in 96% of the patients. Although this study is limited, as it lacked a reference standard, and sensitivity and specificity were not obtained, it further emphasizes the importance of perfusion imaging for diagnosis of pulmonary emboli.

Based on these studies it is apparent that when using state-of-the-art technology, CE-MRA is comparable to CTA in assessing for acute pulmonary embolism. MRA has advantages over CTA in its ability to provide an assessment of pulmonary and right heart function (as discussed earlier) without the need for ionizing radiation and with less allergenic and nephrotoxic contrast agents. However, CTA does have several advantages including widespread availability on a 24-hour basis and is less costly. In addition, CT is quicker and easier for technologists to perform and provides an easier environment for monitoring of ill patients. Thus, it is unlikely that CE-MRA will replace CTA as the primary diagnostic test ordered in patients with suspected acute pulmonary embolism. Nonetheless, in experienced hands a roughly equivalent accuracy of state-of-the-art MRA and CTA can be achieved. Thus, we suggest a low threshold for using MR imaging as a first-line examination in patients in whom CTA is contraindicated or undesirable. These instances include allergy or other contraindication to iodinated contrast, inability to obtain intravenous access, and low suspicion for pulmonary embolism in a young female patient. In addition, MRA can be performed secondarily if the results of CTA are equivocal. Accordingly, CE-MRA ought not to be viewed as an up-and-coming technique for diagnosis of acute pulmonary embolism with potential for future use, but rather as a developed technique with clinical relevance for patient management at the present time. Indeed, a large multicenter trial, the Prospective Investigation of Pulmonary Embolism III (PIOPED), is currently in progress and aims to assess the diagnostic accuracy of CE-MRA (and MR venography) for the diagnosis of acute pulmonary embolism.

Chronic Thromboembolic Disease/Secondary Pulmonary Hypertension

Although the thromboembolic material resolves completely in most patients with an acute episode of pulmonary embolism, a fraction will proceed to develop chronic thromboembolic pulmonary hypertension (CTEPH). The incidence of symptomatic CTEPH is estimated to be about 4% after 2 years, significantly higher than previously reported.[79] The underlying mechanism of this process remains unclear, but likely involves recurrent episodes of occlusion and recanalization of thromboembolic material, in combination with in situ thrombosis and pulmonary small-vessel arteriopathy. The natural history of CTEPH entails a progressive rise in pulmonary pressure with subsequent progressive right heart failure and poor outcome. In patients with CTEPH and mean pulmonary arterial pressure greater than 30 mm Hg who are managed with anticoagulation, survival is estimated to be 50% after an average follow-up time of 18.7 months.[80]

Pulmonary endarterectomy (PEA) entails removal of organized thrombus that is adherent to the vessel well and can be of immediate and dramatic benefit in patients with CTEPH. This surgery restores flow to previously nonperfused segments, allowing for significant long-term improvements in pulmonary hemodynamics and right heart function, with concomitant improvements in quality of life and survival. Although PEA is being performed at an increasing rate as a result of improvements in surgical technique and increased awareness of the condition, not all patients are candidates for this surgery. The critical issue in determining the feasibility of PEA is the location of the thromboembolic material. Specifically, thrombus must be present within the main, lobar, or proximal segmental pulmonary arteries to be surgically accessible.[81]

The diagnostic workup of patients with CTEPH has traditionally been performed with CT and conventional angiography. MDCT provides for the localization of organized thrombus within the pulmonary arterial system, the central issue in assigning patients to medical or surgical management. Angiography with right heart catheterization and selective pulmonary angiography provides assessment of right heart function and pulmonary pressures.

MR can potentially provide the equivalent information in a single noninvasive test. By combining high spatial 3D CE-MRA with time-resolved acquisitions and ECG-gated flow-sensitive phase-contrast MR with cine MR, analysis of arterial morphology, perfusion, and cardiac function may be performed in a single study. Morphologic features of CTEPH include eccentric mural-based filling defects, intraluminal webs, stenoses, and abnormal vessel tapering and cut-offs (**Fig. 9**). Perfusion MR can identify perfusion defects that result from the small-vessel disease of distal pulmonary arteries and also play a role in the pathogenesis of CTEPH. However, at the present time this small vessel component of the disease process is not amenable to surgical correction. Finally, flow-sensitive phase-contrast MRA can provide estimates of pulmonary arterial pressure and function, whereas cine MR imaging permits assessment of right heart function, thereby evaluating the multiple key features of the disease process in a single examination.

Kreitner and colleagues[82] evaluated 34 patients with CTEPH before and after PEA using CE-MRA, phase-contrast MR, and cardiac cine MR, with correlation with DSA. MRA identified typical findings of CTEPH in all patients and performed better than DSA in identifying the precise proximal extent of thromboembolic material, which was found to correspond with surgical findings in all cases. Postoperatively, MRA demonstrated a reduction in diameter of the central pulmonary arteries and re-opening of segmental branches, as well as significant improvements in a number of hemodynamic parameters including right ventricular ejection fraction and pulmonary arterial peak velocity.

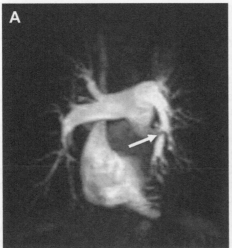 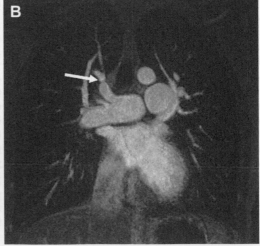

Fig. 9. Coronal MIP of (*A*) a time-resolved MRA and (*B*) a coronal image from a high-resolution MRA in a patient with CTEPH demonstrating webs and bands stenoses (*arrows*) and abnormal vessel tapering in the right upper and left lower lobes with associated well-defined perfusional defects. (*Courtesy of* Henrik J Michaely, Mannheim, Germany.)

Other studies have also demonstrated the ability of MR imaging to accurately identify the proximal extent of thromboembolic material compared with surgical findings[83] and to demonstrate post-operative improvements in hemodynamic parameters such as pulmonary peak velocity and right ventricular ejection fraction following PEA using phase-contrast and cine imaging.[84] Given the ability of MR imaging to answer the important clinical questions pre- and postoperatively, MR imaging has been suggested as a first-line test in the management of patients with CTEPH.[83,84]

Pulmonary Arterial Hypertension

In the revised 2003 World Health Organization (WHO) Clinical Classification of Pulmonary Hypertension, pulmonary arterial hypertension (PAH) is classified separately from CTEPH as well as from pulmonary hypertension associated with left heart disease, lung disease, or hypoxemia. PAH is subclassified as idiopathic, familial, or associated with other diseases that include collagen vascular disorders, portal hypertension, HIV infection, medications, toxins, and congenital pulmonary-systemic shunts.[85] The incidence of idiopathic PA is about 2 to 3 individuals per 1 million per year and has a female predominance.[86] Although not entirely understood, the pathophysiology of PAH is currently believed to entail a pathway that begins with constriction of the distal pulmonary vessels, which over time leads to irreversible remodeling of the vessel walls and increased pulmonary vascular resistance and arterial pressure. As with CTEPH, this increased pulmonary pressure in turn leads to worsening right heart function with associated impaired function and ultimately death. The presenting symptom is typically dyspnea with minimal activity.[87] Patients are primarily managed medically with vasodilatory agents, as prostacyclin therapy has been found to lead to improved functional status and survival.[88]

The role of imaging in the setting of PAH is twofold: first, it is essential to accurately distinguish PAH from CTEPH, as these conditions are primarily treated medically and surgically respectively; second, it is important to be able to perform a reliable functional evaluation to assess response to medical therapy. While right-heart catheterization is the gold-standard for diagnosing PAH, echocardiography has served as the routine noninvasive test for following patients.[87] MR imaging may play a role not just in both of these tasks, but also in assessing the distal pulmonary vessels using perfusion imaging in a way that is not possible with echo, DSA, or MDCT. This information is of particular importance in PAH given the

central role of the distal pulmonary vessels in its pathophysiology and the use of vasodilatory agents that target these vessels in its treatment.

Separate sets of imaging findings are described for CE-MRA and perfusion MR in differentiating CTEPH and PAH. On high-resolution CE-MRA, the nonocclusive changes of PAH are demonstrated, including dilatation of the main pulmonary artery, proximal caliber change, peripheral vessel reduction, focal vessel ectasia, or a tortuous course of the peripheral pulmonary arteries, whereas CTEPH may demonstrate any of these changes with at least one additional occlusive change manifested by complete vessel occlusion, free-floating thrombus, wall-adherent thrombus, or intraluminal webs and bands. On perfusion MR, PAH demonstrates diffuse and/or patchy faintly defined perfusion defects, whereas CTEPH demonstrates segmental and/or well-circumscribed focal defects. Multiple studies have shown the ability to accurately distinguish patients with PAH and CTEPH using a combination of these two MRA approaches.[89,90]

Prior attempts to correlate hemodynamic data obtained using phase-contrast MR with data from right heart catheterization in patients with PAH have had limited success.[91-93] Two more recent studies tried instead to correlate the results of a 3D quantitative perfusion technique with DSA, with more moderate success.[29,40] Although MR currently performs well in differentiating PAH and CTEPH, its ability to provide quantitative functional measurements comparable to DSA and echocardiography remains preliminary, with a number of approaches continuing to evolve. At present, MR can supplement but not replace the data obtained from invasive measures.

Pulmonary Arteriovenous Malformation

Pulmonary arteriovenous malformation (PAVM) represents an abnormal communication between a feeding pulmonary artery and draining pulmonary vein through a thin-walled aneurysm that is prone to slow growth over time. Approximately 70% of cases occur in patients with hereditary hemorrhagic telangiectasia (HHT), whereas approximately 15% to 35% of patients with HHT have PAVM.[94] Patients are at risk of massive hemorrhage as well as of serious neurologic events such as stroke, seizures, and brain abscesses. Because these complications may occur in previously asymptomatic patients, it is critical to be able to accurately screen for PAVM in patients with HHT and their first-degree relatives. Early detection allows for treatment via transcatheter embolization. Currently, embolization is recommended for all PAVMs with a feeding artery 3 mm or larger in size, regardless of the presence of symptoms, which has been found effective in reducing the risk of neurologic complications.[95]

No single screening test for PAVM is currently universally accepted. CT is considered the gold standard with a sensitivity of about 98% and the ability to accurately depict the morphology of PAVMs for treatment planning.[96] However, current recommendations call for extended surveillance of PAVMs given the possibility of slow growth over time of small PAVMs to a size that will ultimately require treatment.[95] This need for routine imaging follow-up makes the ionizing radiation of CT a particular concern in young patients. Some guidelines alternatively suggest the use of contrast echocardiography, perfusion scintigraphy, or blood gas exchange methods, all of which only indirectly indicate the presence of PAVM by identifying a right-to-left shunt.[94] DSA is an invasive test with an estimated sensitivity for PAVM of about 70% and therefore is only performed for the purpose of embolotherapy.[96] MR imaging may therefore prove to be the best single test for achieving the multiple aims of screening for PAVM, depicting their architecture for guiding embolization, and following those that are detected over an extended period without ionizing radiation.

Typically, the imaging appearance of PAVM on CE-MRA is that of an aneurismal sac of contrast that connects a dilated feeding artery and draining vein (**Fig. 10**). PAVMs are frequently multiple and predominantly found in the lower lobes.[97] Important imaging features to report include the number, location, and size of any PAVMs, as well as the size and number of feeding vessels. PAVMs may be classified as simply (single feeding artery and single draining vein) or complex (at least two feeding arteries or at least two draining veins). MIP and volumetric images should routinely be performed for guiding embolization.

A study from 2008 in 203 patients with known HHT or a first-degree relative with HHT found that high-resolution CE-MRA was suitable in screening for HHT, properly selecting patients for embolization, and accurately depicting the morphology of PAVMs for planning embolization.[98] MRA depicted significantly more PAVMs than angiography, including many lesions smaller than 5 mm in size (see **Fig. 10**). In an earlier study, MRA including MR perfusion was performed before and after embolization and compared with MDCT and DSA.[99] MRA identified all PAVMs 3 mm or larger and showed residual enhancement in some PAVMs that decreased in size after embolization, a finding that was not detected by angiography. This residual enhancement is important for follow-up purposes, as it is indicative of bronchial artery–to–pulmonary artery collateral flow that could lead to recanalization and possible delayed rupture of an embolized PAVM.

Given its accuracy in identifying PAVMs and their morphology without ionizing radiation, MR imaging should be considered as a primary test for initial screening and follow-up of PAVMs in young patients in whom it is desired to avoid the ionizing radiation of CT.

Pulmonary Sequestration

Pulmonary sequestration is a rare lung mass consisting of dysplastic lung tissue that lacks normal communication with the tracheobronchial tree and receives systemic arterial blood supply.

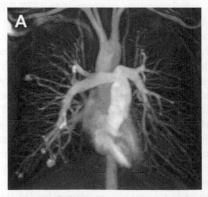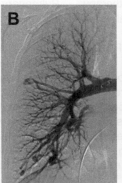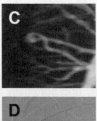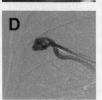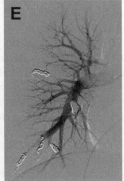

Fig. 10. (*A–E*) A 16-year-old male patient suffering from hereditary hemorrhagic telangiectasia (HHT) or Osler's disease. Maximum intensity projection of a CE-MRA (*A*) demonstrates multiple pulmonary AVMs of the right lung confirmed by selective catheter angiography of the right main pulmonary (*B*) and better delineated by superselective pulmonary angiography (*D*). The multiple AVMS were successfully treated with coil embolization (*E*). (*Courtesy of* Günther Schneider, Homburg/Saar, Germany.)

Sequestration is typically divided into two separate forms: approximately 25% of cases are the extralobar form, characterized by its own pleural lining, systemic venous return, and classic presentation during infancy from association with other congenital anomalies; approximately 75% of cases are the intralobar form, characterized by a lack of a separate pleura, pulmonary venous drainage, and presentation during late childhood or adulthood from recurrent infections.[100] Treatment for both forms is surgical, with intralobar sequestration often requiring lobectomy given its ill-defined margins.

Imaging has a role in documenting the presence of systemic arterial supply to confirm that a mass is indeed a sequestration (Fig. 11), as well as in presurgical planning. CTA and CE-MRA have both been used for this purpose and can obviate the need for angiography to confirm systemic supply.[101,102] Over 95% of intralobar sequestrations are located in the lower lobes, with most occurring in the left lower lobe.[103] Sequestration typically appears as a well-defined or irregular solid mass, with varying degrees of necrotic and cystic change. As a sequestration may have multiple feeding vessels, all arteries that supply the lesion should be documented, including their size, origin, and course.[104] In addition, the venous drainage and any abnormalities of adjacent lung, such as consolidation or atelectasis, should be noted. Several reports with small numbers of patients have demonstrated the ability of CE-MRA to document the presence of systemic arterial supply and to correlate well with surgical

findings.[105–107] One limitation of MR imaging compared with CT in this setting is its poorer performance in depicting gas from possible emphysematous change.

Pulmonary Artery Aneurysm

There are a myriad of causes of pulmonary artery aneurysms and pseudoaneurysms, including trauma, neoplasm, septic emboli, infection such as tuberculosis or invasive aspergillosis, and vasculitis. Behcet disease is the most common nonspecific vasculitis to cause pulmonary artery aneurysms, and warrants special consideration.[108]

Behcet disease is a rare multisystem disorder that is classically characterized by the triad of recurrent apthous oral ulcers, genital ulcers, and uveitis. Underlying vascular inflammation and necrosis are central in disease pathogenesis, with possible involvement of essentially any arterial or venous bed within the body, manifested by venous and arterial occlusions, as well as arterial aneurysms. Although only a small fraction of patients develop pulmonary artery aneurysms, this development is a poor prognostic sign, with such aneurysms at risk of rupture and life-threatening hemoptysis. Patients may undergo sudden death from exsanguination, and approximately half of patients will die within 10 months of onset of hemoptysis.[109] Treatment with resection or embolization has been reported, although not all patients are candidates for embolization, and the

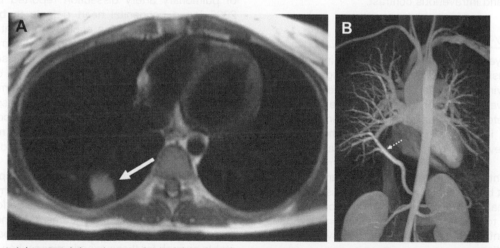

Fig. 11. Axial HASTE (A) and coronal MIP (B) images from a CE-MRA in a 38-year-old patient demonstrates a T2-hyperintense right lower lobe mass (solid arrow) with a large feeding artery (dotted arrow) arising from the celiac axis. Additional images revealed venous drainage via the right inferior pulmonary vein confirming the diagnosis of intralobar pulmonary sequestration.

aneurysms are prone to recur following resection.[108,110]

Numerous reports demonstrate the ability to visualize pulmonary artery aneurysms in the setting of Behcet disease using MR imaging with MRA.[108–112] The aneurysms appear as focal areas of vascular dilatation, most frequently at the level of the descending pulmonary artery, more often on the right.[111] The aneurysms have a tendency to be multiple and bilateral. Pulmonary artery aneurysms are often partially or completely filled with thrombus, with vascular occlusion possible. MR imaging may be the best modality for detecting thrombosed aneurysms; these aneurysms will not enhance on CT and may not be depicted at all on angiography, but will demonstrate intraluminal T1- and T2-hyperintense thrombus on MR.[111] It is also possible to see intramural hematoma within the aneurysm, indicative of prior subadventitial rupture, placing the patient at increased risk for sudden death.[109] Finally, the lungs should be assessed for areas of hemorrhage, infarct, and atelectasis, all of which are possible sequelae of pulmonary artery aneurysms.

The vascular inflammation of Behcet disease places patients at risk from any kind of vascular manipulation, such as arterial or venous puncture. Therefore, catheter angiography, which may lead to venous thrombosis or arterial pseudoaneurysm at the puncture site, may be undesirable in these patients, further increasing the role for noninvasive imaging methods. Even administration of intravenous contrast can incite a vascular response, with one report suggesting that non-gadolinium MRA techniques be used in Behcet disease, rather than CTA, eliminating the need for both venipuncture and intravenous contrast.[110]

Takayasu Arteritis

Takayasu arteritis is a chronic, inflammatory, occlusive vasculitis that, although primarily involving the aorta and its branches, may also involve the pulmonary arteries. One study using catheter angiography found pulmonary involvement in 50% of cases; most of these patients had evidence of moderate pulmonary hypertension, although none were symptomatic.[113] Patients typically present at a young age, with onset before age 40 serving as a possible criterion for making the diagnosis.[114] Therefore, it is valuable to be able to diagnose and follow these patients with a test that does not involve ionizing radiation.

The range of imaging findings of Takayasu arteritis are myriad and include stenosis, occlusion, dilatation, aneurysm, wall thickening, wall enhancement, and mural thrombi.[115–117] One study using pulmonary angiography found that involvement of the pulmonary arteries most commonly has an upper lobe distribution and most frequently impacts segmental and subsegmental branches.[118] The most common abnormality of the pulmonary arteries in a study that used noncontrast MR imaging was a tree-like appearance of the peripheral pulmonary branches, indicative of vascular occlusions.[116] In a later study that compared 3D CE-MRA with angiography in 30 patients with suspected Takayasu arteritis, pulmonary involvement was found in 50% of patients with the disease, with MRA having no false-positives or false-negatives compared with angiography.[117] Peripheral pulmonary arterial branches were poorly visualized, with associated perfusion defects noted on MRA images, again indicative of vascular occlusions.

Pulmonary Artery Dissection

Pulmonary artery dissection is an extremely rare event that occurs in the setting of aneurysmal dilatation of the pulmonary arteries from chronic pulmonary hypertension. The large majority of patients undergo sudden death from rupture into the pericardium leading to acute tamponade, with the diagnosis made at autopsy.[119] In recent years, there have been an increasing number of reports of patients surviving the initial event, with a number of surgical approaches attempted as treatment.[120] In most cases, chronic pulmonary hypertension is attributed to underlying congenital heart disease and in a smaller fraction, primary pulmonary hypertension.[119] A review of 63 cases of pulmonary artery dissection reported before 2005 found congenital heart defects to be the most common underlying etiology, present in 25 of the cases.[120] In such instances, MR imaging can provide not just an evaluation of the dissection (**Fig. 12**) itself, but also an assessment of the congenital heart disease via use of cine imaging and quantitative phase-contrast flow-assessment techniques. More rarely, dissections occur in patients with pulmonary artery aneurysms related to chronic inflammation from underlying collagen vascular disease or infection.[121]

When pulmonary artery dissection is suspected in the emergency setting, echocardiography may be used as an initial fast test that can be performed on an unstable patient, whereas CT and MR imaging may offer a more optimal study in patients stable enough for these examinations when echocardiography is inconclusive.[120,122] The dissection almost always occurs at the site of maximal dilatation,[122] arising within the main pulmonary artery in

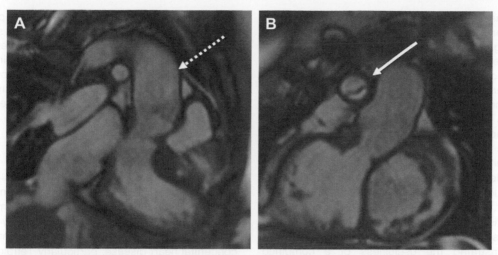

Fig. 12. Cine true FISP images in an 11-year-old patient with congenitally corrected transposition of the great arteries, pulmonary atresia, and VSD, treated with Rastelli procedure with closure of VSD, placement of a conduit from the right ventricle to the main pulmonary artery, and an atrial switch operation. (A) Cine True FISP images reveal patency of the conduit (*white dotted arrow*) as well as a (B) dissection (*solid arrow*) in the main pulmonary artery just distal to the anastamosis with the conduit.

about 80% of cases.[120] A re-entry site of the intimal flap is typically not identified.[122] Important findings to document for surgical planning include the exact location and extent of both the dissection and the underlying pulmonary artery aneurysm, as well as any evidence of rupture into the pericardium, pulmonary regurgitation.[123]

Malignancy Involving the Pulmonary Arteries

Almost all primary tumors of the pulmonary arteries are malignant sarcomas, a rare intravascular tumor that arises from the intima of the central pulmonary arteries.[124] Life expectancy is poor, with patients experiencing progressive right heart failure[125] and having an average survival of 1 year following onset of symptoms.[126] The diagnosis is frequently made at autopsy,[125,126] as patients present with nonspecific symptoms such as progressive dyspnea, and the imaging findings may be mistaken for bland thrombus. Although pulmonary artery sarcoma was previously felt to be universally fatal, the possibility of curative surgery has been more recently suggested, if the diagnosis is made early enough.[127] A number of surgical approaches have been described, including pneumonectomy, endarterectomy, and pulmonary artery resection with reconstruction.[128]

On MR imaging, pulmonary artery sarcoma appears as a polypoid intravascular mass originating in the main, left, or right pulmonary artery that expands and occludes the vessel and

typically shows distal growth into more peripheral arterial branches. The associated expansion of the central arteries can falsely suggest the diagnosis of CTEPH.[129] CE-MR imaging may be considered the ideal imaging study for pulmonary artery sarcoma, because compared with CT and angiography, MRA can best depict the enhancement of the intraluminal filling defect, thereby differentiating bland thrombus from the neovascularity of tumor thrombus.[124,128,130,131] In addition, the intravascular mass may have a heterogeneous appearance with areas of hemorrhage, necrosis, and only peripheral enhancement.[130] In approximately 50% of cases, there is direct transmural extension of tumor outside of the vessel and into surrounding lung, bronchial wall, or lymph node.[131] Mediastinal invasion and proximal growth into the pulmonary valve and right heart are also possible. Peripheral pulmonary nodules may be present, representing distant metastases from embolization of tumor along the pulmonary arteries.[124,125,131,132] Right heart enlargement may be present from the associated increase in pulmonary arterial pressure. MR imaging may not only identify patients for surgery by recognizing the neoplastic nature of an intravascular filling defect, but also assist in selecting the optimal surgical approach by fully characterizing the extent of disease.[133]

The pulmonary arteries may also be secondarily involved by lung cancer. The primary tumor can cause extrinsic vascular compression and luminal narrowing, leading to pulmonary arterial stenosis with associated distal areas of decreased perfusion and infarct (**Fig. 13**). Pulmonary infarct may be suggested when a peripheral pulmonary nodule is detected in the same lobe as a stenotic pulmonary artery that results from a central lung cancer.[134–138] Direct vascular invasion of the pulmonary arteries by lung cancer is also possible (**Fig. 14**).[139] MR imaging has a role in evaluating for secondary involvement of the pulmonary arteries, which aids in lung cancer staging and surgical planning. Imaging findings of tumor involvement include vessel distortion, displacement, stenosis, obstruction, wall irregularity, and intraluminal tumor.[42,140] In addition, perfusion MR may depict peripheral perfusion defects resulting from central stenoses. Two studies with 15 and 18 patients demonstrated the usefulness of a combined approach incorporating CE-MRA and perfusion MR to demonstrate central occlusions and associated perfusion defects, using correlation with

angiography and scintigraphy.[140,141] A separate study found that ECG-gated CE-MRA had a sensitivity of 89% for pulmonary artery involvement, correlated with surgical pathologic specimens, higher than for CE-CT, MR imaging, or conventional CE-CT.[42] MIP and volumetric reconstructed images can be particularly helpful for preoperative planning.[140]

Complex Congenital Heart Disease with Pulmonary Artery Stenosis or Atresia

A spectrum of abnormalities of the pulmonary arteries ranging from mild hypoplasia to complete absence of the main pulmonary artery may frequently be seen in the setting of complex congenital heart disease, particularly Tetralogy of Fallot. Such patients may be cyanotic and develop systemic pulmonary arterial supply, as demonstrated by aorto-pulmonary collaterals (APCs).[142]

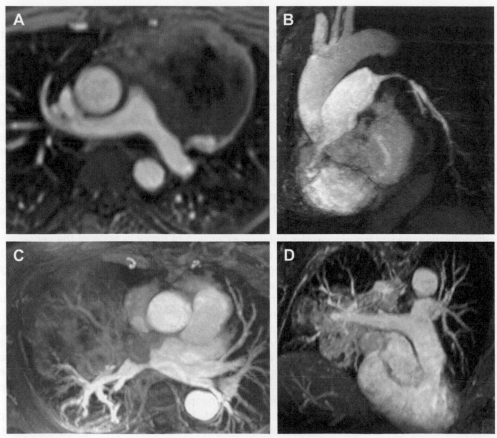

Fig. 13. Axial 2D T1 GRE volume-interpolated breath hold (VIBE) image from a patient with an anterior mediastinal B-cell lymphoma (*A*) and another with a cavitary primary lung cancer (*B*) with varying degrees of compression of the pulmonary artery without frank invasion. However, the third patient below (*C, D*) also suffering from primary lung cancer demonstrates encasement of the right pulmonary artery and invasion of pulmonary artery branches, right pulmonary veins, and the right atrium.

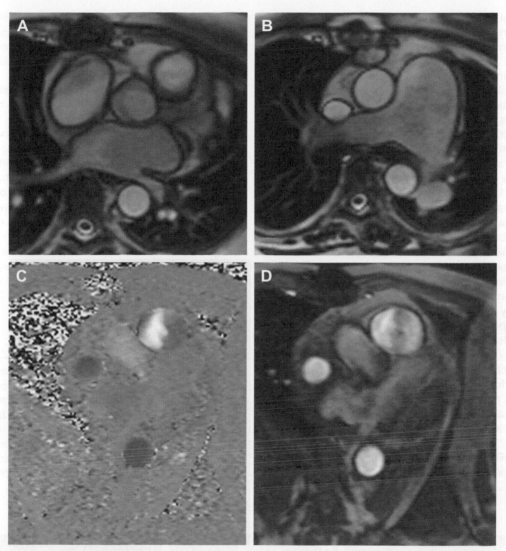

Fig. 14. Axial cine true FISP images (*A, B*), and phase-contrast (*C, D*) magnitude imaging and velocity map at the level of the pulmonic valve in a 56-year-old female patient with fusion of the anterior and left cusps of the pulmonic valve leading to a functionally bicuspid valve with associated enlargement of the pulmonary artery. Phase-contrast images reveal no significant pulmonic stenosis but moderate pulmonic regurgitation with a calculated regurgitant fraction of 40%.

Before corrective or palliative surgery, it is important to be able to identify all collaterals as well as their size and course as precisely as possible. In addition, patients require continued postoperative assessment to evaluate for patency of surgical shunts, residual pulmonary arterial abnormalities, and growth of reperfused distal pulmonary arterial branches.[143] This assessment can be technically challenging given the complex altered anatomy that may be encountered as well as the young age of the patients.

MR imaging should be viewed as a primary imaging test to provide the anatomic and functional evaluation needed in these patients. Ionizing radiation is a major limitation of angiography and CTA, as these patients are very young and likely to get multiple examinations to allow for pre- and postoperative assessment. Although MR may require sedation in young patients, a comprehensive examination including MR perfusion imaging and PC and cine MR can be performed to permit morphologic assessment and quantitative measurements of flow and function in a single comprehensive examination avoiding the need for multiple separate studies (**Fig. 14**). Time-resolved imaging in these patients is very useful, as timing of the contrast bolus may be challenging in young patients and only small quantities of contrast can be used in the pediatric population. More importantly, multiphase high temporal rate imaging is helpful to assess the hemodynamic of complex cardiac anomalies including vascular shunting, global and regional perfusional differences, and anomalous vasculature. The reader should assess for atresia, hypoplasia, stenosis, or discontinuity of the main pulmonary artery and its branches and also evaluate the anatomy of all APCs and the patency of surgical shunts (**Fig. 15**).[144] Right heart and pulmonary valve function should be assessed as well, including the pressure gradient across the valve. The lungs can be evaluated for areas of hypoplasia from diminished perfusion. A broad field of view should be used, as APCs may arise anywhere from the subclavian arteries to the abdominal aorta.[144]

Numerous studies have demonstrated the ability of MR imaging to provide a reliable pre- and postoperative assessment of the pulmonary arteries. For instance, in one study, MRA had 100% sensitivity and specificity for main and branch pulmonary artery stenosis or hypoplasia and for absent or discontinuous branch pulmonary arteries; furthermore, MRA diagnosed not only all APCs that were seen using angiography, but identified additional APCs missed by angiography.[144] A separate study also noted the ability of MR imaging to depict the pulmonary arterial anatomy with better detail than angiography in some congenital heart disease patients.[145] MR imaging has also been found to be more sensitive than echocardiography in the evaluation of branch pulmonary artery abnormalities following operative repair of Tetralogy of Fallot.[146] Also, phase-contrast MR has been used in this setting to accurately assess differential pulmonary blood flow compared with scintigraphy, although technical errors such as MR artifacts, dephasing from turbulent flow, and incorrectly prescribed site of data acquisition, occurred in a significant fraction of patients.[147] Finally, cine MR imaging can provide a simultaneous assessment of the right ventricle. Indeed, MR imaging is viewed as the gold standard for this purpose, whereas echocardiography faces technical challenges in optimally visualizing the right ventricular free wall and is considered less reliable and overall of limited value in this setting.[148,149]

FUTURE DIRECTIONS
High-Field Imaging

Magnets of 3.0 T have become widely available in the clinic. MRA in general benefits from higher field strength because of the higher baseline signal to noise that can be used in exchange for higher spatial or temporal resolution imaging when combined with multielement coils and parallel imaging. In addition, at high field there is prolongation of the T1 of unenhanced blood leading to

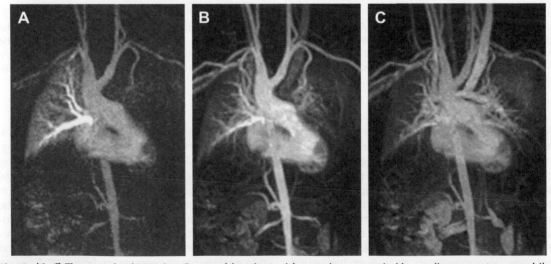

Fig. 15. (A–C) Time-resolved MRA in a 2-year-old patient with complex congenital heart disease post surgery bilateral bidirectional Glenn shunts from the bilateral superior vena cavae to the right and left pulmonary arteries and creation of an atrial septal defect demonstrates relatively early enhancement of the right lung compared with the left due to right arm injection of contrast, consistent with the patient's operative history.

better background suppression with only minimal decrease in T1 relaxivity of gadolinium chelates,[150] potentially resulting in improved tissue contrast. For pulmonary MRA, however, there are expected challenges particular to thoracic imaging. With increasing field strength, radiofrequency inhomogeneity and magnetic susceptibility effects are substantially increased. As discussed above, lung tissue has a very short T2 and T2* and at higher field strength the inhomogeneities expected at air/tissue interfaces are even more pronounced, potentially leading to vessel blurring, overestimation of stenosis, and mismapping. Therefore, it is essential to minimize echo time for gradient-echo imaging and to limit voxel size. Initial studies on volunteers and patients with PAH demonstrated feasibility of high-resolution morphologic imaging and high temporal rate quantitative perfusion assessment using a split bolus technique at 3.0.[7] In a study by the same group, a comparison of pulmonary perfusion at 1.5 versus 3.0 T was performed with higher SNR achieved in the vasculature at 3.0 T but lower SNR in the parenchyma likely a result of T2* effects with no change in the flow measurements performed with PC-MRA.[151] A subsequent study by the same group combined 3.0 T with a 32-channel coil and high T1 relaxivity contrast agent gadobenate dimeglumine (gadolinium-BOPTA) in an effort to increase signal to noise such that higher parallel Imaging acceleration factors could be achieved. In this study, parallel imaging with generalized autocalibrating partially parallel acquisition and an acceleration factor of 6 (3 in the phase-encoding × 2 in the slice-encoding directions) was performed and spatial resolution was increased compared with prior studies to 1 mm³ with the breath hold maintained at 20 seconds. Pulmonary arterial anatomy was well delineated up to fifth order branches with high confidence and excellent interobserver agreement.[152] The increase in SNR at 3.0 T is likely not only to benefit CE-MRA but also NCE techniques as they are often signal poor although SSFP imaging is more challenging at 3.0 T because of field inhomogeneities.

Alternative Exogenous Contrast Agents

Standard extracellular contrast agents permit high-contrast first-pass imaging, but rapid distribution of the contrast leads to a rapid decline in vascular enhancement and appropriate timing of the bolus can be challenging. Recently, a blood pool contrast agent (BPA) has become available in Europe.[153] The unique characteristic of this type of contrast agent is that it is an intravascular agent that remains in the intravascular space with a prolonged plasma half-life permitting prolonged imaging of the vessels with the potential to visualize small vessels with slow or complex flow by basing signal intensity on the shortened T1 of blood rather than flow. These agents may be used for angiography but also for perfusion. BPAs include gadolinium-based small molecules with reversible protein binding, larger gadolinium-based molecules, and super paramagnetic ultra small iron oxides (USPIOs). None of these agents, however, are presently approved for use in the United States and only one agent is approved in Europe, gadofosveset trisodium (Vasovist, Bayer Schering Pharma, Germany). One of the major pitfalls of blood pool agents is the concomitant enhancement of venous blood leading to a challenge separating arterial from venous structures such that segmentation or complex subtraction algorithms may be needed. Another potential advantage of these agents is that when these agents reversibly bind to larger proteins their tumbling rate is slowed, which leads to enhanced paramagnetic effectiveness and allows for administration of lower doses of contrast agent (eg, 0.03 mmol/kg for gadofosveset trisodium) compared with conventional contrast agents (0.1 to 2.0 mmol/kg for MRA) (Fig. 16).[70,153,154] In addition to blood pool agents, targeted agents are being developed with specific binding affinity for fibrln, for example, which are currently being explored for atherosclerotic plaque imaging and show promise for pulmonary emboli imaging.[155–157]

Nongadolinium-Enhanced Imaging Using ECG-Gated Fast Spin Echo

Using ECG-gated spin-echo sequences for angiography were first described in theory by Meuli and colleagues[158] and Wedeen and colleagues[159] in the 1980s, but it was not until 2000 that Miyazaki and colleagues[160] demonstrated the feasibility and potential clinically utility of using an ECG-gated partial Fourier fast spin-echo sequence for non–gadolinium-enhanced MRA. This technique takes advantage of the expected differences in arterial and venous signal on FSE sequence during diastole and signal. Specifically, there is low arterial signal during systole from high flow-related signal loss, and high arterial signal during diastole from the T2-related fluid signal of slow flow. Slow flow in the veins leads to high signal on both systole and diastole. Subtraction of systole from diastole leads to cancellation of the venous signal and high signal in the arterial system free of venous contamination. This type of sequence can be combined with ASL and this combination of techniques shows promise for pulmonary MRA with

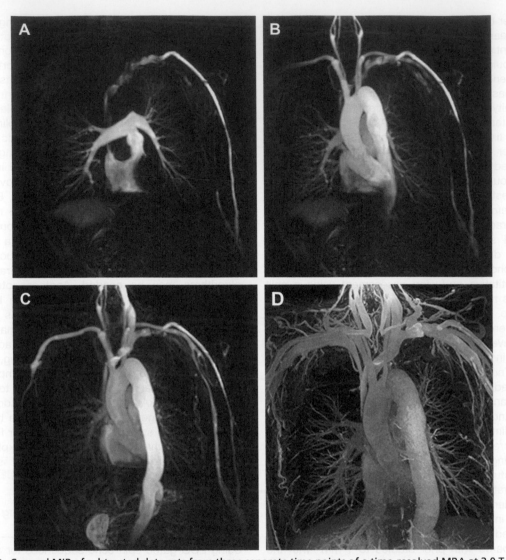

Fig. 16. Coronal MIP of subtracted data sets from three separate time points of a time-resolved MRA at 3.0 T (*A–C*) with a temporal resolution of 1.5 seconds using a gadolinium blood pool agent (Gadofosveset) in a patient with emphysema and elongation of the aorta. Note the paucity of perfusion in the right upper lobe due to cystic changes at the apex related to emphysema. On the steady-state image (*D*), the properties of blood pool agents are demonstrated, note the persistent enhancement in the arteries and veins and opacification of small branch vessels. (*Courtesy of* Henrik J. Michaely, Mannheim, Germany.)

imaging triggering in diastole.[161] Finally, time-resolved MRA is not necessarily limited to CE-MRA techniques and could also potentially be performed without gadolinium contrast using ECG-gated FSE techniques with sequentially varying trigger delay times but further optimization of such a technique is required.

Ventilation

MR is capable of using real-time imaging to visualize diaphragmatic and lung parenchymal motion as well as imaging ventilation. There are several approaches to imaging and quantifying ventilation including using aerosolized gadolinium, hyperpolarized inert gases such as helium, xenon, and most interestingly oxygen because of its low cost and ease of availability and administration. When 100% molecular oxygen is inhaled, T1 shortening and signal changes are observed in the lungs over time, which can be quantified.[162,163] Ventilation can be combined with perfusion imaging (gadolinium enhanced or ASL perfusion) for a more comprehensive assessment of the global and regional pulmonary function particularly in the setting of pulmonary embolism (**Fig. 17**).[19,52,164]

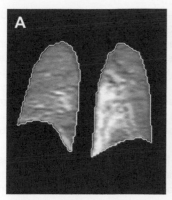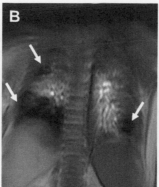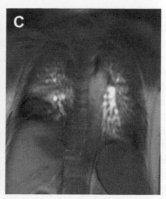

Fig. 17. Oxygen Ventilation MR (*A*) and gadolinium-DTPA-enhanced MR (*B, C*) perfusion imaging in a 63-year-old female patient with shortness of breath and suspected pulmonary embolism. Normal ventilation is demonstrated but perfusion MR demonstrates perfusion defects in the right upper lobe and both lower lobes highly suggestive of bilateral pulmonary emboli. (*Courtesy of* Quen Chen, PhD, New York, NY.)

SUMMARY

Pulmonary MRA continues to rapidly improve in spatial and temporal resolution, making it possible in the clinical setting to examine the anatomic changes that can occur secondary to diverse disease processes as well as the consequences of these anatomic changes through perfusion, flow, and cardiac functional imaging. Although further validation of quantitative perfusion is warranted, the potential for describing hemodynamic changes at the microscopic level is clear. Even more intriguing is combining perfusion with ventilation in the clinical setting, permitting a more comprehensive assessment of pulmonary function. High field combined with multielement coils and parallel imaging is likely to permit further improvements in spatial and temporal resolution of CE and NCE-MRA, whereas more potent contrast agents with prolonged blood half lives and/or more specific contrast agents may increase sensitivity and specificity of pulmonary vascular imaging.

REFERENCES

1. Hoffmann U, Schima W, Herold C. Pulmonary magnetic resonance angiography. Eur Radiol 1999;9(9):1745–54.
2. Siegelman ES, Charafeddine R, Stolpen AH, et al. Suppression of intravascular signal on fat-saturated contrast-enhanced thoracic MR arteriograms. Radiology 2000;217(1):115–8.
3. Axel L, Kolman L, Charafeddine R, et al. Origin of a signal intensity loss artifact in fat-saturation MR imaging. Radiology 2000;217(3):911–5.
4. Oudkerk M, van Beek EJ, Wielopolski P, et al. Comparison of contrast-enhanced magnetic resonance angiography and conventional pulmonary angiography for the diagnosis of pulmonary embolism: a prospective study. Lancet 2002;359(9318):1643–7.
5. Sodickson DK, Manning WJ. Simultaneous acquisition of spatial harmonics (SMASH): fast imaging with radiofrequency coil arrays. Magn Reson Med 1997;38(4):591–603.
6. Pruessmann KP, Weiger M, Scheidegger MB, et al. SENSE: sensitivity encoding for fast MRI. Magn Reson Med 1999;42(5):952–62.
7. Nael K, Michaely HJ, Kramer U, et al. Pulmonary circulation: contrast-enhanced 3.0-T MR angiography–initial results. Radiology 2006;240(3):858–68.
8. Nael K, Saleh R, Nyborg GK, et al. Pulmonary MR perfusion at 3.0 Tesla using a blood pool contrast agent: Initial results in a swine model. J Magn Reson Imaging 2007;25(1):66–72.
9. Korosec FR, Frayne R, Grist TM, et al. Time-resolved contrast-enhanced 3D MR angiography. Magn Reson Med 1996;36(3):345–51.
10. Du J, Bydder M. High-resolution time-resolved contrast-enhanced MR abdominal and pulmonary angiography using a spiral-TRICKS sequence. Magn Reson Med 2007;58(3):631–5.
11. Barger AV, Block WF, Toropov Y, et al. Time-resolved contrast-enhanced imaging with isotropic resolution and broad coverage using an undersampled 3D projection trajectory. Magn Reson Med 2002;48(2):297–305.
12. Mistretta CA, Wieben O, Velikina J, et al. Highly constrained backprojection for time-resolved MRI. Magn Reson Med 2006;55(1):30–40.

13. Hatabu H, Gaa J, Kim D, et al. Pulmonary perfusion: qualitative assessment with dynamic contrast-enhanced MRI using ultra-short TE and inversion recovery turbo FLASH. Magn Reson Med 1996;36(4):503–8.

14. Amundsen T, Kvaerness J, Jones RA, et al. Pulmonary embolism: detection with MR perfusion imaging of lung–a feasibility study. Radiology 1997;203(1):181–5.

15. Amundsen T, Torheim G, Kvistad KA, et al. Perfusion abnormalities in pulmonary embolism studied with perfusion MRI and ventilation-perfusion scintigraphy: an intra-modality and inter-modality agreement study. J Magn Reson Imaging 2002; 15(4):386–94.

16. Goyen M, Laub G, Ladd ME, et al. Dynamic 3D MR angiography of the pulmonary arteries in under four seconds. J Magn Reson Imaging 2001;13(3): 372–7.

17. Schoenberg SO, Bock M, Floemer F, et al. High-resolution pulmonary arterio- and venography using multiple-bolus multiphase 3D-Gd-mRA. J Magn Reson Imaging 1999;10(3):339–46.

18. Matsuoka S, Uchiyama K, Shima H, et al. Detectability of pulmonary perfusion defect and influence of breath holding on contrast-enhanced thick-slice 2D and on 3D MR pulmonary perfusion images. J Magn Reson Imaging 2001;14(5):580–5.

19. Nakagawa T, Sakuma H, Murashima S, et al. Pulmonary ventilation-perfusion MR imaging in clinical patients. J Magn Reson Imaging 2001;14(4): 419–24.

20. wasawa T, Saito K, Ogawa N, et al. Prediction of postoperative pulmonary function using perfusion magnetic resonance imaging of the lung. J Magn Reson Imaging 2002;15(6):685–92.

21. Fink C, Puderbach M, Bock M, et al. Regional lung perfusion: assessment with partially parallel three-dimensional MR imaging. Radiology 2004;231(1): 175–84.

22. Nikolaou K, Schoenberg SO, Brix G, et al. Quantification of pulmonary blood flow and volume in healthy volunteers by dynamic contrast-enhanced magnetic resonance imaging using a parallel imaging technique. Invest Radiol 2004;39(9):537–45.

23. Fink C, Ley S, Kroeker R, et al. Time-resolved contrast-enhanced three-dimensional magnetic resonance angiography of the chest: combination of parallel imaging with view sharing (TREAT). Invest Radiol 2005;40(1):40–8.

24. Molinari F, Fink C, Risse F, et al. Assessment of differential pulmonary blood flow using perfusion magnetic resonance imaging: comparison with radionuclide perfusion scintigraphy. Invest Radiol 2006;41(8):624–30.

25. Hatabu H, Tadamura E, Levin DL, et al. Quantitative assessment of pulmonary perfusion with dynamic contrast-enhanced MRI. Magn Reson Med 1999; 42(6):1033–8.

26. Berthezene Y, Croisille P, Wiart M, et al. Prospective comparison of MR lung perfusion and lung scintigraphy. J Magn Reson Imaging 1999;9(1):61–8.

27. Kluge A, Gerriets T, Stolz E, et al. Pulmonary perfusion in acute pulmonary embolism: agreement of MRI and SPECT for lobar, segmental and subsegmental perfusion defects. Acta Radiol 2006;47(9): 933–40.

28. Ohno Y, Murase K, Higashino T, et al. Assessment of bolus injection protocol with appropriate concentration for quantitative assessment of pulmonary perfusion by dynamic contrast-enhanced MR imaging. J Magn Reson Imaging 2007;25(1):55–65.

29. Ley S, Mereles D, Risse F, et al. Quantitative 3D pulmonary MR-perfusion in patients with pulmonary arterial hypertension: correlation with invasive pressure measurements. Eur J Radiol 2007;61(2): 251–5.

30. Amundsen T, Torheim G, Waage A, et al. Perfusion magnetic resonance imaging of the lung: characterization of pneumonia and chronic obstructive pulmonary disease. A feasibility study. J Magn Reson Imaging 2000;12(2):224–31.

31. Ohno Y, Hatabu H, Higashino T, et al. Dynamic perfusion MRI versus perfusion scintigraphy: prediction of postoperative lung function in patients with lung cancer. AJR Am J Roentgenol 2004; 182(1):73–8.

32. Jang YM, Oh YM, Seo JB, et al. Quantitatively assessed dynamic contrast-enhanced magnetic resonance imaging in patients with chronic obstructive pulmonary disease: correlation of perfusion parameters with pulmonary function test and quantitative computed tomography. Invest Radiol 2008;43(6):403–10.

33. Eichinger M, Puderbach M, Fink C, et al. Contrast-enhanced 3D MRI of lung perfusion in children with cystic fibrosis–initial results. Eur Radiol 2006; 16(10):2147–52.

34. Fenchel M, Saleh R, Dinh H, et al. Juvenile and adult congenital heart disease: time-resolved 3D contrast-enhanced MR angiography. Radiology 2007;244(2):399–410.

35. Kluge A, Dill T, Ekinci O, et al. Decreased pulmonary perfusion in pulmonary vein stenosis after radiofrequency ablation: assessment with dynamic magnetic resonance perfusion imaging. Chest 2004;126(2):428–37.

36. Weisskoff RM, Chesler D, Boxerman JL, et al. Pitfalls in MR measurement of tissue blood flow with intravascular tracers: which mean transit time? Magn Reson Med 1993;29(4):553–8.

37. Ostergaard L, Weisskoff RM, Chesler DA, et al. High resolution measurement of cerebral blood flow using intravascular tracer bolus passages.

Part I: Mathematical approach and statistical analysis. Magn Reson Med 1996;36(5):715–25.

38. St Lawrence KS, Lee TY. An adiabatic approximation to the tissue homogeneity model for water exchange in the brain: I. Theoretical derivation. J Cereb Blood Flow Metab 1998;18(12): 1365–77.

39. Fink C, Risse F, Buhmann R, et al. Quantitative analysis of pulmonary perfusion using time-resolved parallel 3D MRI - initial results. Rofo 2004;176(2):170–4.

40. Ohno Y, Hatabu H, Murase K, et al. Primary pulmonary hypertension: 3D dynamic perfusion MRI for quantitative analysis of regional pulmonary perfusion. AJR Am J Roentgenol 2007;188(1):48–56.

41. Dumoulin CL, Yucel EK, Vock P, et al. Two- and three-dimensional phase contrast MR angiography of the abdomen. J Comput Assist Tomogr 1990; 14(5):779–84.

42. Ohno Y, Adachi S, Motoyama A, et al. Multiphase ECG-triggered 3D contrast-enhanced MR angiography: utility for evaluation of hilar and mediastinal invasion of bronchogenic carcinoma. J Magn Reson Imaging 2001;13(2):215–24.

43. Boss A, Schaefer S, Martirosian P, et al. Magnetic resonance imaging of lung tissue: influence of body positioning, breathing and oxygen inhalation on signal decay using multi-echo gradient-echo sequences. Invest Radiol 2008;43(6):433–8.

44. Stock KW, Chen Q, Hatabu H, et al. Magnetic resonance T2* measurements of the normal human lung in vivo with ultra-short echo times. Magn Reson Imaging 1999;17(7):997–1000.

45. Hatabu H, Alsop DC, Listerud J, et al. T2* and proton density measurement of normal human lung parenchyma using submillisecond echo time gradient echo magnetic resonance imaging. Eur J Radiol 1999;29(3):245–52.

46. Grobner T. Gadolinium–a specific trigger for the development of nephrogenic fibrosing dermopathy and nephrogenic systemic fibrosis? Nephrol Dial Transplant 2006;21(4):1104–8.

47. Kluge A, Muller C, Hansel J, et al. Real-time MR with TrueFISP for the detection of acute pulmonary embolism: initial clinical experience. Eur Radiol 2004;14(4):709–18.

48. Kluge A, Luboldt W, Bachmann G. Acute pulmonary embolism to the subsegmental level: diagnostic accuracy of three MRI techniques compared with 16-MDCT. AJR Am J Roentgenol 2006;187(1):W7–14.

49. Hui BK, Noga ML, Gan KD, et al. Navigator-gated three-dimensional MR angiography of the pulmonary arteries using steady-state free precession. J Magn Reson Imaging 2005;21(6):831–5.

50. Detre JA, Leigh JS, Williams DS, et al. Perfusion imaging. Magn Reson Med 1992;23(1):37–45.

51. Detre JA, Zhang W, Roberts DA, et al. Tissue specific perfusion imaging using arterial spin labeling. NMR Biomed 1994;7(1-2):75–82.

52. Mai VM, Bankier AA, Prasad PV, et al. MR ventilation-perfusion imaging of human lung using oxygen-enhanced and arterial spin labeling techniques. J Magn Reson Imaging 2001;14(5):574–9.

53. Mai VM, Liu B, Polzin JA, et al. Ventilation-perfusion ratio of signal intensity in human lung using oxygen-enhanced and arterial spin labeling techniques. Magn Reson Med 2002;48(2):341–50.

54. Oger E. Incidence of venous thromboembolism: a community-based study in Western France. EPI-GETBP Study Group. Groupe d'Etude de la Thrombose de Bretagne Occidentale. Thromb Haemost 2000;83(5):657–60.

55. Stein PD, Henry JW. Prevalence of acute pulmonary embolism among patients in a general hospital and at autopsy. Chest 1995;108(4): 978–81.

56. Goldhaber SZ, Visani L, De Rosa M. Acute pulmonary embolism: clinical outcomes in the International Cooperative Pulmonary Embolism Registry (ICOPER). Lancet 1999;353(9162): 1386–9.

57. Barritt DW, Jordan SC. Clinical features of pulmonary embolism. Lancet 1961;1(7180):729–32.

58. Dalen JE, Alpert JS. Natural history of pulmonary embolism. Prog Cardiovasc Dis 1975;17(4): 259–70.

59. Diffin DC, Leyendecker JR, Johnson SP, et al. Effect of anatomic distribution of pulmonary emboli on interobserver agreement in the interpretation of pulmonary angiography. AJR Am J Roentgenol 1998;171(4):1085–9.

60. Stein PD, Athanasoulis C, Alavi A, et al. Complications and validity of pulmonary angiography in acute pulmonary embolism. Circulation 1992; 85(2):462–8.

61. British Thoracic Society guidelines for the management of suspected acute pulmonary embolism. Thorax 2003;58(6):470–83.

62. Remy-Jardin M, Pistolesi M, Goodman LR, et al. Management of suspected acute pulmonary embolism in the era of CT angiography: a statement from the Fleischner Society. Radiology 2007; 245(2):315–29.

63. Ravenel JG, Costello P, Schoepf UJ. CT in the diagnosis of pulmonary embolism. AJR Am J Roentgenol 2005;184(5):1707–8, 1707, author reply.

64. Schoepf UJ, Costello P. CT angiography for diagnosis of pulmonary embolism: state of the art. Radiology 2004;230(2):329–37.

65. Meaney JF, Weg JG, Chenevert TL, et al. Diagnosis of pulmonary embolism with magnetic resonance angiography. N Engl J Med 1997;336(20): 1422–7.

66. Greenspan RH. Pulmonary angiography and the diagnosis of pulmonary embolism. Prog Cardiovasc Dis 1994;37(2):93–105.

67. Wittram C, Kalra MK, Maher MM, et al. Acute and chronic pulmonary emboli: angiography-CT correlation. AJR Am J Roentgenol 2006;186 (6 Suppl 2):S421–9.

68. Coche E, Verschuren F, Keyeux A, et al. Diagnosis of acute pulmonary embolism in outpatients: comparison of thin-collimation multi-detector row spiral CT and planar ventilation-perfusion scintigraphy. Radiology 2003;229(3):757–65.

69. Grist TM, Sostman HD, MacFall JR, et al. Pulmonary angiography with MR imaging: preliminary clinical experience. Radiology 1993;189(2): 523–30.

70. Grist TM, Korosec FR, Peters DC, et al. Steady-state and dynamic MR angiography with MS-325: initial experience in humans. Radiology 1998; 207(2):539–44.

71. Loubeyre P, Revel D, Douek P, et al. Dynamic contrast-enhanced MR angiography of pulmonary embolism: comparison with pulmonary angiography. AJR Am J Roentgenol 1994;162(5):1035–9.

72. Ogasawara N, Suga K, Zaki M, et al. Assessment of lung perfusion impairment in patients with pulmonary artery-occlusive and chronic obstructive pulmonary diseases with noncontrast electrocardiogram-gated fast-spin-echo perfusion MR imaging. J Magn Reson Imaging 2004;20(4):601–11.

73. Stein PD, Woodard PK, Hull RD, et al. Gadolinium-enhanced magnetic resonance angiography for detection of acute pulmonary embolism: an in-depth review. Chest 2003;124(6):2324–8.

74. Gupta A, Frazer CK, Ferguson JM, et al. Acute pulmonary embolism: diagnosis with MR angiography. Radiology 1999;210(2):353–9.

75. Blum A, Bellou A, Guillemin F, et al. Performance of magnetic resonance angiography in suspected acute pulmonary embolism. Thromb Haemost 2005;93(3):503–11.

76. Pleszewski B, Chartrand-Lefebvre C, Qanadli SD, et al. Gadolinium-enhanced pulmonary magnetic resonance angiography in the diagnosis of acute pulmonary embolism: a prospective study on 48 patients. Clin Imaging 2006;30(3):166–72.

77. Ohno Y, Higashino T, Takenaka D, et al. MR angiography with sensitivity encoding (SENSE) for suspected pulmonary embolism: comparison with MDCT and ventilation-perfusion scintigraphy. AJR Am J Roentgenol 2004;183(1):91–8.

78. Ersoy H, Goldhaber SZ, Cai T, et al. Time-resolved MR angiography: a primary screening examination of patients with suspected pulmonary embolism and contraindications to administration of iodinated contrast material. AJR Am J Roentgenol 2007; 188(5):1246–54.

79. Pengo V, Lensing AW, Prins MH, et al. Incidence of chronic thromboembolic pulmonary hypertension after pulmonary embolism. N Engl J Med 2004; 350(22):2257–64.

80. Lewczuk J, Piszko P, Jagas J, et al. Prognostic factors in medically treated patients with chronic pulmonary embolism. Chest 2001;119(3):818–23.

81. Auger WR, Kerr KM, Kim NH, et al. Chronic thromboembolic pulmonary hypertension. Cardiol Clin 2004;22(3):453–66, vii.

82. Kreitner KF, Ley S, Kauczor HU, et al. Chronic thromboembolic pulmonary hypertension: pre- and postoperative assessment with breath-hold MR imaging techniques. Radiology 2004;232(2): 535–43.

83. Ley S, Kauczor HU, Heussel CP, et al. Value of contrast-enhanced MR angiography and helical CT angiography in chronic thromboembolic pulmonary hypertension. Eur Radiol 2003;13(10): 2365–71.

84. Ley S, Kramm T, Kauczor HU, et al [Pre- and postoperative assessment of hemodynamics in patients with chronic thromboembolic pulmonary hypertension by MR techniques]. Rofo 2003;175(12): 1647–54.

85. Simonneau G, Galie N, Rubin LJ, et al. Clinical classification of pulmonary hypertension. J Am Coll Cardiol 2004;43(12 Suppl S):5S–12S.

86. Chatterjee K, De Marco T, Alpert JS. Pulmonary hypertension: hemodynamic diagnosis and management. Arch Intern Med 2002;162(17):1925–33.

87. Ley S, Kreitner KF, Fink C, et al. Assessment of pulmonary hypertension by CT and MR imaging. Eur Radiol 2004;14(3):359–68.

88. Barst RJ, Rubin LJ, Long WA, et al. A comparison of continuous intravenous epoprostenol (prostacyclin) with conventional therapy for primary pulmonary hypertension. The Primary Pulmonary Hypertension Study Group. N Engl J Med 1996; 334(5):296–302.

89. Nikolaou K, Schoenberg SO, Attenberger U, et al. Pulmonary arterial hypertension: diagnosis with fast perfusion MR imaging and high-spatial-resolution MR angiography–preliminary experience. Radiology 2005;236(2):694–703.

90. Ley S, Fink C, Zaporozhan J, et al. Value of high spatial and high temporal resolution magnetic resonance angiography for differentiation between idiopathic and thromboembolic pulmonary hypertension: initial results. Eur Radiol 2005;15(11): 2256–63.

91. Ley S, Mereles D, Puderbach M, et al. Value of MR phase-contrast flow measurements for functional assessment of pulmonary arterial hypertension. Eur Radiol 2007;17(7):1892–7.

92. Roeleveld RJ, Marcus JT, Boonstra A, et al. A comparison of noninvasive MRI-based methods of

estimating pulmonary artery pressure in pulmonary hypertension. J Magn Reson Imaging 2005;22(1): 67–72.

93. Sanz J, Kuschnir P, Rius T, et al. Pulmonary arterial hypertension: noninvasive detection with phase-contrast MR imaging. Radiology 2007;243(1):70–9.

94. Gossage JR, Kanj G. Pulmonary arteriovenous malformations. A state of the art review. Am J Respir Crit Care Med 1998;158(2):643–61.

95. White RI Jr, Pollak JS, Wirth JA. Pulmonary arteriovenous malformations: diagnosis and transcatheter embolotherapy. J Vasc Interv Radiol 1996;7(6): 787–804.

96. Remy J, Remy-Jardin M, Wattinne L, et al. Pulmonary arteriovenous malformations: evaluation with CT of the chest before and after treatment. Radiology 1992;182(3):809–16.

97. Guttmacher AE, Marchuk DA, White RI Jr. Hereditary hemorrhagic telangiectasia. N Engl J Med 1995;333(14):918–24.

98. Schneider G, Uder M, Koehler M, et al. MR angiography for detection of pulmonary arteriovenous malformations in patients with hereditary hemorrhagic telangiectasia. AJR Am J Roentgenol 2008;190(4):892–901.

99. Ohno Y, Hatabu H, Takenaka D, et al. Contrast-enhanced MR perfusion imaging and MR angiography: utility for management of pulmonary arteriovenous malformations for embolotherapy. Eur J Radiol 2002;41(2):136–46.

100. Lee EY, Boiselle PM, Cleveland RH. Multidetector CT evaluation of congenital lung anomalies. Radiology 2008;247(3):632–48.

101. Frush DP, Donnelly LF. Pulmonary sequestration spectrum: a new spin with helical CT. AJR Am J Roentgenol 1997;169(3):679–82.

102. Hang JD, Guo QY, Chen CX, et al. Imaging approach to the diagnosis of pulmonary sequestration. Acta Radiol 1996;37(6):883–8.

103. Felker RE, Tonkin IL. Imaging of pulmonary sequestration. AJR Am J Roentgenol 1990;154(2): 241–9.

104. Ko SF, Ng SH, Lee TY, et al. Noninvasive imaging of bronchopulmonary sequestration. AJR Am J Roentgenol 2000;175(4):1005–12.

105. Zhang M, Zhu J, Wang Q, et al. Contrast enhanced MR angiography in pulmonary sequestration. Chin Med J (Engl) 2001;114(12):1326–8.

106. Au VW, Chan JK, Chan FL. Pulmonary sequestration diagnosed by contrast enhanced three-dimensional MR angiography. Br J Radiol 1999;72(859):709–11.

107. Sancak T, Cangir AK, Atasoy C, et al. The role of contrast enhanced three-dimensional MR angiography in pulmonary sequestration. Interact Cardiovasc Thorac Surg 2003;2(4):480–2.

108. Tunaci A, Berkmen YM, Gokmen E. Thoracic involvement in Behcet's disease: pathologic,

clinical, and imaging features. AJR Am J Roentgenol 1995;164(1):51–6.

109. Greene RM, Saleh A, Taylor AK, et al. Non-invasive assessment of bleeding pulmonary artery aneurysms due to Behcet disease. Eur Radiol 1998; 8(3):359–63.

110. Berkmen T. MR angiography of aneurysms in Behcet disease: a report of four cases. J Comput Assist Tomogr 1998;22(2):202–6.

111. Numan F, Islak C, Berkmen T, et al. Behcet disease: pulmonary arterial involvement in 15 cases. Radiology 1994;192(2):465–8.

112. Puckette TC, Jolles H, Proto AV. Magnetic resonance imaging confirmation of pulmonary artery aneurysm in Behcet's disease. J Thorac Imaging. Summer 1994;9(3):172–5.

113. Lupi E, Sanchez G, Horwitz S, et al. Pulmonary artery involvement in Takayasu's arteritis. Chest 1975;67(1):69–74.

114. Arend WP, Michel BA, Bloch DA, et al. The American College of Rheumatology 1990 criteria for the classification of Takayasu arteritis. Arthritis Rheum 1990;33(8):1129–34.

115. Park JH, Chung JW, Im JG, et al. Takayasu arteritis: evaluation of mural changes in the aorta and pulmonary artery with CT angiography. Radiology 1995;196(1):89–93.

116. Yamada I, Numano F, Suzuki S. Takayasu arteritis: evaluation with MR imaging. Radiology 1993; 188(1):89–94.

117. Yamada I, Nakagawa T, Himeno Y, et al. Takayasu arteritis: diagnosis with breath-hold contrast-enhanced three-dimensional MR angiography. J Magn Reson Imaging 2000;11(5):481–7.

118. Yamada I, Shibuya H, Matsubara O, et al. Pulmonary artery disease in Takayasu's arteritis: angiographic findings. AJR Am J Roentgenol Aug 1992;159(2):263–9.

119. Song EK, Kolecki P. A case of pulmonary artery dissection diagnosed in the Emergency Department. J Emerg Med 2002;23(2):155–9.

120. Khattar RS, Fox DJ, Alty JE, et al. Pulmonary artery dissection: an emerging cardiovascular complication in surviving patients with chronic pulmonary hypertension. Heart 2005;91(2):142–5.

121. Senbaklavaci O, Kaneko Y, Bartunek A, et al. Rupture and dissection in pulmonary artery aneurysms: incidence, cause, and treatment–review and case report. J Thorac Cardiovasc Surg 2001; 121(5):1006–8.

122. Neimatallah MA, Hassan W, Moursi M, et al. CT findings of pulmonary artery dissection. Br J Radiol 2007;80(951):e61–3.

123. Wunderbaldinger P, Bernhard C, Uffmann M, et al. Acute pulmonary trunk dissection in a patient with primary pulmonary hypertension. J Comput Assist Tomogr 2000;24(1):92–5.

124. Weinreb JC, Davis SD, Berkmen YM, et al. Pulmonary artery sarcoma: evaluation using Gd-DTPA. J Comput Assist Tomogr 1990;14(4): 647–9.

125. Madu EC, Taylor DC, Durzinsky DS, et al. Primary intimal sarcoma of the pulmonary trunk simulating pulmonary embolism. Am Heart J 1993;125(6): 1790–2.

126. Shmookler BM, Marsh HB, Roberts WC. Primary sarcoma of the pulmonary trunk and/or right or left main pulmonary artery–a rare cause of obstruction to right ventricular outflow. Report on two patients and analysis of 35 previously described patients. Am J Med 1977;63(2):263–72.

127. Mattoo A, Fedullo PF, Kapelanski D, et al. Pulmonary artery sarcoma: a case report of surgical cure and 5-year follow-up. Chest 2002;122(2): 745–7.

128. Anderson MB, Kriett JM, Kapelanski DP, et al. Primary pulmonary artery sarcoma: a report of six cases. Ann Thorac Surg 1995;59(6):1487–90.

129. Smith WS, Lesar MS, Travis WD, et al. MR and CT findings in pulmonary artery sarcoma. J Comput Assist Tomogr 1989;13(5):906–9.

130. Kacl GM, Bruder E, Pfammatter T, et al. Primary angiosarcoma of the pulmonary arteries: dynamic contrast-enhanced MRI. J Comput Assist Tomogr 1998;22(5):687–91.

131. Bressler EL, Nelson JM. Primary pulmonary artery sarcoma: diagnosis with CT, MR imaging, and transthoracic needle biopsy. AJR Am J Roentgenol 1992; 159(4):702–4.

132. Bleisch VR, Kraus FT. Polypoid sarcoma of the pulmonary trunk: analysis of the literature and report of a case with leptomeric organelles and ultrastructural features of rhabdomyosarcoma. Cancer 1980;46(2):314–24.

133. Velebit V, Christenson JT, Simonet F, et al. Preoperative diagnosis of a pulmonary artery sarcoma. Thorax 1995;50(9):1014–5, discussion 1016–7.

134. Nomori H, Horio H, Morinaga S, et al. Multiple pulmonary infarctions associated with lung cancer. Jpn J Clin Oncol 2000;30(1):40–2.

135. Held BT, Siegelman SS. Pulmonary infarction secondary to bronchogenic carcinoma. Am J Roentgenol Radium Ther Nucl Med 1974;120(1): 145–50.

136. Marriott AE, Weisbrod G. Bronchogenic carcinoma associated with pulmonary infarction. Radiology 1982;145(3):593–7.

137. Horio H, Nomori H, Morinaga S, et al [A case of bronchogenic carcinoma associated with pulmonary infarction which showed a tumorous shadow]. Kyobu Geka 1996;49(2):163–6.

138. Yoshida N, Sugita H, Nakajima Y, et al [Relations between chest CT and pathologic findings in pulmonary infarction associated with lung cancer].

Nihon Kyobu Shikkan Gakkai Zasshi 1995;33(10): 1064–72.

139. Yamaguchi T, Suzuki K, Asamura H, et al. Lung carcinoma with polypoid growth in the main pulmonary artery: report of two cases. Jpn J Clin Oncol 2000;30(8):358–61.

140. Kauczor HU, Layer G, Schad LR, et al. Clinical applications of MR angiography in intrathoracic masses. J Comput Assist Tomogr 1991;15(3): 409–17.

141. Lehnhardt S, Thorsten Winterer J, Strecker R, et al. Assessment of pulmonary perfusion with ultrafast projection magnetic resonance angiography in comparison with lung perfusion scintigraphy in patients with malignant stenosis. Invest Radiol 2002;37(11):594–9.

142. Powell AJ, Chung T, Landzberg MJ, Geva T. Accuracy of MRI evaluation of pulmonary blood supply in patients with complex pulmonary stenosis or atresia. Int J Card Imaging 2000;16(3): 169–74.

143. Boechat MI, Ratib O, Williams PL, Gomes AS, Child JS, Allada V. Cardiac MR imaging and MR angiography for assessment of complex tetralogy of Fallot and pulmonary atresia. Radiographics 2005;25(6):1535–46.

144. Geva T, Greil GF, Marshall AC, et al. Gadolinium-enhanced 3-dimensional magnetic resonance angiography of pulmonary blood supply in patients with complex pulmonary stenosis or atresia: comparison with x-ray angiography. Circulation 2002;106(4):473–8.

145. Choe YH, Ko JK, Lee HJ, et al. MR imaging of non-visualized pulmonary arteries at angiography in patients with congenital heart disease. J Korean Med Sci 1998;13(6):597–602.

146. Greenberg SB, Crisci KL, Koenig P, et al. Magnetic resonance imaging compared with echocardiography in the evaluation of pulmonary artery abnormalities in children with tetralogy of Fallot following palliative and corrective surgery. Pediatr Radiol 1997;27(12):932–5.

147. Roman KS, Kellenberger CJ, Farooq S, et al. Comparative imaging of differential pulmonary blood flow in patients with congenital heart disease: magnetic resonance imaging versus lung perfusion scintigraphy. Pediatr Radiol 2005; 35(3):295–301.

148. Greil GF, Beerbaum P, Razavi R, et al. Imaging the right ventricle: non-invasive imaging. Heart 2008; 94(6):803–8.

149. Puchalski MD, Williams RV, Askovich B, et al. Assessment of right ventricular size and function: echo versus magnetic resonance imaging. Congenit Heart Dis 2007;2(1):27–31.

150. Rohrer M, Bauer H, Mintorovitch J, et al. Comparison of magnetic properties of MRI contrast media

solutions at different magnetic field strengths. Invest Radiol 2005;40(11):715–24.

151. Nael K, Michaely HJ, Lee M, et al. Dynamic pulmonary perfusion and flow quantification with MR imaging, 3.0T vs. 1.5T: initial results. J Magn Reson Imaging 2006;24(2):333–9.

152. Nael K, Fenchel M, Krishnam M, et al. 3.0 Tesla high spatial resolution contrast-enhanced magnetic resonance angiography (CE-MRA) of the pulmonary circulation: initial experience with a 32-channel phased array coil using a high relaxivity contrast agent. Invest Radiol 2007;42(6):392–8.

153. Bremerich J, Bilecen D, Reimer P. MR angiography with blood pool contrast agents. Eur Radiol 2007; 17(12):3017–24.

154. Lauffer RB, Parmelee DJ, Dunham SU, et al. MS-325: albumin-targeted contrast agent for MR angiography. Radiology 1998;207(2):529–38.

155. Spuentrup E, Katoh M, Buecker A, et al. Molecular MR imaging of human thrombi in a swine model of pulmonary embolism using a fibrin-specific contrast agent. Invest Radiol 2007;42(8):586–95.

156. Spuentrup E, Buecker A, Katoh M, et al. Molecular magnetic resonance imaging of coronary thrombosis and pulmonary emboli with a novel fibrin-targeted contrast agent. Circulation 2005;111(11): 1377–82.

157. Spuentrup E, Katoh M, Wiethoff AJ, et al. Molecular magnetic resonance imaging of pulmonary emboli with a fibrin-specific contrast agent. Am J Respir Crit Care Med 2005;172(4):494–500.

158. Meuli RA, Wedeen VJ, Geller SC, et al. MR gated subtraction angiography: evaluation of lower extremities. Radiology. 1986;159(2):411–8.

159. Wedeen VJ, Meuli RA, Edelman RR, et al. Projective imaging of pulsatile flow with magnetic resonance. Science 1985;230(4728):946–8.

160. Miyazaki M, Sugiura S, Tateishi F, et al. Non-contrast-enhanced MR angiography using 3D ECG-synchronized half-Fourier fast spin echo. J Magn Reson Imaging 2000;12(5):776–83.

161. Miyazaki M, Lee VS. Nonenhanced MR angiography. Radiology 2008;248(1):20–43.

162. Edelman RR, Hatabu H, Tadamura E, et al. Noninvasive assessment of regional ventilation in the human lung using oxygen-enhanced magnetic resonance imaging. Nat Med 1996;2(11):1236–9.

163. Hatabu H, Tadamura E, Chen Q, et al. Pulmonary ventilation: dynamic MRI with inhalation of molecular oxygen. Eur J Radiol 2001;37(3): 172–8.

164. Chen Q, Levin DL, Kim D, et al. Pulmonary disorders: ventilation-perfusion MR imaging with animal models. Radiology 1999;213(3):871–9.

Pediatric Body MR Angiography

Rajesh Krishnamurthy, MD[a],*, Raja Muthupillai, PhD[b],
Taylor Chung, MD[c]

KEYWORDS

- Pediatric MR angiography • Children
- MR angiography • Congenital heart disease
- Vasculitis • Vascular malformations • Keyhole
- Three-dimensional steady-state free precession

Vascular pathology in children is commonplace and involves every organ system. MR angiography has made significant inroads in the diagnosis of adult vascular conditions; however, there is relative underutilization of the powerful, noninvasive, rapid three-dimensional (3D) imaging capability offered by MR angiography in children. One potential reason is the difference between pediatric and adult MR angiography, which is not limited to clinical indications but also involves sedation, coil selection for patients of different size, contrast administration, choice of MR scan parameters, and image processing. This article provides an overview of general pediatric MR angiography techniques, common indications for body MR angiography in children, and the complementary role of MR angiography to other vascular imaging modalities in children, including CT angiography, Doppler ultrasound, and catheter angiography.

PEDIATRIC MR ANGIOGRAPHY TECHNIQUE
Gadolinium Contrast-Enhanced MR Angiography

The most common and widely available technique is contrast-enhanced MR angiography (CEMRA). The basic pulse sequence on a 1.5-T system is a 3D T1-weighted fast gradient echo sequence using the shortest repetition time and echo time available, with a flip angle of 30° to 45°. A bolus of gadolinium contrast agent is administered intravenously, and the acquisition sequence is initiated when the contrast bolus arrives at the vessel of interest. Some form of centric-order filling of k-space is usually implemented as a dynamic scan or is timed to match optimal enhancement of the target vasculature.

Challenges of Pediatric MR Angiography

The technical aspects and requirements of body MR angiography in children vary depending on the child's age and ability to cooperate with the study. Adult techniques can be easily applied to the older adolescent patient; however, younger adolescents, children, and infants cannot hold still for the duration of the study and require sedation. Children have faster heart rates and respiratory rates. Moreover, their vessels are smaller and have more rapid circulations. Therefore, the need for high spatial and temporal resolution is critical. The volume of administered contrast agent is limited by the child's weight and can be small, even when double-dose gadolinium is used. Hence, the test bolus technique is not routinely used. Optimal intravenous (IV) access is not always available, and hand injections may have to be performed by way of small-bore IVs or peripherally inserted central venous catheters. Timing the contrast to the vessel of interest can be difficult under such circumstances.

Sedation and Control of Respiration

In the authors' experience, most patients younger than 8 years need some form of sedation or general

[a] Departments of Radiology and Pediatrics (Cardiology), Baylor College of Medicine, Edward B. Singleton Department of Diagnostic Imaging, Texas Children's Hospital, Houston, TX, USA
[b] Department of Diagnostic Radiology, St. Luke's Episcopal Hospital, Houston, TX, USA
[c] Department of Diagnostic Imaging, Children's Hospital and Research Center Oakland, Oakland, CA, USA
* Corresponding author.
E-mail address: rxkrishn@texaschildrenshospital.org (R. Krishnamurthy).

Magn Reson Imaging Clin N Am 17 (2009) 133–144
doi:10.1016/j.mric.2008.12.004
1064-9689/08/$ – see front matter © 2009 Elsevier Inc. All rights reserved.

anesthesia. Endotracheal intubation with general anesthesia allows for the acquisition of breath-held sequences and yields the highest-quality images without blurring. Breath holding increases the visualization of peripheral vessel branches and is indispensable in the setting of older hardware and lower-gradient strengths, which result in long dynamic times; however, intravenous sedation without intubation with data acquisition during free breathing is preferred by parents and anesthesiologists for its convenience, less-invasive nature, and rapid recovery from sedation.

In most current machines equipped with strong gradients, phased-array coils, and parallel imaging, very short dynamic times can be achieved, resulting in a time-resolved MR angiography that is fairly insensitive to motion artifact from breathing, and can also yield diagnostic results with spatial resolution of 1 mm and a dynamic time of 4 to 8 seconds.[1–3] With the advent of various sparsely sampled k-space filling schemes[4–6] and parallel imaging reconstructions,[7,8] the CEMRA sequence acquisition time can be very short. Such techniques provide a time-resolved study with separation of the arterial, venous, and parenchymal enhancement phases, even in small children who have rapid circulations (**Figs. 1A, B**).

In the authors' practice, free-breathing studies are performed under intravenous sedation for most routine indications, restricting the use of endotracheal intubation and breath holding to small neonates who have high heart rates or to indications that require reliable evaluation of higher-order branches (such as distal branch renal artery stenosis), aortopulmonary collaterals, or small postsurgical shunts. For example, submillimeter in-plane resolution is needed in a newborn infant for the evaluation of systemic arterial connections to the pulmonary arterial system.[9]

Timing of Bolus and Temporal Resolution

Bolus timing becomes unnecessary using these rapid CEMRA sequences, which can be an advantage in the clinical implementation of CEMRA in a young patient who has rapid hemodynamics and a small volume of available contrast. Multiple rapid CEMRA sequences (dynamics) can be programmed to run consecutively, and almost "real-time" MR angiography can be achieved. This type of real-time MR angiography allows for the study of hemodynamics that, in the past, could only be achieved by invasive digital subtraction angiography.[10,11] The trade-off is temporal resolution versus spatial resolution. Even with these new techniques, the temporal resolution of MR angiography (1 dynamic per second) lags behind that of conventional digital angiography (14 frames per second). Alternatively, a bolus tracking technique may be used to time the onset of acquisition to arrival of contrast within the vessel of interest (**Fig. 2**). This methodology is helpful when breath holding is desired and the patient is unable to cooperate with a long period of breath holding.

Gadolinium in Children

The typical dose of gadolinium for MR imaging is 0.1 mmol/kg. For MR angiography, higher doses (0.2–0.3 mmol/kg) of gadodiamide or gadopentetate are often used. Although six gadolinium-based contrast agents have received approval by the Food and Drug Administration (FDA) for use in MRI in adults, none of these agents has received trial-based approval by the FDA for pediatric MR angiography; however, it is a common "off-label" practice in the United States.

The recent recognition of an association between the administration of gadolinium-based contrast agents and subsequent development of nephrogenic systemic fibrosis in patients who have moderate renal disease (glomerular filtration rate <60 mL/min/1.73 m^2) to end-stage renal disease (glomerular filtration rate <15 mL/min/1.73 m^2 or on dialysis) has sparked renewed interest in noncontrast angiographic techniques.[12,13] Nephrogenic systemic fibrosis is characterized by progressive tissue fibrosis, usually starting in the skin of the lower extremities and advancing over the course of days or weeks to the trunk and extracutaneous structures such as skeletal muscle, heart, lung, and esophagus. Several pediatric cases have been reported, although it is unclear whether the immature kidney function of neonates and infants poses an additional risk factor. In the authors' practice, MR angiographic sequences not using gadolinium contrast are used in patients who have even mild renal insufficiency.

MR Angiographic Sequences Without Gadolinium Contrast

The more commonly used noncontrast angiographic techniques include 3D steady-state free precession (SSFP) with respiratory navigator gating (**Figs. 1C and 1D**), and two-dimensional and 3D phase-contrast sequences (**Fig. 3B**). These techniques are also indispensable in the setting of lack of vascular access. They usually have very specific applications such as coronary MR angiography (**Fig. 4A**) with 3D SSFP.[14,15]

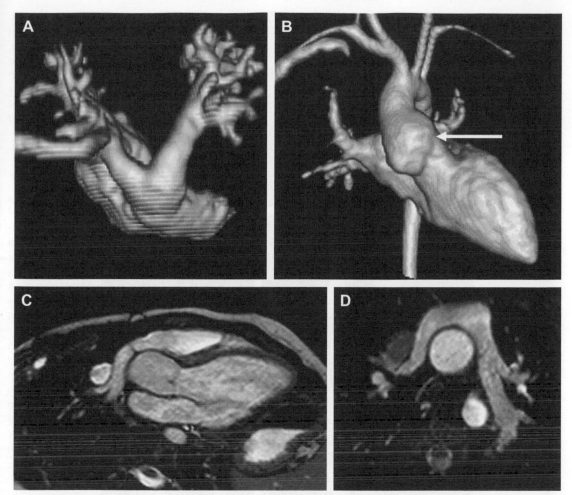

Fig. 1. (*A, B*) Volume-rendered images of 3D gadolinium CEMRA in a patient who has *d*-transposition of the great arteries, status post arterial switch procedure. (*A*) Superior view of an early phase of the angiogram, demonstrating unobstructed branch pulmonary arteries and their characteristic location after an arterial switch procedure. (*B*) Aortic phase of the MR angiography, demonstrating moderately severe aortic root dilatation (*arrow*), a common complication of this procedure. (*C, D*) Oblique reformatted images in the same patient from a respiratory navigator 3D SSFP sequence, an alternative 3D MR angiographic sequence performed without intravenous contrast. (*C*) Right ventricular outflow tract. (*D*) Branch pulmonary arteries straddling the aorta.

Because the acquisition times of most of these noncontrast MR angiography techniques are long, breath holding is not possible. These techniques are therefore designed for free-breathing patients. When the motion compensation schemes are not optimal, however, the resultant MR angiography images are nondiagnostic. The trade-off is acquisition time versus spatial resolution. The longer the acquisition time, the greater the possibility that gross motion will occur, which is difficult to compensate for. There have been no reports of large clinical series of pediatric body MR angiography performed using noncontrast techniques. Limited clinical application of 3D SSFP sequence for MR angiography of the chest in congenital heart disease patients has

been successful.[16] More clinical experience is needed to determine the robustness of this and other noncontrast body MR angiography sequences for the pediatric population.

Black Blood Imaging of the Vasculature

Black blood sequences used for vascular imaging include gated sequences such as double (or triple) inversion recovery fast spin echo, and spin echo T1 with echo planar imaging readout. The use of EKG gating reduces pulsation artifact and flow artifacts within the lumen. The inversion recovery sequences are sensitive to edema and are helpful in the diagnosis and follow-up of vasculitis. The triple inversion recovery sequence provides

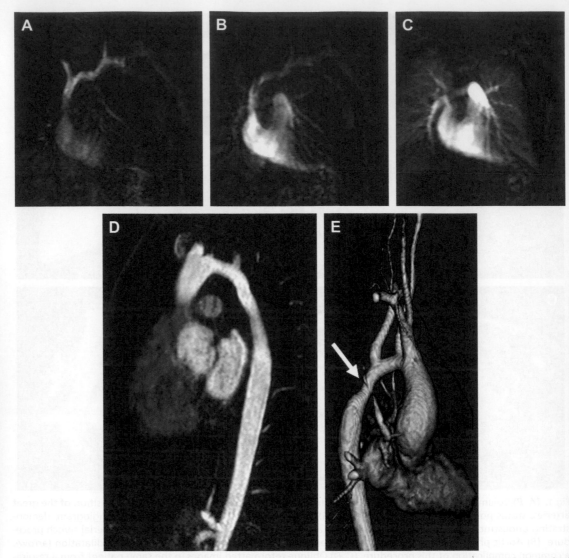

Fig. 2. Use of a bolus tracking sequence to time the contrast bolus to the vessel of interest. (*A–C*) Arrival of contrast to the superior vena cava, right ventricle, and pulmonary arteries, respectively, on the subsecond MR angiography technique. (*D*) The high-resolution 3D MR angiography sequence is initiated at this point, allowing optimal visualization of the aortic coarctation. (*E*) Posterior view of a volume-rendered MR angiography. Arrow points to the coarctation.

additional fat suppression (**Fig. 4B**). The black blood sequences provide a quick cross-sectional overview of the relevant anatomy and the information regarding the vessel wall, which is lacking on the bright blood sequences. Postgadolinium T1-weighted sequences are helpful to look for wall enhancement and to evaluate the perivascular soft tissues and parenchymal organs in the setting of vasculitis.

Postprocessing of MR Angiography

Commonly used postprocessing techniques in pediatric MR angiography include multiplanar reformat, volume rendering, and maximum-intensity projection. The first dynamic is usually obtained without intravenous contrast and serves as a mask that is subtracted from the later dynamics. Currently available 3D post processing software has significantly diminished the time taken to process angiographic data sets. Although a number of automated processing tools are available for adult use, dedicated templates for pediatric applications are still unavailable, and most of the processing steps and measurements are performed manually. Examples of 3D postprocessing are seen on almost all the images in this article.

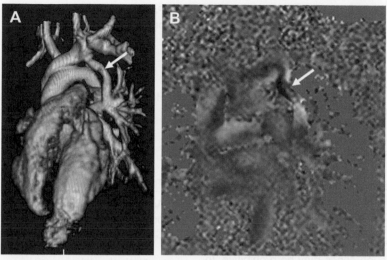

Fig. 3. (*A*) Volume-rendered image from 3D gadolinium MR angiography in a 10-year-old girl showing dual drainage of the left upper lobe pulmonary vein to the left innominate vein (*white arrow*) and to the left atrium (*black arrow*). (*B*) A phase-contrast sequence showed that most of the flow was directed to the innominate vein (*white arrow*), with a Qp:Qs of 1.3:1.

Extensions of volume rendering, such as virtual angioscopy, have served to increase the appeal of this technology to clinicians and surgeons.

THE USE OF MR ANGIOGRAPHY VERSUS DOPPLER ULTRASONOGRAPHY AND CT ANGIOGRAPHY IN CHILDREN

MR angiography may be used as a first-line imaging tool for a number of thoracic and abdominal vascular pathologies.[17] For example, it may be used to screen for vascular rings, midaortic syndrome, renal artery stenosis in the setting of unexplained hypertension in a child, and systemic aneurysms in Kawasaki disease, or to evaluate vascular anatomy before a renal or hepatic transplant. MR angiography is more commonly used as a problem-solving modality after initial Doppler ultrasonography. For example, it is commonly used when echocardiography is unsuccessful in screening the extracardiac vasculature in congenital heart disease. Echocardiographic windows typically diminish in older, larger patients and in the postoperative setting. Although CT

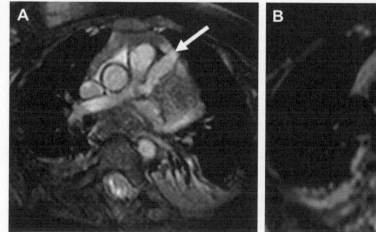

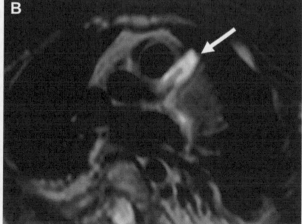

Fig. 4. A 3-month-old boy who has Kawasaki's disease. (*A*) 3D segmented k-space turbo field echo sequence showing long-segment aneurysmal dilatation of the left anterior descending artery (*arrow*). (*B*) Black blood triple inversion recovery sequence showing high signal within the wall of the left anterior descending artery (*arrow*), consistent with active inflammation versus mural thrombus.

angiography and MR angiography may appear as competing modalities in a number of instances because they accomplish similar objectives, they have different strengths and weaknesses. CT angiography is more often performed without sedation due to the short duration of the study. CT angiography provides higher spatial resolution, which may increase diagnostic accuracy in the setting of higher-order branch arterial stenosis or coronary stenosis. In children, CT angiography is typically not performed as a multiphasic study due to radiation concerns and therefore lacks the temporal data available on the MR angiography. Also, indications that require a large field of view (eg, screening for systemic aneurysms in Kawasaki disease) benefit more from MR angiography because the radiation dose associated with a CT angiography in such cases may be prohibitive. In the authors' practice, the risks associated with sedation for MR angiography are weighed more favorably against the risk of ionizing radiation associated with CT.

CLINICAL APPLICATIONS OF PEDIATRIC MR ANGIOGRAPHY

The following are examples of common applications of MR angiography in the pediatric chest, abdomen, and extremities. This list is not meant to be exhaustive but is intended to provide insight into the extensive potential of MR angiography in children. A few applications are discussed later in greater detail.

Chest

1. Evaluation of extracardiac vasculature in congenital heart disease
   a. Systemic arteries
      Diagnosis of aortic coarctation and follow-up after therapy
      Supravalvular aortic stenosis
      Vascular rings
   b. Pulmonary arteries
      Branch pulmonary artery stenosis
      Pulmonary sling
   c. Pulmonary veins
      Anomalous pulmonary venous return
      Pulmonary vein stenosis
   d. Systemic veins
      Systemic venous anatomy in heterotaxy
2. Systemic vein thrombosis
3. Arteritis

Abdomen

1. Mapping abdominal vascular anatomy before surgery

2. Pathology of the abdominal aorta and its branches
      Midaortic syndrome
      Renal artery stenosis
      Aneurysms
      Arterial thromboembolism
3. Hepatic and portal vasculature
      Etiology of portal hypertension
      Screening before and after hepatic transplantation

Extremities

1. Acute arterial occlusion due to trauma, emboli, or arteritis
2. Chronic arterial insufficiency
      Thoracic outlet syndrome
      Radiation injury
3. Deep venous thrombosis of the upper and lower extremities

Miscellaneous

1. Vascular malformations
2. Evaluation of the systemic vasculature in vasculitis
      Screening for arterial aneurysms and Kawasaki disease

Evaluation of the Extracardiac Vasculature in Congenital Heart Disease

Echocardiography is the mainstay of diagnosis of congenital heart disease in the preoperative period; however, there is a small but significant subgroup of patients in the newborn period in whom the acoustic windows are inadequate for delineation of the extracardiac vasculature, including the aorta and its branches, pulmonary arteries, pulmonary veins, and the systemic veins.[18] Examples include atypical coarctation, anomalous pulmonary venous return (see **Fig. 3**), scimitar syndrome, vascular rings, pulmonary sling, aortopulmonary collaterals, anomalous coronaries, systemic and pulmonary venous anatomy in heterotaxy, and status of the main pulmonary artery and branch pulmonary arteries in the setting of pulmonary atresia. MR angiography is used as a problem-solving tool in these situations. Acoustic windows for echocardiography diminish in the postoperative period, and gadolinium-enhanced MR angiography is an integral part of the MR imaging surveillance protocol for a number of conditions. Examples include pulmonary vein stenosis after total anomalous pulmonary venous connection repair, screening for recurrent coarctation, branch pulmonary artery stenosis after Tetralogy of Fallot repair, and screening for venous collaterals after bidirectional Glenn and Fontan procedures (**Fig. 5**).

The MR angiography technique in the setting of congenital heart disease depends on the age of the patient, hemodynamic status, and the vessel of interest. In children, a time-resolved technique with short dynamic times is preferred,[1–3] which achieves selective contrast opacification of the right-sided structures (right atrium, right ventricle, and pulmonary arteries), left-sided structures (pulmonary veins, left atrium, left ventricle, and aorta), and the systemic veins (innominate veins, superior vena cava, hepatic veins, and inferior vena cava [IVC]). The coverage should extend from the neck to the level of the renal vessels because involvement of the vasculature in congenital heart disease frequently extends outside the chest (eg, infradiaphragmatic total anomalous pulmonary venous return, aortopulmonary collaterals in scimitar syndrome, abnormal hepatic venous, and IVC anatomy in heterotaxy). The rate of contrast injection is adjusted for age to ensure a tight contrast bolus. Hand injection may be used in newborns with a saline flush, but an automatic dual injector is preferred in older neonates, infants, and children. Spatial resolution is determined by the application. For instance, a very high spatial resolution is required to screen

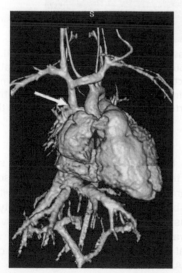

Fig. 5. Volume-rendered image of gadolinium-enhanced 3D MR angiography in a 24-year-old man who has tricuspid atresia, status post right atrium–main pulmonary artery Fontan connection (*black arrow*), who developed severe right atrial dilatation and atrial fibrillation, resulting in severe dilatation of the hepatic veins. A bidirectional Glenn shunt was performed to relieve volume overload of the right atrium (*white arrow*), with subsequent reduction in right atrial size.

for aortopulmonary collaterals in the setting of pulmonary atresia, whereas a lower spatial resolution is adequate to screen for systemic venous thrombosis. The most commonly used postprocessing techniques include volume rendering, oblique multiplanar reformat, and maximum-intensity projection. Vessel measurements are made in orthogonal planes on the 3D workstation.

Arterial Stenosis or Occlusion

A number of vascular conditions in children involve stenosis or occlusion of the arterial tree. Aortic coarctation is the most common example (see **Fig. 2**). The best estimate of the extent and severity of reduction in luminal caliber of the aorta is obtained from a high-resolution 3D angiographic data set. Although discrete coarctation of the aortic isthmus is the most common type, it is important to detect the presence of associated hypoplasia of the transverse aortic arch. Conventional treatment for aortic coarctation by resection of the stenotic segment or by percutaneous balloon dilatation fails in the setting of transverse arch hypoplasia, which has to be treated by arch augmentation. A number of atypical presentations of coarctation, including the presence of aneurysms, midthoracic involvement, or associated stenosis of the head and neck arteries, may potentially be missed by echocardiography and are apparent on the MR angiogram. MR angiography is also extremely useful in the postoperative setting to screen for recurrent coarctation when acoustic windows are severely limited. The accuracy of MR angiography has obviated the need for a conventional diagnostic angiogram in this setting.

Midaortic syndrome,[19] also known as abdominal coarctation, is characterized by segmental narrowing of the proximal abdominal aorta and its major branches and should be included in the differential diagnoses of unexplained hypertension in a child. It may occur as an isolated entity or in association with genetic conditions such as neurofibromatosis, Alagille syndrome (**Fig. 6**), Williams syndrome, or fibromuscular dysplasia. Due to the need for serial follow-up imaging and because of the involvement of large vessels, MR angiography is preferred to CT angiography as the primary noninvasive imaging modality in this setting.

Systemic Vein Thrombosis

The incidence of venous thrombosis in pediatrics is 5.3 per 10,000 hospital admissions.[20] In children, two thirds of thrombosis occurs in the upper extremities,[21] whereas in adults, 90% occurs in the lower extremities. In children, 78% of

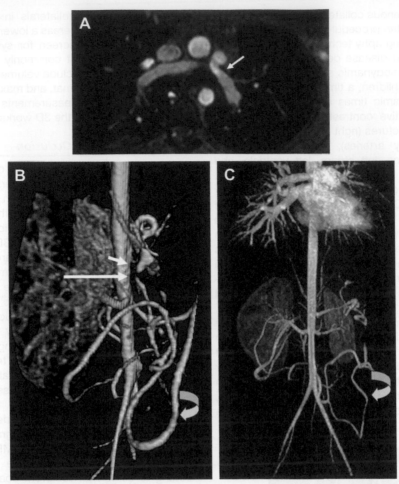

Fig. 6. A 2-year-old girl who has Alagille syndrome. (A) Axial cine fast gradient echo image (nongadolinium MR angiography technique) showing stenosis of the origin of the left pulmonary artery (*arrow*). (B) Lateral volume-rendered view and (C) anteroposterior maximum-intensity projection image of the abdomen from CEMRA showing occlusion of the celiac artery (*small arrow*) and superior mesenteric artery (*long arrow*), with a large circuitous collateral (*curved arrow*) from the inferior mesenteric artery supplying the distribution of the celiac artery and superior mesenteric artery in retrograde fashion.

upper-extremity thrombosis is catheter related. Children who have low birth weight and prematurity are at particular risk for central venous thrombosis. Cancer and congenital heart disease are the most common predisposing factors for thrombosis.

Although the superior vena cava, innominate veins, internal jugular veins, and subclavian veins are commonly affected by thrombosis (**Fig. 7**), IVC thrombosis may also occur in a number of settings, including extension of ileofemoral thrombosis (frequently as a result of idiopathic deep venous thrombosis), previous cardiac catheterization/central venous line placement, extension of renal tumor thrombus into the renal veins and IVC, direct compression of the IVC by abdominal masses, or hypercoagulable states. Collateral pathways include the paravertebral venous

system, the azygos and hemiazygos systems, and the thoracic and abdominal wall vasculature. Venograms are usually best performed with simultaneous bilateral upper- or lower-extremity venous injections of dilute gadolinium, which provide first-pass evaluation of the affected veins and the collateral pathways without any arterial contamination. Axial black blood images, time of flight bright blood images, and postgadolinium T1-weighted images provide complementary information by delineating thrombosed vessels and the perivascular soft tissues, shedding further light on the etiology of thrombosis.

Portal Hypertension

MR angiography is used frequently in a problem-solving role in portal hypertension to evaluate the

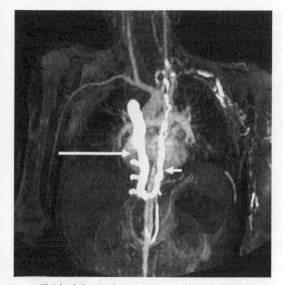

Fig. 7. Thick-slab maximum-intensity projection image from CEMRA in a patient who has extensive thrombosis of the central veins in the chest. Contrast injected into the left arm drains by way of collaterals into the hemiazygos (*short arrow*) and azygos (*long arrow*) system, ultimately returning to the heart by way of the infraazygos segment of the superior vena cava.

status of the hepatic vasculature after a Doppler ultrasound has been performed.[17,22] Common indications include (1) suboptimal ultrasound studies due to patient body habitus; (2) characterization of unusual forms of portal vein thrombosis (eg, isolated intrahepatic portal vein thrombosis, portal vein tumor thrombus, and so forth); (3) determination of the presence and extent of portosystemic varices (**Fig. 8**), especially around the gastroesophageal junction, which may predict the risk for life-threatening hematemesis; (4) screening for the presence and adequacy of a spontaneous splenorenal shunt; (5) mapping the portal circulation to determine feasibility of bypass procedures; and (6) determining patency of portal bypass procedures or surgically created portosystemic shunts. It has also been used in the preoperative evaluation of liver transplant recipients[23] to determine patency of the portal venous system, IVC anatomy, and variations in hepatic arterial anatomy. In the postoperative period after hepatic transplantation, MR angiography is helpful to screen for hepatic artery thrombosis or stenosis and for portal vein thrombosis,

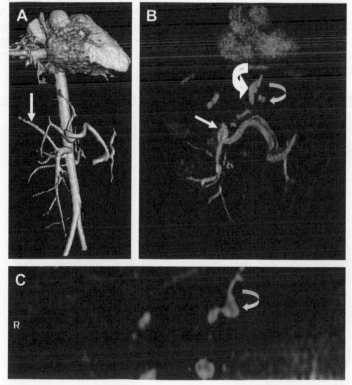

Fig. 8. A 12-year-old girl who has portal hypertension secondary to thrombosis of the main portal vein. (*A*) Arterial phase of CEMRA showing a replaced right hepatic artery arising from the superior mesenteric artery (*arrow*). (*B*) The portal venous phase shows thrombosis of the main portal vein (*straight arrow*), an enlarged left gastric vein (*large curved white arrow*), and a prominent gastric varix (*small curved blue arrow*). (*C*) Axial image of the large intramural varix along the lesser curvature of the stomach.

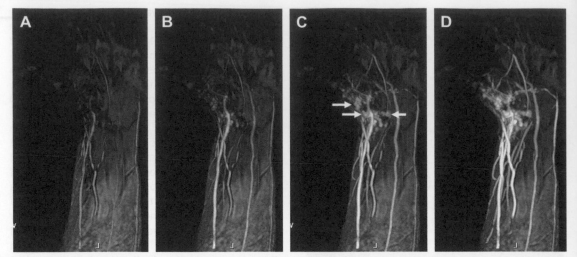

Fig. 9. (A–D) Four consecutive images of high-resolution keyhole-SENSE MR angiography in a patient who has an arteriovenous malformation of the hand, showing major arterial supply from the radial artery, multiple areas of arteriovenous communication in the thenar aspect of the hand (arrows), and multiple early draining veins. The temporal resolution for this study was 1.8 seconds. A bolus tracking technique was used to time the onset of acquisition to contrast arrival within the axillary artery. Thirty dynamics were performed.

especially in the setting of an indeterminate ultrasound.

Mapping Vascular Anatomy Prior to Surgery

MR angiography is commonly used to evaluate vascular anatomy in the following settings:[17]

1. Evaluating IVC and hepatic venous anatomy in the setting of heterotaxy due to the high incidence of IVC interruption with azygos continuation and aberrant hepatic venous drainage to the atria. Accurate mapping of IVC and hepatic venous drainage can be challenging by ultrasound but is easily accomplished by MR

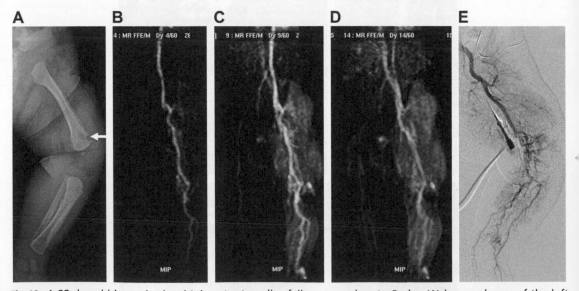

Fig. 10. A 28-day-old boy who has high output cardiac failure secondary to Parkes Weber syndrome of the left lower extremity. (A) Lateral radiograph of the left lower extremity showed evidence of bony involvement (arrow). (B–D) Maximum-intensity projection images from CEMRA obtained at the early arterial, late arterial, and early venous filling phases, respectively, showing extensive muscular involvement by the diffuse arteriovenous malformation (note muscle enhancement) but no large arteriovenous communication that would be amenable to embolization. (E) These findings were confirmed on the contrast angiogram.

angiography and helps surgical planning as to the development of optimal techniques to incorporate the hepatic veins into the Fontan circuit.

2. Mapping hepatic vasculature to determine the feasibility and type of segmental resection of liver tumors.[24,25]

3. Determining variations in renal arterial and venous anatomy before renal transplantation; screening for renal vessel involvement in abdominal neoplasms.[26]

Peripheral MR Angiography and Vascular Malformations

Peripheral MR angiography is a well-established indication in adults but is an infrequent procedure in pediatrics because of the rarity of limb-threatening ischemia or chronic arterial occlusion in children. The most common indications for peripheral MR angiography in children are high-flow vascular malformations (**Figs. 9** and **10**), embolic disease, trauma, iatrogenic vascular injury (**Fig. 11**), and extrinsic compression of the vessels related to anatomic abnormalities such as thoracic outlet syndrome or to neoplasms. In the setting of high-flow vascular malformations such as arteriovenous malformation or fistula, a very high temporal resolution along with high spatial resolution is required

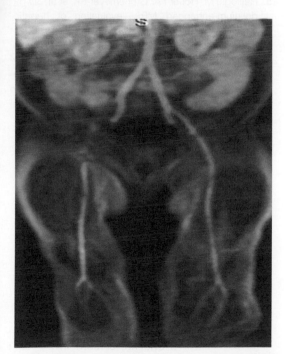

Fig. 11. Maximum-intensity projection image from CEMRA on a 10-day-old boy showing right external iliac and right common femoral artery occlusion due to placement of an arterial line.

for selective visualization of the nidus and to demonstrate the early draining veins. In the authors' practice, this is achieved by using a combination of keyhole MR angiography with parallel imaging. **Fig. 9** demonstrates the application of this technique in a patient who has an arteriovenous malformation of the hand that had multiple sites of arteriovenous communication.

SUMMARY

The vast potential of MR angiography in children remains unfulfilled in most pediatric practices, with CT assuming a large proportion of the noninvasive vascular imaging workload. The success of pediatric MR angiography depends on modifying the MR angiography on the basis of patient size, hemodynamic status, and clinical indications in children, and requires an adequate understanding of pediatric-specific hardware, software, and equipment requirements. The challenge of equipment manufacturers and educators in radiology is to streamline and demystify the process to enhance acceptance of the technique by the mainstream imaging community so that more children may benefit from the versatility and safety of this technique.

REFERENCES

1. Chung T, Krishnamurthy R. Contrast-enhanced MR angiography in infants and children. Magn Reson Imaging Clin N Am 2005;13(1):161–70.

2. Chung T. Magnetic resonance angiography of the body in pediatric patients: experience with a contrast-enhanced time-resolved technique. Pediatr Radiol 2005;35:3–10.

3. Muthupillai R, Vick GW III, Flamm SD, et al. Free breathing time resolved contrast enhanced MRA in pediatric patients with sensitivity encoding. Magn Reson Imaging 2003;17:559–64.

4. Du J, Carroll TJ, Wagner HJ, et al. Time-resolved, undersampled projection reconstruction imaging for high resolution CE-MRA of the distal runoff vessels. Magn Reson Med 2002;48:516–22.

5. Tsao J, Boesiger, Pruessmann KP, et al. k-t BLAST and k-t SENSE: dynamic MRI with high frame rate exploiting spatiotemporal correlations. Magn Reson Med 2003;50:1031–42.

6. Willinek WA, Hadizadeh DR, von Falkenhausen M, et al. 4D time-resolved MR angiography with keyhole (4D-TRAK): more than 60 times accelerated MRA using a combination of CENTRA, keyhole, and SENSE at 3.0T. J Magn Reson Imaging 2008;27(6):1455–60.

7. Sodickson DK, Manning WJ. Simultaneous acquisition of spatial harmonics (SMASH): fast imaging

with radiofrequency coil arrays. Magn Reson Med 1997;38:591–603.

8. Pruessmann KP, Weiger M, Scheidegger MB, et al. SENSE: sensitivity encoding for fast MRI. Magn Reson Med 1999;42:952–62.

9. Kellenberger CJ, Yoo SJ, Buchel ER, et al. Cardiovascular MR imaging in neonates and infants with congenital heart disease. Radiographics 2007; 27(1):5–18.

10. Korperich H, Gieseke J, Esdom H, et al. Ultrafast time-resolved contrast-enhanced 3D pulmonary venous cardiovascular magnetic resonance angiography using SENSE combined with CENTRA-keyhole. J Cardiovasc Magn Reson 2007;9(1): 77–87.

11. Goo HW, Yang DH, Park IS, et al. Time-resolved three-dimensional contrast-enhanced magnetic resonance angiography in patients who have undergone a Fontan operation or bi-directional cavopulmonary connection: initial experience. J Magn Reson Imaging 2007;25:727–36.

12. Mendichovzky IA, Marks SD, Simcock CM, et al. Gadolinium and nephrogenic systemic fibrosis: time to tighten practice. Pediatr Radiol 2008;38:489–96.

13. Broome DR. Nephrogenic systemic fibrosis associated with gadolinium based contrast agents: a summary of the medical literature reporting. Eur J Radiol 2008;66:230–4.

14. Weber OM, Martin AJ, Higgins CB, et al. Whole-heart steady state free precession coronary artery magnetic resonance angiography. Magn Reson Med 2003;50:1223–8.

15. Takemura A, Suzuki A, Inaba R, et al. Utility of coronary MR angiography in children with Kawasaki disease. AJR Am J Roentgenol 2007;188:534–9.

16. Sorensen TS, Korperich H, Greil GF, et al. Operator-independent isotropic three-dimensional magnetic resonance imaging for morphology in congenital heart disease: a validation study. Circulation 2004; 110(2):163–9.

17. Krishnamurthy R, Guillerman RP. Pediatric abdominal magnetic resonance angiography. Semin Roentgenol 2008;43(1):60–71.

18. Krishnamurthy R. Pediatric cardiac MRI: anatomy and function. Pediatr Radiol 2008;38(suppl 2): S192–9.

19. Panayiotopoulos YP, Tyrrell MR, Koffman G, et al. Mid-aortic syndrome presenting in childhood. Br J Surg 1996;83:235–40.

20. Petaja J, Peltola K. Venous thrombosis in pediatric cardiac surgery. J Cardiothorac Vasc Anesth 1997; 11:889–94.

21. Male C, Kuhle S, Mitchell L, et al. Diagnosis of venous thromboembolism in children. Semin Thromb Hemost 2003;29:377–89.

22. Teo EHJ, Strouse PJ, Prince MR, et al. Applications of magnetic resonance imaging and magnetic resonance angiography to evaluate the hepatic vasculature in the pediatric patient. Pediatr Radiol 1999;29: 238–43.

23. Ng KK, Cheng YF, Wong HF, et al. Gadolinium-enhanced magnetic resonance portography: application in paediatric liver transplant recipients. Transplant Proc 2000;21:2099–100.

24. Haliloglu M, Hoffer FA, Groemeyer SA, et al. Applications of 3D contrast enhanced MR angiography in pediatric oncology. Pediatr Radiol 1999;29:863–8.

25. Haliloglu M, Hoffer FA, Gronemeyer SA, et al. 3D gadolinium-enhanced MRA: evaluation of hepatic-vasculature in children with hepatoblastoma. J Magn Reson Imaging 2000;11:65–8.

26. Pfluger T, Czekalla R, Hundt C, et al. MR angiography versus color Doppler sonography in the evaluation of renal vessels and the inferior vena cava in abdominal masses of pediatric patients. AJR Am J Roentgenol 1999;173:103–8.

Coronary MR Imaging: Lumen and Wall

Sebastian Kelle, MD[a,b], Robert G. Weiss, MD[b,c], Matthias Stuber, PhD[b,c,d,*]

KEYWORDS

- Coronary MR imaging • Vessel wall • Imaging
- Atherosclerosis • Vessel lumen

Coronary artery disease remains the leading cause of death for men and women in the United States.[1] The current gold standard for the diagnosis of hemodynamically significant coronary artery disease in vivo is selective x-ray coronary angiography. X-ray coronary angiography, however, has a few disadvantages. X-ray coronary angiography identifies lesions that impede on the vessel lumen but offers relatively little relevant information about the coronary artery vessel wall. Furthermore, a small but significant risk of complications exists and these are related to the invasive nature of the procedure, radiation exposure for both the patient and physician, and iodinated contrast agents.[2,3] In addition, up to 40% of patients who undergo invasive x-ray coronary angiography are found to have no significant coronary artery lumen stenosis.[4] For these reasons, there is a strong need for an alternative technique that is noninvasive, more cost effective, and which provides not only information about the vessel lumen but also the vessel wall without the need for ionizing radiation and nephrotoxic contrast agents.

Coronary MR imaging offers several advantages. It has a relatively high spatial resolution, high soft-tissue contrast, and the ability to generate images in any three-dimensional plane without the need for ionizing radiation. Other advantages of coronary MR imaging are the possibility for repeated measurements and the ability to assess cardiac anatomy, function, viability, and coronary artery blood flow in a single examination.

TECHNICAL CONSIDERATIONS FOR CORONARY MR IMAGING

For accurate coronary MR imaging, images must be obtained rapidly and with high spatial and temporal resolution. Acquisition of the whole coronary artery tree with sufficient spatial resolution can take 10 to 15 minutes, however, compared with seconds with multislice CT. There might be a greater chance for motion artifacts the longer the data acquisition lasts. Two sources of motion are associated with coronary MR imaging: motion related to intrinsic cardiac contraction-relaxation, and motion attributable to diaphragmatic and chest wall movement during respiration.[5]

CARDIAC MOTION

For the assessment of all coronary artery segments with coronary MR imaging, three-dimensional volumes covering the whole coronary

---

Dr. Kelle is supported by a scholarship from the German Cardiac Society. This work was supported by National Institutes of Health grant R01-HL084186; R01-HL61912 and by the Donald W. Reynolds Foundation. Dr. Stuber was compensated as a consultant by Philips Medical Systems, The Netherlands, the manufacturer of the equipment described in this article. The terms of this agreement have been approved by the Johns Hopkins University in accordance with its conflict of interest policies.

a Division of Cardiology, Department of Medicine, German Heart Institute, Berlin, Germany
b Division of Magnetic Resonance Research, Department of Radiology, Johns Hopkins University School of Medicine, Baltimore, MD, USA
c Division of Cardiology, Department of Medicine, Johns Hopkins University, Baltimore, MD, USA
d Department of Electrical and Computer Engineering, Johns Hopkins University, Baltimore, MD, USA
* Corresponding author. Department of Radiology, Johns Hopkins University School of Medicine, Park Building, Room 338, 600 North Wolfe Street, Baltimore, MD 21287, USA.
E-mail address: mstuber@mri.jhu.edu (M. Stuber).

Magn Reson Imaging Clin N Am 17 (2009) 145–158
doi:10.1016/j.mric.2008.12.003
1064-9689/08/$ – see front matter © 2009 Published by Elsevier Inc.

artery tree (whole-heart imaging) can be acquired.[6] With such contemporary methods, however, volumetric high-resolution MR imaging data acquisition cannot be performed in real time. The collection of data over multiple cardiac cycles is mandatory (k-space segmentation). Segmented data acquisition is commonly performed using R-wave triggering during up to 300 consecutive cardiac cycles.[7] Typically, data acquisition is performed in a short time-window (<100 milliseconds) and during a period of minimal motion. The period of minimal myocardial motion is typically assessed visually by inspecting a cine MR imaging scan that precedes coronary MR imaging.[8] A period of minimal myocardial motion is commonly found in late diastole.[9] In patients with tachycardia, end-systolic imaging also may be beneficial.[10]

RESPIRATORY MOTION

With the advent of segmented k-space acquisition techniques that permitted coronary MR imaging data acquisition in less than 15 seconds, breath-holding strategies were used to suppress respiratory motion.[7] Two-dimensional and more recently also three-dimensional breath-hold techniques for coronary MR imaging have been implemented.[11] Breath-holding is fraught, however, with several limitations. First, the spatial resolution of this method depends on the patient's ability to hold his or her breath. In addition, during a sustained breath-hold, a cranial diaphragmatic drift of up to 1 cm has been reported.[12] The development of respiratory navigators[13] for the suppression of respiratory motion enabled free-breathing coronary MR imaging data collection.[14–16] A navigator signal is typically obtained from a moving structure, such as the lung-liver interface. Then, a computer algorithm detects the position of that interface in real time. If that interface position falls within an end-expiratory gating window of user-defined width, the immediately afterward acquired image data are accepted for reconstruction. Otherwise, they are rejected, do not contribute to the final image, and have to be remeasured during a subsequent RR interval. In combination with steady-state free-precession techniques, navigator technology supports high diagnostic accuracy with better image quality than that obtained with breath-holding.[17] In addition, free-breathing navigator-gated coronary MR imaging offers improved patient comfort as compared with breath-holding techniques and does not require significant patient and operator involvement. Typical examination times for free-breathing whole-heart three-dimensional navigator coronary MR imaging, however, are still in the order of 7 to 15 minutes.[5]

CONTRAST ENHANCEMENT IN CORONARY MR IMAGING

Most commonly, coronary MR imaging is performed without intravenous administration of contrast agents. Contrast between the coronary artery lumen and the surrounding myocardium and epicardial fat can be achieved by exploiting the inflow effect[18] or by the application of MR imaging prepulses to suppress signal from the surrounding tissue.[19] With the implementation of steady-state free-precession imaging sequences,[20] in combination with fat saturation and T2Prep (a magnetization-prepared, T2-weighted sequence that is used to suppress muscle and venous structures),[21] improved image quality with a high coronary blood pool contrast and vessel sharpness can be achieved (**Fig. 1**).[22] The lack of exposure to ionizing radiation and the absence of exogenous contrast agents facilitate repeat MR imaging studies when clinically warranted.[5] Another method to visualize the coronary lumen is black-blood coronary MR imaging, in which the coronary lumen appears signal-attenuated while the surrounding tissue shows high signal intensity.[23]

As an alternative to endogenous contrast enhancement, which takes advantage of naturally occurring T1 and T2 differences of blood, the myocardium, and fat, extracellular T1-lowering contrast agents in combination with inversion-recovery magnetization preparation[24] can be used for contrast generation. However, these agents quickly extravasate into the extracellular space, thereby reducing the contrast between the lumen blood pool and the surrounding tissue.[25] Because of this and the need for a bolus injection, these agents are not particularly well suited for contrast enhancement in high-resolution coronary MR imaging with large volumetric coverage and prolonged imaging times. More recently, however, a slow gadolinium contrast infusion whole-heart protocol, with accelerated parallel imaging and a slightly reduced spatial resolution,[26] has received considerable attention, although its value for the identification of luminal narrowing remains to be defined (**Fig. 2**).

Alternatively, intravascular or so-called "blood pool contrast agents" offer the advantage of adequate equilibrium-phase visualization of the coronary vasculature with high signal-to-noise ratio because of their greater T1 relaxivity and longer plasma half-life time than extracellular agents. The plasma half-life times for blood pool contrast agents range between 10 minutes and

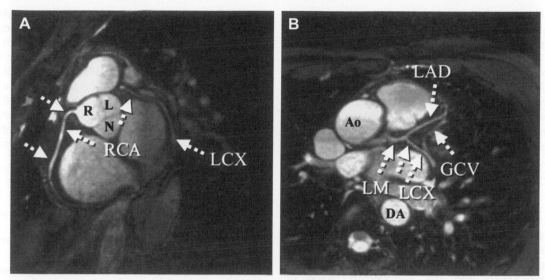

Fig.1. Navigator-gated and corrected free-breathing MR coronary angiography (MRCA) data acquired in a healthy subject using a segmented three-dimensional balanced fast field echo imaging sequence (TR = 4 milliseconds, TE = 2 milliseconds). (*A*) Image displays a double-oblique view of the right coronary artery (RCA) and a left circumflex (LCX) with a high visual vessel definition (*arrows*). (*B*) Transverse imaging plane demonstrating a left coronary system including the left main (LM), left anterior descending (LAD), the left circumflex (LCX), and a great cardiac vein (GCV) (*arrows*). These images were obtained without any exogenous contrast agent. (*From* Spuentrup E, Bornert P, Botnar RM, et al. Navigator-gated free-breathing three-dimensional balanced fast field echo (TrueFISP) coronary magnetic resonance angiography. Invest Radiol 2002;37:637; with permission.)

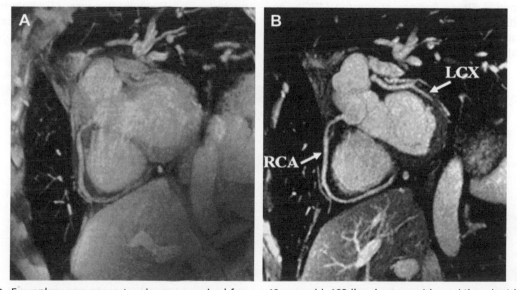

Fig. 2. Exemplary coronary artery images acquired from a 40-year-old, 192-lb volunteer without (*A*) and with (*B*) slow infusion of contrast agent. Note that the depiction of the RCA is markedly improved with administration of contrast agent. The proximal and middle sections of the LCX are clearly visualized as well in the postcontrast image. (*From* Bi X, Carr J, Li D. Whole-heart coronary magnetic resonance angiography at 3 Tesla in 5 minutes with slow infusion of Gd-BOPTA, a high-relaxivity clinical contrast agent. Magn Reson Med 2007;58:1; with permission of John Wiley & Sons, Inc.)

4 hours.[27–30] Until now, no blood pool contrast agent is clinically available for MR coronary angiography (MRCA).

When using either extracellular or intravascular contrast agents for MRCA, concomitant signal enhancement of the venous system has to be considered. This may be particularly disadvantageous for the identification of disease in the left circumflex, which often runs in close proximity to the great cardiac vein.

CORONARY ARTERY LUMEN IMAGING FOR DETECTION OF SIGNIFICANT STENOSES

Sufficient volumetric coverage and high spatial resolution are needed for coronary artery lumen imaging. For adequate visualization of the coronary arteries, a high contrast between the coronary lumen and the surrounding tissue is crucial.[31] The ability to visualize and rule out critical stenosis of coronary artery segments of more than 2 mm in diameter would allow the identification of most patients with invasively treatable coronary artery disease.[32]

The only MRCA multicenter trial to date, now 7 years after publication, clearly demonstrated a high sensitivity and negative predictive value for the identification of any significant coronary artery disease. The sensitivity (100%), specificity (85%), and negative predictive value (100%) were particularly high for the identification of left main stem or multivessel coronary artery disease.[33] Those findings suggested MRCA, as of 2001, however, had not yet reached an adequate quality for routine clinical use for symptomatic patients suspected of having hemodynamically significant coronary artery disease.[33] In a subsequent single center study the use of a whole-heart technique to cover the entire coronary artery tree (similar to multislice CT) in combination with parallel imaging (SENSE) and steady-state free-precession technique was investigated (Fig. 3).[34] In that study, a sensitivity of 82% and a specificity of 90% were obtained for the identification of significant coronary artery disease when compared with invasive x-ray coronary angiography (Table 1).[34]

IMAGING OF CORONARY ARTERY BYPASS GRAFTS

A recent study in 38 subjects with coronary artery bypass grafts demonstrated a sensitivity of 83% and specificity of 98% for the definition of graft occlusion with MR imaging (Fig. 4).[35] Practical limitations, however, include artifacts and focal signal loss attributable to metallic clips and sternal wires.

ANOMALOUS CORONARY ARTERIES

The visualization of anomalous coronary arteries with x-ray angiography can sometimes be difficult or unsuccessful. For these reasons, coronary MR imaging is the preferred test in patients in whom an anomalous origin of a coronary artery is suspected.[5,36–38] Recently, the use of whole-heart 3-T coronary MR imaging for the identification of coronary anomalies and variants has also been described (Fig. 5).[39]

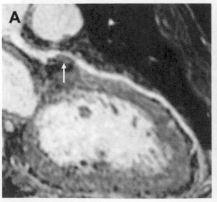 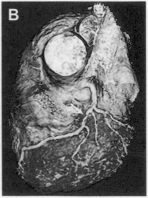 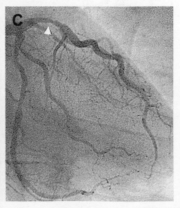

Fig. 3. Visualization of a stenosis in the left anterior descending artery (LAD) with whole-heart coronary MR angiography. (A) Curved multiplanar reconstruction image shows a stenosis in LAD (arrow). (B) Volume-rendering method demonstrates three-dimensional view of LAD with stenosis (white arrows). (C) X-ray coronary angiography reveals a stenosis of proximal LAD (arrowhead). (From Sakuma H, Ichikawa Y, Chino S, et al. Detection of coronary artery stenosis with whole-heart coronary magnetic resonance angiography. J Am Coll Cardiol 2006;48:1946; with permission.)

Table 1
Diagnostic accuracy of coronary MR angiography to detect stenoses ≥50%

Study (y)	Patients (N)	Sensitivity	Specificity
Huber et al (1999)[80]	20	73	50
Lethimonnier et al (1999)[81]	20	65	93
Sandstede et al (1999)[82]	30	81	89
Sardanelli et al (2000)[83]	39	82	89
Ikonen et al (2000)[84]	14	84	70
Kim et al (2001)[33,a]	109	93	42
Sommer T et al (2002)[85]	77	88	91
Jahnke et al (2005)[6]	32	78	91
Sakuma et al (2005)[86]	34	82	91
Sakuma et al (2006)[34]	113	82	90
			average of all studies
Total	488	81	80

Overview of the literature: studies comparing MR coronary angiography with invasive coronary angiography.
[a] First multicenter trial.

CORONARY ARTERY ANEURYSMS

Coronary MR imaging has been shown to be a clinically useful tool for patients with coronary artery aneurysms or Kawasaki disease.[40–42] This method offers the opportunity of long-term follow-up examination with repeated quantitative measurements.

CORONARY ARTERY FLOW MEASUREMENT

Magnetic resonance flow mapping was initially validated as a measure of absolute coronary artery flow in animals by comparison with Doppler ultrasound recordings.[43,44] These cine velocity-encoded phase-contrast MR imaging techniques

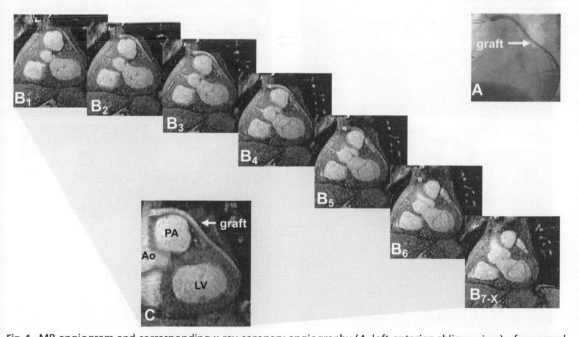

Fig. 4. MR angiogram and corresponding x-ray coronary angiography (*A*, left-anterior-oblique view) of a normal vein graft to the obtuse marginal branch of the left circumflex coronary artery. (*B*) Selection of individual slices of the MR angiogram in the oblique coronal plane. (*C*) Multiplanar-reconstruction of the three-dimensional scan revealed the graft in a single imaging plane. Ao, ascending aorta; LV, left ventricle; PA, pulmonary artery. (*From* Langerak SE, Vliegen HW, de Roos A, et al. Detection of vein graft disease using high-resolution magnetic resonance angiography. Circulation 2002;105:328; with permission.)

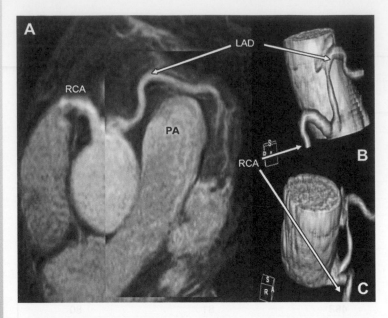

Fig. 5. Common origin of the right coronary artery (RCA) and the left anterior descending artery (LAD) in a 62-year-old man with chest pain. (*A*) Composite image generated by overlaying two reformatted images to create one multiplanar reformatted transaxial image shows the common origin of the LAD and the RCA from the right sinus of Valsalva. The LAD passes anteriorly around the pulmonary artery (PA). (*B*) Anterior oblique view of the volume-rendered coronary MR angiogram reveals the LAD and the RCA have a common origin. (*C*) Right anterior oblique view of the volume-rendered coronary MR angiogram shows the RCA. (*From* Gharib AM, Ho VB, Rosing DR, et al. Coronary artery anomalies and variants: technical feasibility of assessment with coronary MR angiography at 3 T. Radiology 2008;247:220; with permission.)

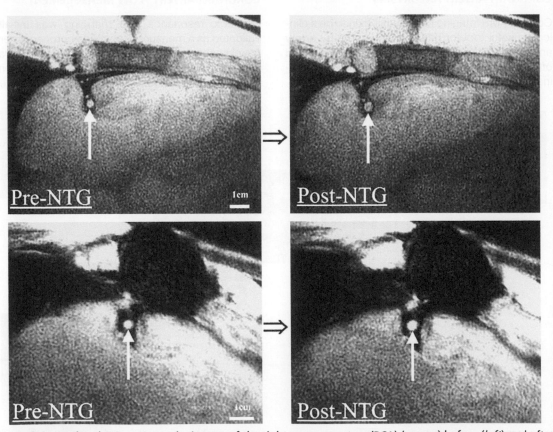

Fig. 6. Cross-sectional MR angiography images of the right coronary artery (RCA) (*arrows*) before (*left*) and after (*right*) nitroglycerin (NTG), showing vasodilation in a healthy volunteer (*top*) and a heart transplant patient (*bottom*). In this study, by using this endothelial-independent vasodilator, the difference in vasodilation between healthy subjects and patients who had coronary artery disease was not significant. (*From* Terashima M, Meyer CH, Keeffe BG, et al. Noninvasive assessment of coronary vasodilation using magnetic resonance angiography. J Am Coll Cardiol 2005;45:104; with permission.)

were extended to noninvasive measures of absolute coronary arterial flow in humans.[45,46] Phase-contrast MR imaging detected pharmacologically induced changes in coronary arterial flow and was able to distinguish between subjects with normal and abnormal coronary arterial flow reserve.[46] MR imaging flow measurements allowed the determination of coronary blood flow velocities after stent deployment and provided results similar to Doppler flow measurements.[47]

CORONARY ENDOTHELIAL FUNCTION

Endothelial-dependent coronary artery vasomotor reactivity is an important indicator of vascular function and can predict cardiovascular events.[48] Changes in coronary artery cross-sectional area and flow velocity occur in response to endothelial-dependent stressors and these can be detected by MR imaging methods.[49] An early study also reported a significant endothelium-independent

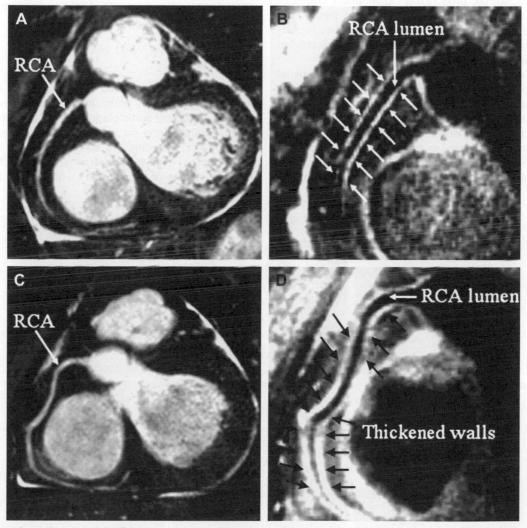

Fig. 7. Three-dimensional reformatted coronary MR image of the proximal RCA in two subjects without coronary luminal stenosis: a 58-year-old man with long-standing type 1 diabetes and normoalbuminuria (A) and a 44-year-old man with long-standing type 1 diabetes and diabetic nephropathy (C). The corresponding three-dimensional black-blood vessel wall scan (B) shows no coronary MR imaging evidence of atherosclerotic plaque (average and maximum vessel wall thickness, 1.1 and 1.3 mm, respectively), however, an increased atherosclerotic plaque burden in (D) (average and maximum vessel wall thickness, 2.3 and 3 mm, respectively). The anterior and posterior RCA walls are indicated by arrows. (*From* Kim WY, Astrup AS, Stuber M, et al. Subclinical coronary and aortic atherosclerosis detected by magnetic resonance imaging in type 1 diabetes with and without diabetic nephropathy. Circulation 2007;115:228; with permission.)

increase in coronary diameter in response to sublingual nitroglycerin (**Fig. 6**).[50] Its prognostic information and its feasibility for follow-up of progression of different stages of disease have yet to be determined.

CORONARY VESSEL WALL IMAGING

Rupture of high-risk atherosclerotic plaques commonly leads to myocardial infarction or sudden cardiac death.[51] Current imaging methodologies cannot identify such high-risk lesions. Identification of these lesions could alter systemic therapies (ie, prescribing higher statin doses or adjunctive treatments despite target serum lipid levels), and possibly guide local therapies (eg, intracoronary stenting of high-risk lesions) in patients at very high risk.[51,52]

Current state-of-the-art MR imaging spatial resolution is too low to distinguish or characterize accurately coronary plaque components (eg, the thickness of the fibrous cap or the lipid core). Early studies demonstrated, however, that coronary vessel wall thickness can be quantified noninvasively using black-blood MR imaging.[18,53] In a study comparing patients with x-ray–defined

mild-moderate coronary artery disease with healthy adult subjects, increased coronary artery wall thickness with preservation of normal lumen size was reported in the patient cohort. This means that MR imaging is a noninvasive tool for the quantification of Glagov-type[54] positive arterial remodelling (**Fig. 7**).[55] A study in patients with type 1 diabetes demonstrated the ability of coronary MR imaging to visualize different stages of diabetes by measuring of coronary vessel wall thickness.[56] In addition, the use of black-blood free-breathing three-dimensional MR imaging in conjunction with semiautomated analysis software allows for reproducible measurements of right coronary arterial vessel-wall thickness.[57]

CORONARY VESSEL WALL DELAYED ENHANCEMENT

Delayed contrast-enhanced MR imaging of the vascular wall is a very promising method for evaluating carotid and aortic plaque and inflammatory vasculopathies, and for identifying some plaque components, including the fibrous cap.[58–61] The first human delayed contrast-enhanced MR imaging studies of the coronary wall showed the

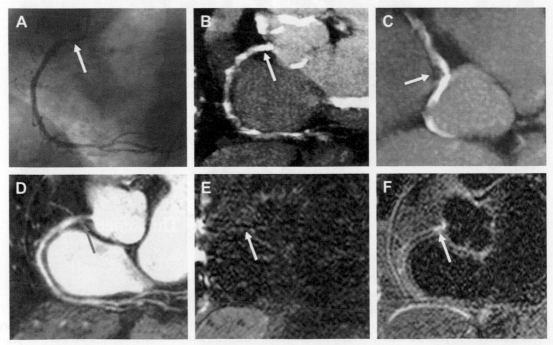

Fig. 8. Detection of coronary artery plaque enhancement. High-grade ostial stenosis of the RCA as demonstrated by x-ray coronary angiography (*A*) and MR angiography (*D*). Multislice CT (*B*) shows that the underlying plaque is not only severely calcified, but also has noncalcified components (*C*). Inversion recovery coronary MR imaging before (*E*) and after (*F*) gadolinium administration demonstrates strong focal enhancement of the plaque and diffuse enhancement of the RCA wall. (*From* Maintz D, Ozgun M, Hoffmeier A, et al. Selective coronary artery plaque visualization and differentiation by contrast-enhanced inversion prepared MRI. Eur Heart J 2006;27:1732; with permission.)

potential for coronary artery plaque visualization and characterization using a T1-weighted coronary MR imaging technique (**Fig. 8**).[62,63] The authors concluded that delayed contrast-enhanced MR imaging contrast uptake might be associated with increased vascular permeability (as may occur with inflammation) or with an increased distribution volume (as with fibrosis and neovascularization) in the altered vessel wall.

MOLECULAR TARGETED IMAGING

A number of recently described molecular imaging strategies have been proposed to detect inflamed atherosclerotic plaque noninvasively, using targeted gadolinium agents[64,65] and superparamagnetic nanoparticles.[66] Currently, the development of contrast agents that highlight specific plaque components seems to be very promising. So far, molecular contrast agents targeted to fibrin, macrophages, or high-density lipoprotein have been tested at the preclinical level.[67–69]

Arterial and venous thrombi contain fibrin, making fibrin a target for noninvasive thrombosis imaging. Early studies demonstrated that molecular MR imaging using the fibrin-targeted contrast agent EP-2104R allowed selective visualization of human clot material in a model of coronary thrombosis in swine[70] and of thrombi in the arterial vasculature and the ventricular chambers in humans.[71]

Macrophages, key inflammatory cells in atherosclerosis,[52] abound in coronary plaques that have caused sudden cardiac death.[72] In a recently published study, a positive contrast off-resonance imaging sequence (inversion recovery with ON-resonant water suppression)[73] was combined with superparamagnetic nanoparticles (monocrystalline iron-oxide nanoparticles) to generate positive contrast for atherosclerotic plaque macrophage imaging.[74] Using this methodology, areas of macrophage-rich plaques were highlighted and the magnitude of enhancement was significantly related to the histology-confirmed number of macrophages.[74]

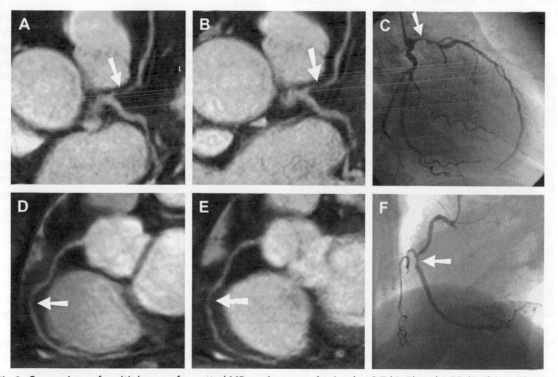

Fig. 9. Comparison of multiplanar reformatted MR angiograms obtained at 3 T (*A, D*) and 1.5 T (*B, E*) in a 59-year-old male patient with severe disease in the LAD (*A–C*) and moderate disease in the RCA (*D–F*), including stenoses in the LAD artery (*arrow* in *A* and *B*) and the RCA (*arrow* in *D* and *E*). (*C, F*) X-ray coronary angiography. At quantitative analysis, the LAD artery and RCA stenoses (*arrow*) were calculated to be 83% and 52%, respectively. At both field strengths, there is good correlation between the MR angiograms and the corresponding x-ray coronary angiography. (*From* Sommer T, Hackenbroch M, Hofer U, et al. Coronary MR angiography at 3.0 T versus that at 1.5 T: initial results in patients suspected of having coronary artery disease. Radiology 2005;234:718; with permission.)

HIGH-FIELD CORONARY ARTERY IMAGING

Most published coronary artery MR imaging studies were performed on clinical 1.5-T MR imaging systems. Higher signal-to-noise ratio afforded by high-field 3-T MR imaging, however, promises images with higher spatial resolution, higher temporal resolution, or shorter acquisition times. An early study of coronary MR imaging in healthy adult volunteers demonstrated that a superior spatial resolution can be obtained at 3 T when compared with 1.5 T.[75] Although a study in patients suspected of having coronary artery disease demonstrated the feasibility of MRCA at 3 T along with a significant increase in signal-to-noise ratio and contrast-to-noise ratio compared with 1.5 T, the diagnostic accuracy for the detection of coronary artery stenoses (sensitivity and specificity 82% and 89%, respectively, at 3 T versus 82% and 88% at 1.5 T) was almost identical at both field strengths (Fig. 9).[76] The development of high-field specific technical modifications including higher order shimming,[77] adiabatic T2Prep,[78] has since been pursued. These high-field specific adaptations lead to significantly improved image quality and enhanced diagnostic performance is now expected (Fig. 10). Early studies demonstrated the use of black-blood vessel wall imaging at 3 T.[79] Simultaneously, commercial 7-T human whole-body systems have recently been introduced. Although the current focus at that field strength is clearly on neurologic applications, its use for cardiovascular applications including coronary MR imaging remains to be determined.

SUMMARY

Coronary MR imaging is a promising noninvasive technique for the combined assessment of coronary artery anatomy (coronary artery lumen and vessel wall) and function (coronary artery flow, endothelial function, contrast agent uptake). Anomalous coronary arteries and aneurysms can reliably be assessed in clinical practice using coronary MR imaging and the presence of significant left main or proximal multivessel coronary artery disease detected. Two great advantages of coronary MR imaging as compared with x-ray angiography and multislice CT are the absence of ionizing radiation and no need for iodinated contrast agents.

So far, only limited multicenter MRCA experience is available and there are still no data on the prognostic value of coronary MR imaging. Technical challenges that need to be addressed are further improvements in motion suppression and abbreviated scanning times aimed at improving spatial resolution and patient comfort. The development of new and specific contrast agents, high-field MR imaging with improved spatial resolution, and continued progress in MR imaging methods development will undoubtedly lead to further progress toward the noninvasive and comprehensive assessment of coronary atherosclerotic disease.

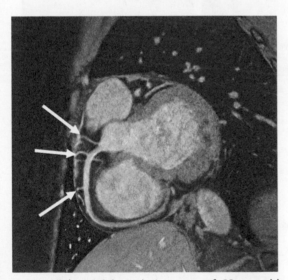

Fig. 10. High spatial resolution scan of 23-year-old healthy man acquired at 3 T using navigator-gated and navigator-corrected double oblique three-dimensional segmented k-space gradient-echo imaging sequence (3 T, TR/TE = 7.5/2.3, α = 20 degrees, resolution = 0.35 × 0.35 × 1.5 mm, field of view = 270 × 216 mm, 800 × 610 matrix). Arrows indicate small sidebranches. (*From* Ustun A, Desai M, Abd-Elmoniem KZ, et al. Automated identification of minimal myocardial motion for improved image quality on MR angiography at 3 T. AJR Am J Roentgenol 2007; 188:W283; with permission.)

REFERENCES

1. Rosamond W, Flegal K, Friday G, et al. Heart disease and stroke statistics–2007 update: a report from the American Heart Association Statistics Committee and Stroke Statistics Subcommittee. Circulation 2007;115:e69.
2. Davidson CJ, Mark DB, Pieper KS, et al. Thrombotic and cardiovascular complications related to nonionic contrast media during cardiac catheterization: analysis of 8,517 patients. Am J Cardiol 1990; 65:1481.
3. Omran H, Schmidt H, Hackenbroch M, et al. Silent and apparent cerebral embolism after retrograde catheterisation of the aortic valve in valvular stenosis: a prospective, randomised study. Lancet 2003;361:1241.

4. Dissmann W, de Ridder M. The soft science of German cardiology. Lancet 2002;359:2027.

5. Bluemke DA, Achenbach S, Budoff M, et al. Noninvasive coronary artery imaging: magnetic resonance angiography and multidetector computed tomography angiography: a scientific statement from the american heart association committee on cardiovascular imaging and intervention of the council on cardiovascular radiology and intervention, and the councils on clinical cardiology and cardiovascular disease in the young. Circulation 2008;118:586.

6. Jahnke C, Paetsch I, Nehrke K, et al. Rapid and complete coronary arterial tree visualization with magnetic resonance imaging: feasibility and diagnostic performance. Eur Heart J 2005;26:2313.

7. Edelman RR, Manning WJ, Burstein D, et al. Coronary arteries: breath-hold MR angiography. Radiology 1991;181:641.

8. Kim WY, Stuber M, Kissinger KV, et al. Impact of bulk cardiac motion on right coronary MR angiography and vessel wall imaging. J Magn Reson Imaging 2001;14:383.

9. Hofman MB, Wickline SA, Lorenz CH. Quantification of in-plane motion of the coronary arteries during the cardiac cycle: implications for acquisition window duration for MR flow quantification. J Magn Reson Imaging 1998;8:568.

10. Gharib AM, Herzka DA, Ustun AO, et al. Coronary MR angiography at 3T during diastole and systole. J Magn Reson Imaging 2007;26.921.

11. Stuber M, Botnar RM, Danias PG, et al. Breathhold three-dimensional coronary magnetic resonance angiography using real-time navigator technology. J Cardiovasc Magn Reson 1999;1:233.

12. Danias PG, Stuber M, Botnar RM, et al. Navigator assessment of breath-hold duration: impact of supplemental oxygen and hyperventilation. AJR Am J Roentgenol 1998;171:395.

13. Ehman RL, Felmlee JP. Adaptive technique for high-definition MR imaging of moving structures. Radiology 1989;173:255.

14. Li D, Kaushikkar S, Haacke EM, et al. Coronary arteries: three-dimensional MR imaging with retrospective respiratory gating. Radiology 1996; 201:857.

15. McConnell MV, Khasgiwala VC, Savord BJ, et al. Comparison of respiratory suppression methods and navigator locations for MR coronary angiography. Am J Roentgenol 1997;168:1369.

16. Oshinski JN, Hofland L, Mukundan S Jr, et al. Two-dimensional coronary MR angiography without breath holding. Radiology 1996;201:737.

17. Jahnke C, Paetsch I, Schnackenburg B, et al. Coronary MR angiography with steady-state free precession: individually adapted breath-hold technique versus free-breathing technique. Radiology 2004; 232:669.

18. Edelman RR, Chien D, Kim D. Fast selective black blood MR imaging. Radiology 1991;181:655.

19. Botnar RM, Stuber M, Danias PG, et al. Improved coronary artery definition with T2-weighted, free-breathing, three-dimensional coronary MRA. Circulation 1999;99:3139.

20. Deshpande VS, Shea SM, Laub G, et al. 3D magnetization-prepared true-FISP: a new technique for imaging coronary arteries. Magn Reson Med 2001; 46:494.

21. Brittain JH, Hu BS, Wright GA, et al. Coronary angiography with magnetization-prepared T2 contrast. Magn Reson Med 1995;33:689.

22. Spuentrup E, Bornert P, Botnar RM, et al. Navigator-gated free-breathing three-dimensional balanced fast field echo (TrueFISP) coronary magnetic resonance angiography. Invest Radiol 2002;37:637.

23. Stuber M, Botnar RM, Kissinger KV, et al. Free-breathing black-blood coronary MR angiography: initial results. Radiology 2001;219:278.

24. Kessler W, Laub G, Achenbach S, et al. Coronary arteries: MR angiography with fast contrast-enhanced three-dimensional breath-hold imaging–initial experience. Radiology 1999;210:566.

25. Edelman RR. Contrast-enhanced MR imaging of the heart: overview of the literature. Radiology 2004;232:653.

26. Bi X, Carr J, Li D. Whole-heart coronary magnetic resonance angiography at 3 Tesla in 5 minutes with slow infusion of Gd-BOPTA, a high-relaxivity clinical contrast agent. Magn Reson Med 2007;58:1.

27. Herborn CU, Schmidt M, Bruder O, et al. MR coronary angiography with SH L 643 A: initial experience in patients with coronary artery disease. Radiology 2004;233:567.

28. Kelle S, Thouet T, Tangcharoen T, et al. Whole-heart coronary magnetic resonance angiography with MS-325 (Gadofosveset). Med Sci Monit 2007;13: CR469.

29. Paetsch I, Jahnke C, Barkhausen J, et al. Detection of coronary stenoses with contrast enhanced, three-dimensional free breathing coronary MR angiography using the gadolinium-based intravascular contrast agent gadocoletic acid (B-22956). J Cardiovasc Magn Reson 2006;8:509.

30. Parmelee DJ, Walovitch RC, Ouellet HS, et al. Preclinical evaluation of the pharmacokinetics, biodistribution, and elimination of MS-325, a blood pool agent for magnetic resonance imaging. Invest Radiol 1997;32:741.

31. Stuber M, Weiss RG. Coronary magnetic resonance angiography. J Magn Reson Imaging 2007;26:219.

32. Kelle S, Hug J, Kohler U, et al. Potential intrinsic error of noninvasive coronary angiography. J Cardiovasc Magn Reson 2005;7:401.

33. Kim WY, Danias PG, Stuber M, et al. Coronary magnetic resonance angiography for the detection of coronary stenoses. N Engl J Med 2001;345:1863.

34. Sakuma H, Ichikawa Y, Chino S, et al. Detection of coronary artery stenosis with whole-heart coronary magnetic resonance angiography. J Am Coll Cardiol 2006;48:1946.

35. Langerak SE, Vliegen HW, de Roos A, et al. Detection of vein graft disease using high-resolution magnetic resonance angiography. Circulation 2002;105:328.

36. Hendel RC, Patel MR, Kramer CM, et al. ACCF/ACR/SCCT/SCMR/ASNC/NASCI/SCAI/SIR 2006 appropriateness criteria for cardiac computed tomography and cardiac magnetic resonance imaging: a report of the American College of Cardiology Foundation Quality Strategic Directions Committee Appropriateness Criteria Working Group, American College of Radiology, Society of Cardiovascular Computed Tomography, Society for Cardiovascular Magnetic Resonance, American Society of Nuclear Cardiology, North American Society for Cardiac Imaging, Society for Cardiovascular Angiography and Interventions, and Society of Interventional Radiology. J Am Coll Cardiol 2006;48:1475.

37. McConnell MV, Ganz P, Selwyn AP, et al. Identification of anomalous coronary arteries and their anatomic course by magnetic resonance coronary angiography. Circulation 1995;92:3158.

38. Vliegen HW, Doornbos J, de Roos A, et al. Value of fast gradient echo magnetic resonance angiography as an adjunct to coronary arteriography in detecting and confirming the course of clinically significant coronary artery anomalies. Am J Cardiol 1997;79:773.

39. Gharib AM, Ho VB, Rosing DR, et al. Coronary artery anomalies and variants: technical feasibility of assessment with coronary MR angiography at 3 T. Radiology 2008;247:220.

40. Greil GF, Stuber M, Botnar RM, et al. Coronary magnetic resonance angiography in adolescents and young adults with Kawasaki disease. Circulation 2002;105:908.

41. Mavrogeni S, Papadopoulos G, Douskou M, et al. Magnetic resonance angiography is equivalent to X-ray coronary angiography for the evaluation of coronary arteries in Kawasaki disease. J Am Coll Cardiol 2004;43:649.

42. Takemura A, Suzuki A, Inaba R, et al. Utility of coronary MR angiography in children with Kawasaki disease. AJR Am J Roentgenol 2007;188:W534.

43. Clarke GD, Eckels R, Chaney C, et al. Measurement of absolute epicardial coronary artery flow and flow reserve with breath-hold cine phase-contrast magnetic resonance imaging. Circulation 1995;91:2627.

44. Hofman MB, van Rossum AC, Sprenger M, et al. Assessment of flow in the right human coronary artery by magnetic resonance phase contrast velocity measurement: effects of cardiac and respiratory motion. Magn Reson Med 1996;35:521.

45. Edelman RR, Manning WJ, Gervino E, et al. Flow velocity quantification in human coronary arteries with fast, breath-hold MR angiography. J Magn Reson Imaging 1993;3:699.

46. Hundley WG, Lange RA, Clarke GD, et al. Assessment of coronary arterial flow and flow reserve in humans with magnetic resonance imaging. Circulation 1996;93:1502.

47. Nagel E, Thouet T, Klein C, et al. Noninvasive determination of coronary blood flow velocity with cardiovascular magnetic resonance in patients after stent deployment. Circulation 2003;107:1738.

48. Schachinger V, Britten MB, Zeiher AM. Prognostic impact of coronary vasodilator dysfunction on adverse long-term outcome of coronary heart disease. Circulation 2000;101:1899.

49. Bedaux WL, Hofman MB, de Cock CC, et al. Magnetic resonance imaging versus Doppler guide wire in the assessment of coronary flow reserve in patients with coronary artery disease. Coron Artery Dis 2002;13:365.

50. Terashima M, Meyer CH, Keeffe BG, et al. Noninvasive assessment of coronary vasodilation using magnetic resonance angiography. J Am Coll Cardiol 2005;45:104.

51. Naghavi M, Libby P, Falk E, et al. From vulnerable plaque to vulnerable patient: a call for new definitions and risk assessment strategies: Part I. Circulation 2003;108:1664.

52. Libby P. Inflammation in atherosclerosis. Nature 2002;420:868.

53. Fayad ZA, Fuster V, Fallon JT, et al. Noninvasive in vivo human coronary artery lumen and wall imaging using black-blood magnetic resonance imaging. Circulation 2000;102:506.

54. Glagov S, Weisenberg E, Zarins CK, et al. Compensatory enlargement of human atherosclerotic coronary arteries. N Engl J Med 1987;316:1371.

55. Kim WY, Stuber M, Bornert P, et al. Three-dimensional black-blood cardiac magnetic resonance coronary vessel wall imaging detects positive arterial remodeling in patients with nonsignificant coronary artery disease. Circulation 2002;106:296.

56. Kim WY, Astrup AS, Stuber M, et al. Subclinical coronary and aortic atherosclerosis detected by magnetic resonance imaging in type 1 diabetes with and without diabetic nephropathy. Circulation 2007;115:228.

57. Desai MY, Lai S, Barmet C, et al. Reproducibility of 3D free-breathing magnetic resonance coronary vessel wall imaging. Eur Heart J 2005;26:2320.

58. Cai J, Hatsukami TS, Ferguson MS, et al. Vivo quantitative measurement of intact fibrous cap and

lipid-rich necrotic core size in atherosclerotic carotid plaque: comparison of high-resolution, contrast-enhanced magnetic resonance imaging and histology. Circulation 2005;112:3437.

59. Desai MY, Stone JH, Foo TK, et al. Delayed contrast-enhanced MRI of the aortic wall in Takayasu's arteritis: initial experience. AJR Am J Roentgenol 2005; 184:1427.

60. Wasserman BA, Smith WI, Trout HH III, et al. Carotid artery atherosclerosis: in vivo morphologic characterization with gadolinium-enhanced double-oblique MR imaging initial results. Radiology 2002; 223:566.

61. Yuan C, Kerwin WS, Ferguson MS, et al. Contrast-enhanced high resolution MRI for atherosclerotic carotid artery tissue characterization. J Magn Reson Imaging 2002;15:62.

62. Maintz D, Ozgun M, Hoffmeier A, et al. Selective coronary artery plaque visualization and differentiation by contrast-enhanced inversion prepared MRI. Eur Heart J 2006;27:1732.

63. Yeon SB, Sabir A, Clouse M, et al. Delayed-enhancement cardiovascular magnetic resonance coronary artery wall imaging: comparison with multislice computed tomography and quantitative coronary angiography. J Am Coll Cardiol 2007; 50:441.

64. Amirbekian V, Lipinski MJ, Briley-Saebo KC, et al. Detecting and assessing macrophages in vivo to evaluate atherosclerosis noninvasively using molecular MRI. Proc Natl Acad Sci U S A 2007; 104:961.

65. Botnar RM, Buecker A, Wiethoff AJ, et al. In vivo magnetic resonance imaging of coronary thrombosis using a fibrin-binding molecular magnetic resonance contrast agent. Circulation 2004;110:1463.

66. Ruehm SG, Corot C, Vogt P, et al. Magnetic resonance imaging of atherosclerotic plaque with ultrasmall superparamagnetic particles of iron oxide in hyperlipidemic rabbits. Circulation 2001; 103:415.

67. Corti R. Noninvasive imaging of atherosclerotic vessels by MRI for clinical assessment of the effectiveness of therapy. Pharmacol Ther 2006; 110:57.

68. Cyrus T, Lanza GM, Wickline SA. Molecular imaging by cardiovascular MR. J Cardiovasc Magn Reson 2007;9:827.

69. Frias JC, Williams KJ, Fisher EA, et al. Recombinant HDL-like nanoparticles: a specific contrast agent for MRI of atherosclerotic plaques. J Am Chem Soc 2004;126:16316.

70. Spuentrup E, Katoh M, Wiethoff AJ, et al. Molecular coronary MR imaging of human thrombi using EP-2104R, a fibrin-targeted contrast agent: experimental study in a swine model. Rofo 2007; 179:1166.

71. Spuentrup E, Botnar RM, Wiethoff AJ, et al. MR imaging of thrombi using EP-2104R, a fibrin-specific contrast agent: initial results in patients. Eur Radiol 2008;18:1995–2005.

72. Burke AP, Farb A, Malcom GT, et al. Coronary risk factors and plaque morphology in men with coronary disease who died suddenly. N Engl J Med 1997;336:1276.

73. Stuber M, Gilson WD, Schar M, et al. Positive contrast visualization of iron oxide-labeled stem cells using inversion-recovery with ON-resonant water suppression (IRON). Magn Reson Med 2007; 58:1072.

74. Korosoglou G, Weiss RG, Kedziorek DA, et al. Noninvasive detection of macrophage-rich atherosclerotic plaque in hyperlipidemic rabbits using "positive contrast" magnetic resonance imaging. J Am Coll Cardiol 2008;52:483.

75. Stuber M, Botnar RM, Fischer SE, et al. Preliminary report on in vivo coronary MRA at 3 Tesla in humans. Magn Reson Med 2002;48:425.

76. Sommer T, Hackenbroch M, Hofer U, et al. Coronary MR Angiography at 3.0 T versus That at 1.5 T: Initial Results in Patients Suspected of Having Coronary Artery Disease. Radiology 2005;234:718.

77. Schar M, Kozerke S, Fischer SE, et al. Cardiac SSFP imaging at 3 Tesla. Magn Reson Med 2004;51:799.

78. Nezafat R, Stuber M, Ouwerkerk R, et al. B1-insensitive T2 preparation for improved coronary magnetic resonance angiography at 3 T. Magn Reson Med 2006;55:858.

79. Bansmann PM, Priest AN, Muellerleile K, et al. MRI of the coronary vessel wall at 3 T: comparison of radial and cartesian k-space sampling. AJR Am J Roentgenol 2007;188:70.

80. Huber A, Nikolaou K, Gonschior P, et al. Navigator echo-based respiratory gating for three-dimensional MR coronary angiography: results from healthy volunteers and patients with proximal coronary artery stenoses. AJR Am J Roentgenol 1999; 173:95.

81. Lethimonnier F, Furber A, Morel O, et al. Three-dimensional coronary artery MR imaging using prospective real-time respiratory navigator and linear phase shift processing: comparison with conventional coronary angiography. Magn Reson Imaging 1999;17:1111.

82. Sandstede JJ, Pabst T, Beer M, et al. Three-dimensional MR coronary angiography using the navigator technique compared with conventional coronary angiography. AJR Am J Roentgenol 1999;172:135.

83. Sardanelli F, Molinari G, Zandrino F, et al. Three-dimensional, navigator-echo MR coronary angiography in detecting stenoses of the major epicardial vessels, with conventional coronary angiography as the standard of reference. Radiology 2000; 214:808.

84. Ikonen AE, Manninen HI, Vainio P, et al. Repeated 3D coronary MR angiography with navigator echo gating: technical quality and consistency of image interpretation. J Comput Assist Tomogr 2000;24:375.

85. Sommer T, Hofer U, Hackenbroch M, et al [Submillimeter 3D coronary MR angiography with real-time navigator correction in 107 patients with suspected coronary artery disease]. Rofo 2002;174:459.

86. Sakuma H, Ichikawa Y, Suzawa N, et al. Assessment of coronary arteries with total study time of less than 30 minutes by using whole-heart coronary MR angiography. Radiology 2005;237:316.

Nephrogenic Systemic Fibrosis

Jeffrey C. Weinreb, MD[a,b,*], Phillip H. Kuo, MD, PhD[c,d]

KEYWORDS

- Gadolinium • Nephrogenic systemic fibrosis
- Gadolinium-based contrast agent • MR imaging
- MR contrast agents • Gadolinium chelates

Intravenous gadolinium-based contrast agents (GBCAs) are used commonly for MRI to aid in the detection, characterization, and staging of disease. For magnetic resonance angiography (MRA), many radiologists have become reliant on these agents because their use facilitates production of reliable, high-quality, higher spatial resolution, and time-efficient examinations. Furthermore, because their use previously was considered almost risk-free, GBCA-enhanced MRA often was preferred to contrast-enhanced digital subtraction angiography or CT angiography, which use intravenous iodinated contrast agents.

Until recently, there was general agreement that GBCAs were especially valuable for imaging vascular structures in patients who have compromised renal function, because they are less likely than iodinated agents to cause contrast-induced nephropathy. They commonly were administered generously, and sometimes indiscriminately, with very little concern about adverse events or renal function status, despite cautions from the manufacturers. Screening patients for chronic kidney disease (CKD) was thought to be unnecessary and was not considered the standard of care. In 2006, however, there were reports of an association between GBCAs and a rare, debilitating, and sometimes fatal disease called "nephrogenic systemic fibrosis" (NSF), and it was suggested that intravenous GBCAs might serve as a trigger for NSF.[1–3]

Subsequent publications and self-reported data received by the US Food and Drug Administration (FDA) Medwatch program seemed to validate the epidemiologic association of NSF with the administration of GBCAs in patients who had renal disease, and the FDA issued a Public Health Advisory on June 9, 2006.[4] Since then, the evidence for an association between GBCAs and NSF has continued to build and has had a considerable impact on the use of contrast-enhanced MRA, especially in patients who have kidney disease. Virtually unknown to the radiology community before 2006, NSF has generated concern and confusion among radiologists, clinicians, and their patients. In the relatively brief time since the emergence and recognition of NSF, policies have been developed, modified, and re-modified as the medical and legal communities seek to gain a better understanding of the disease and its apparent association with GBCA administration.

This article addresses the relationship between GBCAs and NSF and answers some common

J.C.W. has received research support and has served as a consultant and speaker for GE Healthcare and Bayer Healthcare Pharmaceuticals.

[a] Department of Diagnostic Radiology, Yale University School of Medicine, 333 Cedar Street, P.O. Box 208042, New Haven, CT 06520-5913, USA
[b] Body Imaging and MRI, Yale-New Haven Hospital, 333 Cedar Street, P.O. Box 208042, New Haven, CT 06520-5913, USA
[c] Department of Medicine, Section of Hematology/Oncology, University of Arizona, 1515 N. Campbell Avenue, P.O. Box 245024, Tucson, AZ 85724-5024, USA
[d] Department of Radiology, Southern Arizona Veterans Administration Hospital, 1515 N. Campbell Avenue, P.O. Box 245024, Tucson, AZ 85724-5024, USA
* Corresponding author. Department of Diagnostic Radiology, Yale University School of Medicine, 333 Cedar Street, P.O. Box 208042, New Haven, CT 06520-5913.
E-mail address: jeffrey.weinreb@yale.edu (J.C. Weinreb).

questions. A more detailed discussion of clinical manifestations, epidemiology, pathogenesis, pathology, and treatment of NSF is beyond the scope of this article.

WHAT IS NEPHROGENIC SYSTEMIC FIBROSIS?

NSF, initially called "nephrogenic fibrosing derm-opathy" (NFD), was observed first in 1997, when patients in a hemodialysis center were noted to suffer progressive dermal hardening and thick-ening and erythema of the limbs, often accompa-nied by pruritus and sometimes pain. The lower extremities were affected more severely than the upper extremities. On histologic examination, the affected skin was characterized by profound fibrosis, sometimes with mucin deposition but no inflammatory infiltrates or paraprotein, one of the main features that distinguished NFD from sclero-myxedema. The first cases were reported in 2000.[5,6]

Over time, as it became apparent that NFD was not merely a cutaneous process but a systemic one involving noncontiguous tissues and organs such as the heart, pericardium, diaphragm, pleura, kidneys, and testes, the disease was renamed "nephrogenic systemic fibrosis." The precise pathophysiology of NSF remains an active area for research and speculation, but it seems to be related to the administration of GBCAs to patients who have renal compromise.

WHAT ARE GADOLINIUM-BASED CONTRAST AGENTS?

Gadolinium is a rare earth metal in the lanthanide series. In the 3+ oxidation state gadolinium has seven unpaired electrons that can interact with nuclear spins and cause a decrease in relaxation times of fluids and tissues. This ability to shorten the T1-relaxation time, or paramagnetism, makes gadolinium attractive for use in MR contrast agents, because its presence increases signal intensity on T1-weighted images. Free gadolinium itself, however, is highly toxic, in part because it is approximately the same size as a calcium ion and can block calcium channels and inhibit calcium-dependent enzymes. Thus, when gadolinium is used in intravenous MR contrast agents, the gado-linium ion is bound to an organic moiety (ligand) to form a metal-chelate complex. This binding results in an adequate safety profile while maintaining the favorable paramagnetic qualities. The gadolinium-chelate complex and varying amounts of chelating agent (depending upon the particular brand) then are dissolved in water to produce the GBCA formulation used in contrast-enhanced MRI/MRA.

In 2008, there were six FDA-approved GBCAs are commercially available in the United States, and several other GBCAs are in use in other parts of the world (Table 1). All these agents contain a gadoli-nium-chelate, but the ligand is different in each. Some have a linear structure, others are macrocyclic, and each has a unique constellation of stability constants and kinetics.

Gadobenate dimeglumine has a higher relaxivity than the extracellular agents that have been in use for MRI/MRA in the United States and may be used in smaller doses for certain applications, especially at a magnetic field strength of 3 T.[7–9] Gadobenate dimeglumine and gadoxetate disodi-um have some specific hepatobiliary uses. Never-theless, the general attributes of the various GBCAs for MRA are comparable (even if they are not approved by the US FDA for this application). There are, however, two properties that have drawn considerable attention because they seem to be related— stability and safety.

Stability refers to how tightly the gadolinium ion is bound to the chelating molecule and the likeli-hood that it will dissociate. When dissociation occurs, the released gadolinium ion is picked up by a variety of competing anions and cation-binding proteins in the circulating blood. Overall, other factors being equal, the rates of dissociation of gadolinium are orders of magnitude slower from macrocyclic ligands than from linear ones, and macrocyclic ligands therefore are the most "stable."[10] There is evidence suggesting that the propensity to dissociate is related in some way to the induction of fibrosis in NSF. The exact mechanism has not been elucidated or firmly established, but circulating fibrocytes[11] and "free gadolinium" have been implicated.[3,12]

WHAT IS THE RELATIONSHIP BETWEEN GADOLINIUM-BASED CONTRAST AGENTS AND NEPHROGENIC SYSTEMIC FIBROSIS?

In 2006, Grobner[2] published the first report of cases of NSF associated with GBCA exposure, and subsequent studies seemed to confirm the association, indicating that the risk of a patient who has renal disease contracting NSF following an exposure to GBCA varies widely, depending on the particular agent used, the dose, patient population, and the methodology of the study. For example, one retrospective study found no cases of NSF in 74,124 patients who were not screened for renal disease and who received a standard (single) dose of GBCA, mostly gadodia-mide and gadopentetate dimeglumin.[13] Another study showed that 0.77% of dialysis patients who underwent GBCA-enhanced MRI developed

Table 1
Gadolinium-based contrast agents (GBCAs)

Generic Name	Brand Name	Acronym	Chemical Structure	Charge
Gadodiamide	Omniscan	Gd-DTPA-BMA	Linear	Non-ionic
Gadoversetamide	OptiMARK	Gd-DTPA-BMEA	Linear	Non-ionic
Gadopentetate dimeglumine	Magnevist	Gd-DTPA	Linear	Ionic
Gadobenate dimeglumine	MultiHance	Gd-BOPTA	Linear	Ionic
Gadoxetate disodium	Eovist (Primovist)	Gd-EOB-DTPA	Linear	Ionic
Gadofosveset trisodium	Vasovist[a]	Gd-DTPA	Linear	Ionic
Gadoteridol	ProHance	Gd-HP-DO3A	Cyclic	Non-ionic
Gadobutrol	Gadovist[a]	Gd-BT-DO3A	Cyclic	Non-ionic
Gadoterate meglumine	Dotarem[a]	Gd-DOTA	Cyclic	Ionic

[a] Approved by the European Medicines Agency (EMEA) for use with MRIs and MRAs in Europe but not approved by the US FDA.

NSF based on clinical and pathology findings.[14] A study in which a minority of cases was proven by biopsy reported that 30% of patients on dialysis who had been exposed to GBCAs developed cutaneous changes of NSF.[15]

As a result of these and many other reports with disparate results, it is unclear whether there is a true understanding of the scope of the disease and the patients at risk, or whether the disease is being vastly underdiagnosed and underreported.

In October 2006, shortly after the presumed relationship between GBCAs and NSF was first established, it seemed that one particular agent, gadodiamide, was responsible for almost all the cases.[4] Updated information from FDA Medwatch in May 2007 presented a somewhat different picture, however.[16] Although there still seemed to be a disproportionate number of cases associated with the use of gadodiamide, many NSF cases were associated with other GBCAs. As of May 2007, there were 513 cases in the FDA database, 73% of which were from the United States. Of the American cases, 68% were associated with gadodiamide, 26% with gadopentetate dimeglumine, and 5% with gadoversetamide. There now are reports of cases of NSF associated with the other two GBCAs that were available in the United States in 2007, gadobenate dimeglumine and gadoteridol (although all but one of the cases associated with gadoteridol were confounded by or exposure to multiple agents). At this time, there are no reported cases of NSF after the sole administration of gadobenate dimeglumine.

Nevertheless, a disproportionate number of reported cases continue to be associated with two of the agents, gadodiamide and gadopentetate

dimeglumine. One retrospective study found an overall incidence of NSF at two academic medical centers using gadodiamide of 0.039% and an incidence at two other academic medical centers with similar patient demographics using gadopentetate dimeglumine of 0.003%.[17]

Looking at all available data, some have concluded that the use of three of these agents (gadodiamide, gadopentetate dimeglumine, and gadoversetamide) is more risky than the use of others, that some of these other agents are safer to use in patients who have severe renal impairment, and that the incidence of NSF can be diminished dramatically simply by using one of these safer agents.

It is important to understand, however, that the reporting of cases of NSF to the FDA does not mean that the cases are fully or even accurately documented. The criteria for the clinical diagnosis of NSF had not been established firmly at the time of reporting, but many of the reported cases depended on clinical diagnosis. Furthermore, many of the reported cases did not have a skin biopsy, which is considered essential for making a confident diagnosis in many (but probably not all) cases. Even when there was a biopsy, there may not have been accurate interpretation.

There are other problems with the historical data. For instance, the case mix for the use of the various agents is not known. It is possible that the GBCAs that have been associated with more NSF cases were used more commonly in patients who had chronic kidney disease or other ailments that put them at greater risk for NSF. In fact, the two agents, gadodiamide and gadopentate dimeglumine, that have been associated with by far the highest number of reported NSF cases also are the two agents that have been used most commonly in the United States and are, unquestionably, the two agents that have undergone the most intense scrutiny.

The data from Europe are even more tenuous, in large part because of inconsistent and unreliable reporting. As of March 2008, there were 104 NSF cases in the European Union database.[18] Two countries, Denmark and Switzerland, with 2% of the total population, reported approximately 50% of all cases. The Danish Medical Authority had received 35 reports, but the European Union database included only 30 of these, and 97% of the cases in Denmark came from one hospital. Some of the larger European countries, which have used gadodiamide and gadopentate dimeglumine extensively, including high doses for MRA, have reported only in single-digit numbers of cases at that time.

In Japan, as of the beginning of 2008, only five NSF cases had been reported, all associated with gadodiamide.[19]

Therefore, although there seem to be significant differences in the NSF-related safety profiles of the various GBCAs, based on the currently available data, both an accurate numerator (ie, the number of cases of NSF) and an accurate denominator (the number of doses administered to patients at risk) are lacking. Therefore, at present, the relative risks associated with each agent have not been elucidated clearly. Until there are better case-controlled and prospective studies, conclusions or inferences are based on imperfect data and "educated guesses," even among the experts.

Although the renal disease may be acute, chronic, or transient, most patients who develop NSF have some form of CKD, and approximately 90% are dialysis dependent.[20] Patients who have non–end-stage renal disease account for about 10% to 18% of cases in the published and registry-reported data.[21–23] These data include two cases of NSF developing in patients who had an estimated glomerular filtration rate (eGFR) of 30 mL/min/1.73 m^2.[23] Both of these patients, however, were experiencing acute kidney injury (AKI) in which the glomerular filtration rate (GFR) was declining at the time of multiple exposures to GBCA, and the GFR probably was overestimated.[24]

Most patients who have renal compromise, even those who have severe or end-stage CKD or who are on hemodialysis, do not develop NSF after exposure to a GBCA. Thus, it is thought that renal compromise is necessary but not sufficient to explain most cases of NSF, and that other co-factors must be involved. Nevertheless, there is general agreement and a plethora of supportive data show that the patients who are at greatest risk for developing NSF following GBCA administration are those on dialysis, those who have stage 4 or 5 CKD, and those who have AKI,[21–23] and these patients frequently are referred for contrast-enhanced MRA.

WHAT ARE OTHER RISK FACTORS?

There seems to be a relationship between the dose of GBCA and the risk of developing NSF, and the patients at highest risk seem to be those exposed to high doses or multiple standard doses.[13,14] This relationship is particularly relevant to any discussion of contrast-enhanced MRA, because MRA is the MRI examination that most commonly used high doses in patients who had severely compromised renal function. This relationship may explain, in part, the low incidence of reported cases in Japan and in selected institutions in Europe, the United States, and elsewhere where high-dose contrast-enhanced MRA never became standard of care in renal-compromised patients.

Several studies indicate that cumulative dose of GBCA over the lifetime of the patient who has renal compromise increases the risk of NSF, but standard doses over many years may pose less of a problem than the single injection of a high dose.[13,14,25] NSF cases, however, have occurred in some patients with a only a single exposure to a single standard dose (0.1 mmol/kg) GBCA,[26,27] an indication that the relationship between dose and response is not a simple one. Whether doses of GBCA administered before the deterioration of renal function play a role in the eventual development of NSF is a controversial subject that is being investigated.

Although there seems to be a disproportionate number of affected patients who have severe liver disease (the FDA has included these patients in its Public Health Advisory), especially those in the peri–liver transplant period, this disproportion probably is related to their renal comorbidity rather than to the liver disease itself.[28,29] Other factors that have been suggested as predisposing to NSF include metabolic acidosis, increased iron, calcium, and/or phosphate levels, high-dose erythropoietin therapy, immunosuppression, vasculopathy (including hypercoagulability and/or vascular injury as a result of surgery or endovascular catheterization), and other proinflammatory conditions.[13] Which of these factors, if any, actually is important is an active area for investigation.

WHAT ARE RECOMMENDATIONS FOR PREVENTING NEPHROGENIC SYSTEMIC FIBROSIS?

The FDA issued a Public Health Advisory for all GBCAs in June and December 2006[4] and then issued an updated alert in May 2007 that requested the addition of a Boxed Warning and new warnings about risk of NSF to the full prescribing information for all GBCAs that are marketed within the United States.[16] The Boxed Warning states that exposure to GBCAs increases the risk for NSF in patients who have acute or chronic severe renal insufficiency (GFR < 30 mL/min/1.73 m^2) or acute renal insufficiency of any severity caused by hepatorenal syndrome or in the perioperative liver transplantation period. It also states that all patients should be screened for renal dysfunction by obtaining a history and/or laboratory tests and that the dose recommended in product labeling should not be exceeded when administering a GBCA.

The European regulatory agencies do not share the FDA's class effect approach to all the GBCAs. The European Pharmacovigilance Working Party and the United Kingdom Commission on Human Medicines have recommended that both gadodiamide and gadopentetate be contraindicated in patients who have an eGFR less than 30 mL/min/1.73 m^2 but that the other agents can be used in these patients "after careful consideration."[30]

In June 2007, an American College of Radiology Committee on MR Safety published a guidance document that delineated recommendations for the administration of GBCAs to patients who have renal failure/disease.[31] The most recent edition of the American College of Radiology *Manual on Contrast Media* in 2008 states that before administration of a GBCA, patients who have an eGFR less than 30 mL/min/1.73 m^2 should be identified by obtaining an eGFR within 6 weeks of the anticipated GBCA-enhanced examination if they are over 60 years of age or have a history of hypertension, diabetes, kidney disease, or severe liver disease, with strong consideration of contemporaneous assessment in this last group as well as in patients who present acutely.[32]

How exactly these recommendations are to be implemented is left to the discretion of the individual MRI facilities. Since the FDA issued its warnings about GBCA and NSF, the number of new cases of NSF has dwindled to a trickle. Whether this decrease resulted from a widespread change in practice (eg, screening of patients at risk, use of lower doses of GBCA, greater use of non–contrast-enhanced MRI/MRA, scanning CKD patients by CT angiography rather than enhanced MRA, and other measures), a change

in the precise type of GBCA used, or other factors is not known at present. When and if one (or more) of the GBCAs is proven with confidence to be less likely to produce NSF (or possibly even to be completely devoid of this complication), then the use of this (or these) agent will limit the number of patients developing NSF even further.

POLICY FOR ADMINISTRATION OF GADOLINIUM-BASED CONTRAST AGENTS

The remainder of this article delineates the policy that has been implemented at Yale-New Haven Hospital to prevent GBCA-associated NSF. The underlying premise is that identification and exclusion of patients on dialysis, who have stage 4 or 5 CKD (ie, eGFR < 30 mL/min/1.73 m^2), or who have AKI should prevent most cases of NSF. As much as possible, the policy is based on evidence rather than anecdote, and it has been flexible and adapted to changes in knowledge. This policy is constantly reassessed and then refined or modified based on credible new evidence. Much of the published data are confusing and contradictory, and it would be counterproductive and ineffective to react to every new presentation or publication by changing the policy. When the evidence is judged to be adequate, however, the policy is changed readily.

The goal has been to develop a policy that is neither too liberal nor too restrictive. Although the desire is to prevent patients from developing NSF, it is not desirable to have policies that restrict patients who would benefit from contrast-enhanced MRI/MRA but do not have any genuine risk for developing NSF.

Some of the elements of the policy can be labeled as "common sense:"

- If an examination is likely to provide adequate diagnostic results without GBCA administration, or if there is a "safer" alternative examination, GBCA administration should be avoided.
- The lowest dose necessary for a diagnostic quality examination should be used.
- Every patient should be weighed before the examination, and the GBCA dose generally should be based on weight.
- The name of the GBCA and the dose should be documented in the report of every examination.

If the free gadolinium hypothesis is correct, and the accumulation of gadolinium ions in the blood and/or other tissues induces NSF, then the risk of the disease should be minimized with the use of one of the more "stable" agents. Although the proof for this hypothesis is, at present, wanting, many already have opted to use this approach. From this point of view, the macrocyclic agents would seem to be the "safest." There may, however, be other considerations such as relaxivity, dose, and the possibility of other adverse events. Until more conclusive data suggest otherwise, the authors believe it is prudent to screen patients and to minimize exposure for those at risk, regardless of the GBCA used.

The authors have endeavored to implement policies that fit into their clinical workflow. As elucidated in the following sections, they use different approaches for inpatients and outpatients. These approaches may or may not be appropriate for other clinical environments.

WHAT CAN BE DONE TO MINIMIZE THE RISK OF NEPHROGENIC SYSTEMIC FIBROSIS BEFORE THE MR IMAGING EXAMINATION IS PERFORMED?

The Yale-New Haven Hospital policy is based on the belief that underlying renal insufficiency is a prerequisite for developing NSF and that the risk seems to be greatest for those exposed to high doses or multiple doses of GBCAs.

When the likely association between GBCAs and NSF first became known, an education and communication plan was developed for Yale-New Haven Hospital radiology personnel and the local health care community, especially health professionals who refer patients to this medical center for MRI. This plan required the active involvement of members of the radiology department and representatives from nephrology, pharmacy, hospital administration, information technology, and risk assessment, as well as from affiliated institutions.

Inpatients

Identifying inpatients scheduled for contrast-enhanced MRI and who are on dialysis proved to be relatively simple. When a contrast-enhanced MRI is ordered through the hospital information system, a message asks the ordering health professional if the patient is on dialysis. If the answer is affirmative, the ordering professional receives a message stating that the examination cannot be scheduled without a nephrology consultation. Since this procedure was implemented, GBCAs rarely have been administered to patients on dialysis, and those patients who do receive an intravenous GBCA are, by pre-arrangement, sent immediately from the MRI examination to hemodialysis.

Identification of inpatients who have CKD also has been relatively simple. For all inpatients, an eGFR must be obtained within 72 hours before a contrast-enhanced MRI examination. This information already is in the records of most inpatients, and it can be accessed remotely. When a contrast-enhanced MRI is ordered through the hospital information system, a message asks if the patient has AKI, an eGFR less than 30 mL/min/1.73 m^2, or severe (unstable) liver disease. If the answer to any of these questions is affirmative, the MRI will not be scheduled without the appropriate nephrology or hepatology consultation. If the eGFR is greater than 30 mL/min/1.73 m^2 and is stable, the contrast-enhanced MRI examination is performed as ordered (assuming it is appropriate). Any concerns about appropriateness or safety can be addressed by direct communication between the ordering physician and radiologist.

Among inpatients at increased risk for NSF, the most problematic are those who have AKI. A number of different studies have shown that patients who have rapidly diminishing renal function are in greater jeopardy, and hospitalized patients, in general, are predisposed to deteriorating renal function. For example, Prince and colleagues[13] found a 19% incidence of NSF in patients who had acute renal failure, who received a high dose of GBCA, and who did not undergo hemodialysis within 2 days. To identify the patients who have AKI, it is not sufficient to look at a single eGFR value, because it may be greater than 30 mL/min/1.73 m^2 but still be substantially decreased compared with earlier values. Thus, for any patient who has an eGFR less than 60 mL/min/1.73 m^2, it is necessary to review a series of eGFRs during the course of the hospitalization to identify a downward trend in renal function that could indicate AKI. A change in eGFR by 50% or more in a 24-hour period is sign of AKI, no matter the level of GFR or of serum creatinine. Except in a dire emergency, these patients will not receive a GBCA until their renal function stabilizes at an adequate level.

There also is increased vigilance for patients who may receive multiple contrast-enhanced MRI examinations over a relatively short period of time. Multiple examinations seem to be most common in patients who have brain tumors or who have had MRA examinations that need to be repeated. Although these examinations may be necessary and unavoidable, increased awareness of the potential risk of NSF has resulted in increased reluctance to use GBCA-MRI for repeat examinations during hospitalization and has increased the use of alternative studies, when possible. In general, higher doses of GBCA are avoided in these patients, even those who have adequate renal function.

Cirrhotic patients are another special case. Although it is believed that cirrhosis itself is unlikely to put a patient at increased risk for NSF, cirrhotic patients often have accompanying varying degrees of renal compromise and may experience acute changes in measured renal function immediately after removal of ascitic fluid for acute hepatic decompensation. Furthermore, in cirrhotics the Modification of Diet in Renal Disease (MDRD) formula can overestimate the eGFR.[33,34] There are a number of equations used to estimate GFR, with the abbreviated MDRD equation being the most commonly used. Because the MDRD is a population-based formula derived from outpatients who have kidney function in steady state, it uses serum creatinine, age, race, and gender. It is not a direct measure of GFR, and it may have limitations when applied to patients not included in the original study population, including those who have decreased muscle mass, injury or recent amputation, or malnutrition, very young pediatric patients, and those over 70 years of age.[35,36] Patients who have hepatic cirrhosis often have diminished muscle mass and therefore have a significantly higher eGFR than true GFR. Thus, for these inpatients a cut-off eGFR of 40 mL/min/1.73 m^2 is used, rather than 30 mL/min/1.73 m^2, and it must be obtained within 24 hours of injection of the GBCA. The hepatologist, radiologist, and patient together weigh the risks versus benefits of contrast-enhanced MRI for liver patients who have eGFR less than 40 mL/min/1.73 m^2. At Yale-New Haven Hospital, It is common for cirrhotic patients who have a low GFR to undergo contrast-enhanced MRI rather than CT to evaluate for hepatocellular carcinoma. The authors have not seen evidence that patients after liver transplantation, who may be on nephrotoxic drugs, are at an increased risk of NSF as long as their renal function is adequate and stable.

In children, the GFR rises above the "CKD" level a few months after birth, but it does not reach adult levels until a few years later. It is not known for certain whether "immature" kidneys render infants at higher risk, but there are no documented cases of NSF in children less than 8 years old despite a very large number of exposures to all types of GBCA. Given the concern about radiation exposure from CT in children, the risk–benefit equation moves even further in the direction of MR than in adults.

Outpatients

For outpatients, schedulers ask every patient, or whoever is ordering the examination, if the patient is on dialysis. If the answer is yes, they are informed that the examination will not be scheduled until a nephrologist caring for the patient in consultation with one of the hospital's radiologists has agreed that the examination is truly necessary and appropriate dialysis immediately after the MRI examination has been pre-arranged.

It would be impractical and unmanageable in this clinical setting, and with the broad and diverse referral base, to require that every patient being scheduled for contrast-enhanced MRI provide an eGFR to identify the outpatients who have severe or end-stage CKD and who are not on dialysis. As an alternative, the schedulers have been trained to ask whether the prospective patient has risk factors for compromised renal function, including a personal or family history of kidney disease, a solitary kidney, a renal transplant, renal tumor, hypertension, or diabetes. If the answer to any of these questions is affirmative or the patient is more than 60 years old, the person ordering the test is informed that the referring physician must provide an eGFR obtained within the prior 6 weeks. Although the examination is scheduled, this information must be faxed or emailed to the scheduler or be available in the Yale-New Haven Hospital information system, for the GBCA to be given. If the patient's eGFR is less than 30 mL/min/1.73 m^2 (< 40 mL/min/1.73 m^2 for patients who have severe liver disease), the examination will not be performed without a documented referring physician consultation with the radiologist.

As with inpatients, cirrhotic outpatients are a special case. If a scheduler identifies a cirrhotic patient, it is necessary to determine if the patient has undergone paracentesis or aggressive diuretic therapy or if the renal status has changed between the time of the reported eGFR and the scheduled MRI examination. If so, another eGFR is obtained within 24 hours of the MRI examination. If the eGFR is less than 40 mL/min/1.73 m^2, a contrast-enhanced MRI is performed only if the referring physician, after consultation with the patient, believes that the potential benefits outweigh the potential risks, and informed consent is obtained by the supervising radiologist.

On the day of the scheduled examination, every patient fills out a safety questionnaire, just as they did in the past. Questions concerning kidney disease, diabetes, hypertension, liver disease, and dialysis have been added. A staff member checks the answers before preparing the patient for the examination. If the patient indicates that he or she has one of the conditions that puts the patient at increased risk for severe or end-stage CKD, and thus for NSF, and the problem was not identified at the time of scheduling, the attending radiologist or his/her designate is consulted about the appropriate course of action to be taken. In some cases the appropriate course of action requires immediately obtaining a serum creatinine level and eGFR, which in Yale-New Haven Hospital requires a venipuncture and takes 1 to 2 hours. Of course, this delay could be very disruptive to the MR scanning schedule as well as an inconvenience and delay for the patient. If the decision is made to proceed and administer the GBCA, the risk of NSF is discussed with the patient, and informed consent is obtained.

WHY IMPLEMENT POINT-OF-SERVICE ESTIMATED GLOMERULAR FILTRATION RATE SCREENING FOR OUTPATIENTS?

Having implemented the policy described in the previous sections and having trained schedulers to screen outpatients verbally for risk factors for CKD, the authors found that, despite an enormous effort by the staff, the process was not 100% foolproof. Patients at risk for NSF occasionally slipped through the screening procedures and received GBCA without appropriate workup and consent. It is not surprising that CKD is common, that awareness is low, and that verbal screening may be insufficient. For these reasons, many thousands of people in the United States who are at risk for NSF will not be identified by verbal screening alone. If Yale-New Haven Hospital had a closed health care system (in which everyone coming for MRI received all their care within the network), or if a national medical health record database were in place, point-of-service eGFR screening might not be worthwhile. But that is not the case. The task of obtaining an eGFR from the referring physician for every patient, without a huge investment of personnel and resources, is extremely challenging. Furthermore, the process is complicated and disruptive to workflow.

Therefore, point-of-care analysis of eGFR was implemented at Yale-New Haven Hospital in February 2008. This approach uses a variety of commercially available devices that make it possible to obtain a serum creatinine level and eGFR within a matter of seconds or minutes at the time and place of care.

Implementation in a hospital environment was not a simple matter. There are federal regulations for point-of-care laboratory testing, and point-of-care laboratory testing devices had to be validated by the Yale-New Haven Hospital laboratory. There were issues about data entry into the various information systems, and there were issues concerning education, personnel, and process changes. Finally there were, of course, associated costs and billing and reimbursement issues.

Although the authors currently are researching the effectiveness and costs of this point-of-care screening process for outpatients, it certainly has eased the complexity and decreased the time needed for scheduling. Furthermore, professional personnel involved with MRI at the hospital feel more confidant that patients who have severe and end-stage CKD are being identified and appropriately triaged. Although occasionally it is necessary to cancel or reschedule a case because it is discovered that a patient who arrives for a contrast-enhanced MRI/MRA is at increased risk for NSF, the authors believe that they are doing both the patient and the referring physician a service by identify CKD and preventing exposure to a GBCA.

INFORMED CONSENT

At Yale-New Haven Hospital, the policy of obtaining informed consent and writing an explicit order for administration of GBCA is applied only to patients considered at increased risk for NSF, including those who have an eGFR below 30 mL/min/1.73 m^2 or who are on dialysis. In these cases only, an explicit order for the GBCA is written and signed by the radiologist, which states the amount and specific type of agent to be administered for a specific MR examination. Policies concerning informed consent, however, often are determined by state regulations or institutional legal counsel.

REFERENCES

1. Grobner T. Gadolinium—a specific trigger for the development of nephrogenic fibrosing dermopathy and nephrogenic systemic fibrosis? Nephrol Dial Transplant 2006;21:1745.
2. Grobner T. Gadolinium—a specific trigger for the development of nephrogenic fibrosing dermopathy and nephrogenic systemic fibrosis? Nephrol Dial Transplant 2006;21:1104–8.
3. Marckmann P, Skov L, Rossen K, et al. Nephrogenic systemic fibrosis: suspected causative role of gadodiamide used for contrast-enhanced magnetic resonance imaging. J Am Soc Nephrol 2006;17:2359–62.
4. Food and Drug Administration Center for Drug Evaluation and Research. Public health advisory. Update on magnetic resonance imaging (MRI) contrast agents containing gadolinium and nephrogenic fibrosing dermopathy. Available at: http://www.fda.gov/cder/drug/infopage/gcca/default/htm. Assessed July 18, 2006.
5. Cowper SE, Robin HS, Steinberg SM, et al. Scleromyxoedema-like cutaneous diseases in renal-dialysis patients. Lancet 2000;356:1000–1.

6. Cowper SE, Su LD, Bhawan J, et al. Nephrogenic fibrosing dermopathy. Am J Dermatopathol 2001; 23:383–93.

7. Schneider G, Mass R, Schultze Kool L, et al. Low-dose gadobenate dimeglumine versus standard dose gadopentetate dimeglumine for contrast-enhanced magnetic resonance imaging of the liver; an intra-individual crossover comparison. Invest Radiol 2003;38:85–94.

8. Volk M, Strotzer M, Lenhart M, et al. Renal time-resolved MR angiography: quantitative comparison of gadobenate dimeglumine and gadopentetate dimeglumine with different doses. Radiology 2001; 220:484–8.

9. Habibi R, Krishnam MS, Lohan DG, et al. High-spatial-resolution lower extremity MR angiography at 3.0 T: contrast agent dose comparison study. Radiology 2008;248:680–92.

10. Rofsky NM, Sherry DA, Lenkinski RE. Nephrogenic systemic fibrosis: a chemical perspective. Radiology 2008;247:608–12.

11. Cowper SE, Bucala R. Nephrogenic fibrosing dermopathy: suspect identified, motive unclear. Am J Dermatopathol 2003;25:358.

12. Sieber MA, Pietsch H, Walter J, et al. A preclinical study to investigate the development of nephrogenic systemic fibrosis: a possible role for gadolinium-based contrast media. Invest Radiol 2008;43:65–75.

13. Prince MR, Zhang H, Morris M, et al. Incidence of nephrogenic systemic fibrosis in two large medical centers. Radiology 2008;248:807–16.

14. Collidge TA, Thomson PC, Mark PB, et al. Gadolinium-enhanced MR imaging and nephrogenic systemic fibrosis: retrospective study of a renal replacement therapy cohort. Radiology 2007;245:168–75.

15. Todd DJ, Kagan An Chibnik LB, Kay J. Cutaneous changes of nephrogenic systemic fibrosis: predictor of early mortality and association with gadolinium exposure. Arthritis Rheum 2007;56(10):3433–41.

16. FDA. Information on gadolinium-containing contrast agents. Available at: http://www.fda.gov/cder/drug/infopage/gcca/default/htm. Accessed April 17, 2008.

17. Wertman R, Altun E, Martin DR, et al. Risk of nephrogenic systemic fibrosis: evaluation of gadolinium chelate contrast agents at four universities. Radiology 2008;248:799–806.

18. Thomsen HS. Presented at the 2nd Annual Scientific Symposium on Nephrogenic Systemic Fibrosis and Gadolinium-Containing Contrast Agents. Yale University School of Medicine, New haven, CT, 2008.

19. Tsushima Y, Takahashi-Taketomi A, Endo K. Nephrogenic systemic fibrosis in Japan: advisability of keeping the administered dose as low as possible. Radiology 2008;247:915–6 [letter to the editor].

20. Cowper SE. Nephrogenic fibrosing dermopathy (NFD/NSF Web site) 2001–2007. Available at: http://www.icnfdr.org. Assessed January 7, 2008.

21. Broome DR, Girguis MS, Baron PW, et al. Gadodiamide-associated nephrogenic systemic fibrosis: why radiologists should be concerned. AJR Am J Roentgenol 2007;188:586–92.

22. Deo A, Fogel M, Cowper SE. Nephrogenic systemic fibrosis: a population study examining the relationship of disease development to gadolinium exposure. Clin J Am Soc Nephrol 2:264–7.

23. Sadowski EA, Bennett LK, Chan MR, et al. Nephrogenic systemic fibrosis: risk factors and incidence estimation. Radiology 2007;243:148–57.

24. Saab G, Abu-Alfa A, Sadowski EA, et al. Are patients with moderate renal failure at risk for developing nephrogenic systemic fibrosis? Radiology 2007; 244:930–2 [Letter to the Editor].

25. Lauenstein TC, Salmon K, Morreira R, et al. Nephrogenic systemic fibrosis; center case review. J Magn Reson Imaging 2007;26: 1198–203.

26. Shabana W, Cohan RH, Ellis JH, et al. Nephrogenic systemic fibrosis: a report of 29 cases. AJR Am J Roentgenol 2008;190:736–41.

27. Pryor JG, Scott SG. Nephrogenic systemic fibrosis: a clinicopathologic study of 6 cases. J Am Acad Dermatol 2007;57:902–3.

28. Mazhar SM, Shiehmorteza M, Kohl CA, et al. Is chronic liver disease an independent risk factor for nephrogenic systemic fibrosis? A comprehensive literature review. Available at: http://www.ismrm.org.

29. Foster ZW, Martin K, Kohl CA, et al. Prevalence of nephrogenic systemic fibrosis in patients with chronic liver disease. Available at: http://www.ismrm.org.

30. Committee for Medicinal Products for Human Use (CHMP). Committee of the European Medicines Agency (EMEA);2004. Available at: http://www.ema.europa.eu. Accessed July 1, 2008.

31. Kanal E, Barkovich AJ, Bell C, et al. ACR guidance document for safe MR practices 2007. AJR Am J Roentgenol 2007;188:1447–74.

32. ACR manual on contrast media 2008, Version 6. Available at: http://www.acr.org. Accessed October 16, 2008.

33. Skluzacek P, Szwec R, Nolan C, et al. Am J Kidney Dis 2004;42:1169–76.

34. Papadakis MA, Arieff AI. Unpredictability of clinical evaluation or renal function in cirrhosis: prospective study. Am J Med 1987;82:945–52.

35. Poggio ED, Nef PC, Wang X, et al. Performance of the Cockcroft-Gault and modification of diet in renal disease equations in estimating GFR in ill hospitalized patients. Am J Kidney Dis 2005;46: 242–52.

36. Stevens LA, Coresh J, Feldman HI, et al. Evaluation of the modification of diet in renal disease study equation in a large diverse population. J Am Soc Nephrol 2007;18:2749–57.

Index

Note: Page numbers of article titles are in **boldface** type.

mri.theclinics.com

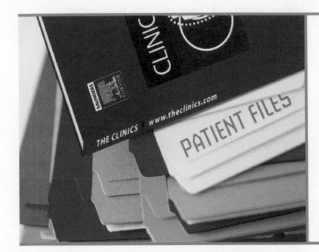
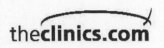

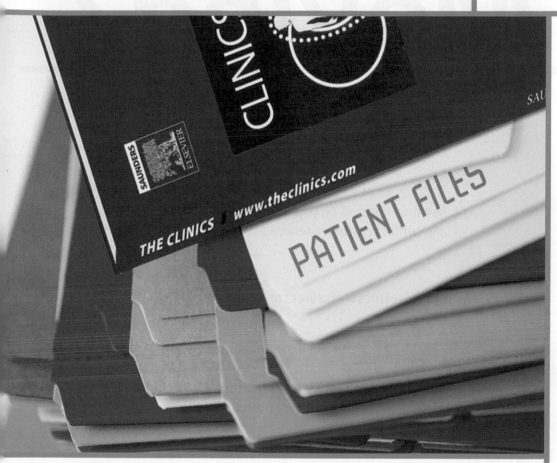

Moving?

Make sure your subscription moves with you!

To notify us of your new address, find your **Clinics Account Number** (located on your mailing label above your name), and contact customer service at:

E-mail: elspcs@elsevier.com

800-654-2452 (subscribers in the U.S. & Canada)
314-453-7041 (subscribers outside of the U.S. & Canada)

Fax number: 314-523-5170

Elsevier Periodicals Customer Service
11830 Westline Industrial Drive
St. Louis, MO 63146

*To ensure uninterrupted delivery of your subscription, please notify us at least 4 weeks in advance of move.

ELSEVIER

Printed and bound by CPI Group (UK) Ltd, Croydon, CR0 4YY

03/10/2024

01040362-0014